BEFORE YOU GIVE UP

FROM AMAZON BEST-SELLING AUTHOR...

REV. JOHN W. ROBERTS

Author Photo Credit: Tim O'Donnell
Cover Photo Credit: Ian Chen

Library of Congress Control Number: 2024922600

Paperback ISBN: 978-1-965092-95-8
Hardcover ISBN: 978-1-965092-96-5

    1. Main Category—Self-Help › Spiritual
    2. Other Category—Religion & Spirituality › General
    3. Other Category—Health, Fitness & Dieting › Mental Health › General

First Edition

Published by: AR PRESS
Roger L. Brooks, Publisher
roger@americanrealpublishing.com
americanrealpublishing.com

TABLE OF CONTENTS

INTRODUCTION

IF I SHOULD WAKE BEFORE I DIE

*Each night, when I go to sleep, I die. And the next morn-
ing, when I wake up, I am reborn.*

—Mahatma Gandhi

MY MOM PRAYED WITH ME for the first sixteen years of my life. Finally, at age sixteen, I said, "I got this, Mom, but thanks!" We always ended with this prayer: "Now I lay me down to sleep; I pray the Lord my soul to keep. If I should die before I wake, I pray the Lord my soul to take."

One night, however, I got the words mixed up and accidentally said, "If I should wake before I die…"

Then I stopped in embarrassment and apologized, "Oh, Mom, I got all mixed up."

Wisely, my mom responded, "Not at all, Son; actually, that's a good prayer. It's a good thing for you to wake up before you die."

I hope you all will wake up before you die. Many people sleepwalk through their relationships, work, dreams, and lives. Some are not even asleep; they have become the real *Walking Dead.*

Do you know the story of Arthur Barry? Arthur Barry is considered the greatest jewel thief of all time. He committed more than 150 robberies, stealing jewelry worth millions of dollars. Interestingly, he only robbed people in high society, resembling a modern-day Robin Hood. He wore a tuxedo while committing his crimes and was said to be so charming that on several occasions, when caught in the act of robbery, he talked his victims out of immediately reporting the crime. However, the law finally caught up with Arthur Barry, and he spent seventeen years in prison for his crimes.

After his release, he worked as a waiter at a restaurant on the East Coast, making fifty dollars a week. Later in life, a reporter tracked Arthur Barry down and asked him about his career as a criminal. Arthur Barry summed up his life: "I'm not very good at drawing morals, but when I was young, I had intelligence, charm, the ability to get along with people, and guts. I could have made something out of my life, but I didn't. So, when you write the story of my life and tell people about all these robberies, don't leave out the big one. You can tell them that Arthur Barry robbed Jessie Livermore, the Wall Street baron. And you can tell them that he robbed the cousin of the King of England. But don't forget to tell them that, most of all, Arthur Barry robbed Arthur Barry."[1]

That is, the most critical person Arthur Barry robbed was himself. Could you come to the end of your life and conclude that you have robbed of all people—yourself? Are you living a life that will count beyond success but of actual significance?

Success dies with you; significance outlives you!

Is there a point in living this life beyond paying the mortgage and having the right brand on your shirt, purse, or car?

Is there a way where we can know that our lives do matter? Maybe you can say the prayer and get it right this time:

Wake me up now, before I die, that I may truly live the life I have dreamed about!

Before you give up your hopes and dreams, can you hear what God wants to speak to your heart? Before you say, "It is what it is," and, "It has to be this way…" can you hear from the one who can do all things?

---

1 Woodward, T. (2011, March 16). "The Man Who Robbed Himself." Albert's Sermon Illustrations. http://aksermonillustrations.blogspot.com/2011/03/man-who-robbed-himself.html

CHAPTER ONE

THE DEEP TRUTH ABOUT YOU

Everyone is struggling. I suppose we must try to understand and learn rather than judge.

—Amish Tripathi

HERE'S THE TRUTH ABOUT YOU: **You need help.**

It's a deep truth, and I'll tell you a little secret about me: I need help.

Live long enough in this world, and you will need some assistance.

Some people need help asking for help.

Take out your phone, grab a random contact, and text them: You need help.

No matter who they are, it will be true of them. We all need help. Only some people seek help, get help, or want help, but we all *need* help.

Have you ever come out of the shower, stood there naked, looked in the mirror, and thought, *I need some help? Anyone over forty should be saying yes at this point!*

Have you ever looked at your relationships and thought, *I need help?*

Have you ever looked at your relationship with God and thought, *I need help?*

Have you ever looked at the doctor's lab results and thought, *I need help?*

Have you ever turned on the news and thought, *This world needs help?*

Everyone needs some life coaching or counseling at some point in their life! Every marriage could benefit from counseling at some point, but only some get the help they need.

You need help, and so do I.

I know your story. I know what you say because after thirty years of counseling people, it's what I hear:

I am only human. I am just me. I am the worrier. I am the one who has this problem. There's nothing I can do. It's just life. I've been like this my whole life! It is all their fault. I wouldn't be this way if this didn't happen. I had a rough childhood. My mom didn't act like a mom. My dad was always at work. My spouse cheated on me. God let me down. God allowed this to happen. It is what it is!

Popeye is your favorite cartoon character. "I yam, what I yam!" You are disappointed, not living the life "appointed" for you. You think others shouldn't get their hopes up for you changing much. *It's not going to happen!* It's so easy to see how others could change, so hard to know how you could change. You've learned to live with what you can't rise above. You have believed those lies for so long, it's become your truth.

Are you finally ready to live as a victor? A victor is a former victim who decided to do something about the thing that victimized them. A victor is someone who decided to do something about their life besides complain about it. Do you feel like you cannot bloom where you are planted? You are not a tree. You can get up and move, your life *can* be different. Your life can be *better*.

I wrote this book to tell you:

- **Your past can be forgiven.**
- **Your present can have a purpose.**
- **Your future can have hope.**

Yes, you are who you are, but that's not *all* you are. You are still determining what you *will* be. Can you believe it, like you believe in gravity?

Is your life the same every day? Is it the same in a positive or negative way?

I wrote this book to tell you some good news. Help is always available, and *it doesn't have to be this way!*

I wrote this book to encourage you with some hope—some real, authentic hope from the source of all hope!

Most people aren't afraid of yesterday; they fear tomorrow. Most of the monsters we face live in our todays and tomorrows. Sometimes a wake-up call from life or God reminds us, "Yes, I do need help!" One of my wake-up calls happened coming out of a car wash.

Jacob, our older child, was in his booster seat. Buckling Zach into his car seat was a process, as always with a three-year-old. First, there's the season where you have to buckle him in. Then there's the season where he wants to buckle himself in, which was the season we were now in. He was not very good at it, fast at it, or thorough about fastening his seatbelt. So that's aggravating, but he would cry if I went back to help him, shouting and screaming: "I can do it myself."

I have often wondered how many times God has wanted to help me, tried to help me through others, and I am there stubbornly shouting:

"I can do it myself!"

How much of my life has been put on pause because I refused help sent from above because of stubborn independence—like a three-year-old?

Whether we are three or fifty-three, we often don't like asking for help.

So there's always the waiting while he tries to do it "himself," and there's always the triple confirmation. Did Zach buckle himself in? Is it done correctly? Is it at his sternum? Is it tight enough? We successfully got confirmation from Jacob, who is older and more detailed. Jacob says, "Yes, Dad, he is buckled in."

We come out of the car wash unbuckled because, during the car wash, everybody's unbuckled.

It's a three-clown circus in our car. Everyone looks at the sunroof and watches the giant hairy octopus attack the vehicle. There's laughter sometimes as the rainbow colors of the soap stream all over the windows, and sometimes there are tears because the "Hairy octopus is going to eat us, right, Dad?" You find yourself saying things as an adult you never thought you would say as you tell your three-year-old that his fears about the hairy octopus are unfounded. Once the octopus is done, we venture out.

Coming out of the car wash and turning left, I spot the opening and hit the gas. As I settle into the lane, Jacob says, "Dad, Dad, Dad." And I say, "What, what, *what*?" He goes, "Zach." I go, "What, Jacob? Did he unbuckle?" He goes, "No, he tipped over." "He did *what*?!" I quickly pulled over to the side of the road, looked back, and saw that Zach had tipped over. He was in his car seat. Oh, that part we got right! His car seat was not buckled into the car, marking the first spiritual epiphany. I heard a chorus of angels singing, *"Zach knows how to unbuckle his car seat!"* It's a new thing we have to confirm. Is he buckled in? Is the car seat buckled in?

So, the second epiphany. This is still a question for which I don't know the answer and will, when I get to heaven, among many other things, seek forgiveness for. *For how many days had his car seat remained unbuckled without anyone making a quick adjustment?* So, I am at Dairy Queen buying Jacob the Blackmail Ice Cream. Not sure what that means? It's called The Hush Blizzard! It's a new flavor they don't advertise. It's what you give to your oldest son when you mess up as a dad with the younger son. I handed it to him and said, "You know, any time you want one of these, let me know, and let's not mention this whole car seat deal to Mom. Cool?" He connected the Dairy Queen dots!

As I continued heading down the road, that's when God began to speak to me and got me thinking, **What areas of my life appear well put together but need a solid foundation or root system deep down? Wake up! I need help!**

You thought your life was all buckled in, but it's not!

So, there you are, buying another self-help book, which is ironic. There is no such thing as self-help books. Your help is coming from another author. It's God's help we need, often given through another.

I can hear it now. People say this all the time:

God helps those who help themselves.

It's in the Bible, right?

Wrong!

"God helps those who help themselves."

Eighty-two percent of Americans, as polled by Gallup, believe this statement is in the Bible.[2]

When Renee and I were newlyweds and I was in Seminary, we had no money. Renee's Aunt Barbara visited us and got into a big argument with me about this saying, and I told her, "Aunt Barbara, trust me. I'm a professional. It's *not* in the Bible," but she knew it was in the Bible. She made a sizable bet with me, 200 dollars, and she stayed up until 1:00 in the morning looking for a verse that was not there. The following day, she tried to get out of paying it off by saying that the Bible says you can't gamble, but I told her that verse isn't in the Bible either. So we went double or nothing, and I got even more money from her.

The saying, "God helps those who help themselves," comes from one of Aesop's fables.

In this fable, a man drives a wagon stuck in mud. He gets out, kneels, and prays to the gods to get it unstuck. Hercules appears to him and tells him to get off his knees and put his shoulder to the wheel. Aesop says that the moral is that the gods help those who help themselves. That saying goes way back, but it's not in the Bible.

It is undoubtedly true that God does not call us to be passive. God has given each of us a mind, a body, and a will, and he wants us to take initiative and take responsibility. That's a good thing.

Faith in God does not mean I get a free pass from studying for tests, exercising to be healthy, or showing up for work on time with a good attitude. God will generally not do for you what he enables you to do yourself. God will generally not do for you what he allows you to do, but our most significant problems in life are in precisely those areas where we cannot help ourselves.

Then, we find we have this strange resistance to asking for help.

---

2   Ortlund, R. (2009, January 6). On Our Watch. *The Gospel Coalition*.
https://www.thegospelcoalition.org/blogs/ray-ortlund/on-our-watch/

Seeking help offends my pride. Everyone wants to buckle their seat belts for the ride of life, but asking for help makes me feel small, incompetent, or three years old.

So, God sends wake-up calls into our lives, but why don't we hear them?

Busyness.

Most people I counsel need help not because they are bad people but because they are busy. The devil knows if he can't make you bad, he will make you busy. Busy and distracted doing a million things a million miles away from your God-driven purposes. You not only wasted opportunities but also wasted your only chance at life.

I bury three or four people a month at funeral homes in Corpus. The funeral directors call me and match me up with strangers, and we gather before the service to talk about their dead mom, aunt, or grandpa who passed. I see dead people every week, and for thirty years, the question has always been: What do we say about our loved ones? Some folks don't need a eulogy. Their whole lives have been a sermon. Let's say we must get creative with the cleanup for others. Others just come right out, and the entire eulogy goes about one inch deep:

"Well, Lydia, she had nice teeth…and ah…great hair." Really? Lydia spent seventy-seven years of her life on this earth, and the most significant thing she did was brush her teeth. She also had a great hairstylist. Is this the sum of our lives? "Well, Bill, Bill was a great dad because he was ahh…busy…always busy at work, he worked non-stop, his whole life…"

I hear these eulogies, and I want to jump and stand up and say, "Busy?"

"Busy at what?" What are you most busy with?

There is nothing wrong with being driven, but who or what is doing the driving? At funerals, people discuss their master passions or lack thereof: What is yours?

What could be more important than spending your life so that one other person can breathe easier and have a better life because you have lived?

Sometimes we need help to quit staring at our belly buttons so much.

It's possible to be so busy in your life that you never stop considering what's happening.

Socrates said, "Beware the barrenness of a busy life."

I want to live for something bigger than myself.

I want to live for something bigger than paying the mortgage and having white at the bottom of my dress shoes.

What are you doing today that will outlive you tomorrow? What are you doing that will give your family something to talk about at your funeral? Do you have a grand funeral resume? Because that's the sign of a life well lived! What will I have to show this world at the end of 3,910 weeks? What have you spent the majority of your weeks doing so far?

Yes, I know you got your seat belt fastened, but what is your seat belt fastened *to*?

Yourself? This world? God?

Strapping into all three is challenging. But have you securely fastened the thing you're strapped into?

What is your life buckled into?

What are you building your life upon?

You can be zipping along but need that anchor, foundation, or something scalable long-term. We don't want to have a good year or even a good decade.

We want to last.

We want to build lives out of marble.

We want eternal impact!

Sometimes, when it's dark, you finally see the light. The light tells you: Today comes with no refunds. Life is a one-time offer. You only get to do this once. Please do it now and do it well. Time isn't your friend.

You need help if you don't want your life to be this way. I need help if I don't want my life to be this way: Shallow, skimming the surface in my relationships, spending all my days gazing at my belly button instead of seeing what other belly buttons I can bless. Am I busy with success, or am I busy with significance? Significance is always about other people!

A great danger (we've all been there) is that if we don't get help, what started as a problem will become a crisis.

What started as going over budget ended up in debt and shame.

What started as a pattern of unresolved conflict ended in divorce.

What started as a bad habit became an addiction.

A problem with flirtation turns into an affair.

A problem with procrastination turns into unemployment.

A problem with sarcasm turns into a life where people don't want to be your friend.

I think about how the most intelligent man once wrote a wake-up call letter for his son. Have you ever had a wake-up call to your children or come to a Jesus talk?

It's been 3,500 years, but I think if you listen closely, you can hear Solomon's son screaming:

"I can do it myself, Dad! I can live my own life. I don't need your help…"

Over time, we have rehearsed this line very well.

Like any wise father, Solomon responds to his son the same way God responds to us, with love and a wake-up call. Solomon talks about an experience he had at Proverbs 24:30-34 (NIV):

> I went past the field of a sluggard,
>
> past the vineyard of someone who has no sense;
>
> thorns had come up everywhere,
>
> the ground was covered with weeds,
>
> and the stone wall was in ruins.
>
> I applied my heart to what I observed
>
> and learned a lesson from what I saw;
>
> A little sleep, a little slumber;
>
> A little folding of the hands to rest-
>
> And poverty will come on you like a thief
>
> And scarcity like an armed man.

Solomon is talking about looking back into his past to deal with future fears, primarily of someone who wastes their life. If he wrote it today, the first line might read: I went past the field of a "busy person…"

When I lived in Escondido, California, my wife kidnapped me and took me to Napa Valley for a romantic overnight getaway for just the two of us. I had never been to Napa Valley before. It's lovely. It was very lovey-dovey, smoochie-smoochie, sippy, sippy, sippy. In Napa Valley, what is striking is all the thought and action that went into the rows of vines. Vineyards don't just spring up by accident. Someone is behind them. A life of significance doesn't just spring up by accident; it takes *intentionality*. No one ever accidentally has a great life, a great marriage, or a great vineyard. No one ever becomes great in their field by accident.

Every fruitful vineyard has some help to produce the finest wine. No fruitful vineyard happens by itself.

Solomon tells his son: I was going past a mess of a vineyard. Thorns littered every-where, weeds covered the grounds, and the walls crumbled. Don't let this be your life. He's telling him: Do you know that to have a piece of land in the Middle East capable of growing crops was one of the most valuable things in the world? To own a vineyard was to be blessed with a lifetime opportunity. Slothfulness, laziness, busyness, and living an unexamined life are wasting the weeks and days God has given you. Solomon says to his son and us, the readers:

Wake up and get to work on your vineyard!

You can complain about your vineyard, but that won't change the fact that someone gave you a vineyard. When you were born, you got a vineyard. You have a body, mind, will, and some relationships. You have financial resources and the chance to do some good work. You have a soul. Everybody gets a vineyard, which is your only shot on this planet. It's a lifetime opportunity; you mustn't care for it alone. God will partner with you.

The message of the Bible is not that God is some cosmic judge to be afraid of because you will never be tall enough to ride the ride to heaven. The message is not, "Hey, good luck with your vineyard."

No, the message is this. The same God who created the sun and the moon and the billions of galaxies thought of you and gave you a unique vineyard and wants to help you tend it, shepherd it, guard it, and help make it fruitful for others. **Here's the key, though— vineyards don't exist for themselves. They exist for others. Life is not about you.** Jesus says you are the salt of the earth. Salt does not exist for itself; it exists to bring flavor to something else. Your master passion, if you want meaning and significance, should always be asking others, "How can I help you? How can I better love you?"

You were created to enrich the lives of others, like grapes destined for fine wine, and preparing your contribution will require some assistance. Of course, to get to the wine, the grapes have to be crushed! You must be willing to let go of your old ways and let the new ways take root! Jesus was crushed in the garden and on the cross, but the wine of forgiveness and abundant and eternal life came out of that.

Wake-up calls happen *before* funerals. They can happen anytime. My last visceral one occurred during the COVID-19 pandemic:

So, I am praying, but it's a usual set of prayers. "Lord help this day go OK. Lord, help my wife teach all those kids for eight hours a day on Zoom. Help my seventeen-year-old son do well this year and improve his career goals from living in a van by the river. Lord, help me forgive my Catholic neighbors who threw fireworks over my fence. Lord, help me get through this day. Lord, help me pay my bills. Lord, help the hurricane to miss Corpus. Lord, help me to be better than I am. Lord, help me be a good dad, a good husband, and a good pastor. Speaking of help at work, Lord, help me write a short sermon or at least a long one. Amen."

I am praying ordinary prayers, and I hear God speak. Now, this doesn't always happen. It's rare, but God stops me in my prayer and says, "John, remember what your mother told you…"

What? Because I am getting a little deaf! God says again, "Remember what your mother told you?" *Huh?* So, I quit praying and started thinking about everything my mom said. My mom said many things. "Wait till I tell your father! If you fall out of that tree and break both legs, don't come running to me. Boys don't have brains until they're twenty-one, and even then, the little head does most of the thinking for the big head. (smile) That's the last time I'm gonna tell you to take out the garbage. You are not listening to me, John. You better start listening to me. I might say something important one day." And my mom often said, "I love you." But none of those seemed to be what God was talking about!

I was a military brat, meaning we moved a lot, like fourteen times. After ten times, you don't count. I remember one time we were going from Virginia to Nebraska. My dad and mom decided to drive both cars. I am a little nine-year-old brat, so I asked my dad, "How will we keep from getting separated?" My dad reassured me, "We'll drive slowly. One car can follow the other." "But what if we *do* get separated?" I persisted. "Well, then, I guess we'll never see each other again," Dad joked. I remember quickly answering, "Then I'm riding with Mom." But I am thinking the whole day, *What is God trying to tell me?* I look to the heavens and say, "Can we stop with the riddles? Does everything have to be a puzzle, God?" Then it's about ten at night, and I am lying in bed, scrolling and trolling on the Facebook feed, and God speaks again. "Remember what your mother told you!"

"Okay, God, I need a little help here."

So, I get up and get my Mom Box. If you have lost your mom, I think everyone should have a Mom Box. After she died, I created a box with everything she ever gave me: birthday cards, letters, mementos, all kinds of stuff, souvenirs, etc. I started digging through it and came across a letter my mom wrote me in 1992.

Ever had a wake-up call from thirty years ago?

I did. God wanted me to hear this letter again, so I opened it. She had written it right after I told her I was going into the ministry, right after I'd told her God had called me to pastor. I won't quote it all to you, but when I read my mom's words in this letter, I knew what God was telling me…

She said, "John, I always knew God was going to use you, even though you were the kid who gave us the most trouble growing up! Believe me, John, you led me to tears and prayers many a night." *Okay…yeah, not good. Sorry, Mom.* She continued, "I prayed, and I prayed, and I prayed every day for you to come around, and you have." Then she wrote these words, and they hit me like she reached into my soul and touched me with thirty-year-old words.

"Make sure you always pray God-sized prayers. Make sure your prayers are always God-sized. Remember, with God, all things are possible! As a gospel song says: 'God's got a bigger thing going on than these little old eyes can see.'[3] Make sure you pray

---

3   NRT Media. (n.d.). *God's got a bigger thing going on song lyrics | greater vision lyrics | Christian music song lyrics, Christian music | newreleasetoday.* New Release Today. https://www.newreleasetoday.com/lyricsdetail.php?lyrics_id=52709

bigger prayers. Keep your eyes on eternity. You've got a role to play in this epic drama. Make sure God can count on you!"

She told me that when I asked for help, I should go big or go home. I noticed she was telling me to ask for help. Don't try to live this life alone. I folded the letter up, and I cried. Then I said, "I am sorry, God. I am sorry, Mom. I forgot what you wrote thirty years ago. My prayers have not always been God-sized prayers!" Don't forget what your mom told you—Pray God-Sized Prayers! When you ask for help, make sure you ask for enough so it's clear to everyone where your help is coming from.

Have you put boundaries on your prayers? Are your prayers in Spanish? *Sin limites*—without limits?

Are you praying God-sized prayers?

Why would my mom say that?

Simple reason: How you pray will determine what kind of life you live.

People who ask for help do better than those who don't. In Robert Putnam's book *Bowling Alone*, he talks about how if you join one social club in the next year, regardless of health, you increase your longevity for that year by more than 60 percent. That's the power of the other. "It's not good for Adam or man to be alone."[4]

Ordinary, get-by prayers mean you will live a small, ordinary, get-by life. But when you boldly ask God for big things, you ask him to open doors that would typically not open. When you ask him to take you further than anyone in your family, you will see the greatness of God's power when you pray God-sized prayers. I think God says to you today:

Ask me for cows with your initials on them. (Huh?) Ask me to turn drug addicts around. Ask me for children who will become history makers. Ask me to part the Red Sea, bring water out of a rock, and show you floods of my favor! Ask me for help; I want to give it to you!

Now, all through the scripture, we see this principle. Elisha prayed that it wouldn't rain. For three and a half years, there was no rain. Joshua prayed for more daylight. God stopped the sun. One prophet prayed for protection. The enemy standing right in front of him didn't recognize him. God made him invisible.

The common denominator is that they asked for the unthinkable. When was the last time you asked God to do something impossible, something out of the ordinary? One reason we don't see God do great things is that we only pray over our food, pray for our protection, and pray for our safe travels. That's all good, but it limits what God can do.

4   Putnam, R. D. (2020). *Bowling alone: The collapse and revival of American community*. Simon & Schuster Paperbacks.

There should be something you're praying about, something that you're asking for that seems far out. Ordinary prayers get ordinary results. God meets us at the level of our faith. If you ask small, you're going to receive small. If you bring God a thimble, he will fill it up. If you bring God a bucket, he will fill it up. A God-sized prayer is, "God, I'm asking you to not only turn my child around but use him in a great way. Let him make a difference in this life!"

An ordinary prayer is, "God, help me to get by this month. God, help me to pay my rent." There's nothing wrong with that, but a God-sized prayer is, "God, I'm asking you to increase *me* so that I cannot only pay my house off but help pay somebody else's house off too!" An ordinary prayer is, "God, just take me as far as my parents. God, help me at least not to lose any ground." A God-sized prayer is, "God, help me to take our family to a new level. Let me set a new standard. When people look back one hundred years from now, God, let them say, 'It was that man, that woman, that made a real difference!'"

But I wonder how many of your prayers are unanswered simply because "Well, God's God. If he wants to bless me, he'll bless me!" Or God helps those who help themselves, so let me do this alone! It says in James 4:2 (NIV), "You do not have because you do not ask!"

If you're not asking big, you are short-changing yourself. You will never reach your destiny if you only pray small prayers. Now, I'm not talking about just making a wish list and praying every whim. I'm talking about asking God for what he's already promised you. Ask God to help your vineyard produce some of the finest wine ever tasted. The Scriptures say, When you walk in God's ways, you will lend and not borrow. With a long life, God will give you peace and satisfy you. Plus, there are specific dreams and desires that God has placed in your heart. They didn't just randomly show up. Those tugs on your heart to make a difference, those little nudges and shoulder taps to pay it forward, the creator of the universe put them in you. They are a part of your divine destiny.

Psalms speaks about the secret petitions of our hearts. One way you know a dream is from God is that the dream is so massive you cannot accomplish it on your own. God does this purposefully, yet it will take enough faith to ask for help. A lot of times, we think: Me? God can use someone holier, a lot better, and a lot more Jesus-like than me. Why would God work through me?

God works through those who always ask for help.

A couple of weeks ago, someone who owns a house on Ocean Drive in Corpus Christi invited me over. This area isn't on the low-rent side of town; it's between million-dollar houses on one side and three-million-dollar houses on the other, all near the water. I was in somebody's home who was quite wealthy. A friend of a friend of a friend invited me, and I went to see how a multi-millionaire lives. With paintings on the wall, that's how. I got some Kohl's clocks and Home Depot decor, but when you have money, you get paintings. This guy has all these paintings on the wall; to me, they weren't imposing. Some of them looked like a child had painted them. But that shows my ignorance—very abstract, modern paint thrown here and there. Later that evening, the homeowner mentioned they had paid over one million dollars for just one of those paintings. Excuse me, a million? Huh. I looked at it again and thought, *Wow, that is beautiful.* I came to find out that it was an original painting by a famous artist who lived in the nineteenth century. I went home, and I was lying in bed that night, and I had this thought, another wake-up call from God:

It's not so much what the painting looks like; it's who the painter is. The painting gets its value from its creator. In the same way, our value doesn't come because of what we look like, what we do, or who we know. Our value comes from the fact that Almighty God is our painter.

Now, let's not criticize what God has painted. In Ephesians 2:10 (NLT) the Bible says, "For we are God's masterpiece." Ever woke up and looked in the mirror and saw the Picasso? Some art pieces may appear abstract, much like others I know. (smile) Accept yourself. Approve yourself. You are not an accident. "I praise you because I am fearfully and wonderfully made!" (Psalm 139:14, NIV) And fearfully here means with a sense of awe and wonder. I wonder what would happen if all through the day, instead of putting ourselves down, instead of dwelling and complaining about our lives, we would think, "I'm a masterpiece. I'm wonderfully made. I'm talented. I'm original. I have everything that I need!"

See, the enemy doesn't want you to feel good about yourself. He would love for you to go through life listening to the nagging voices reminding you of everything you're not. I dare you to get up each day and say, "Good morning. You are a wonderful thing. You are fearfully and wonderfully made!" David said in Psalm 139:14 (NLT) "Thank you for making me so wonderfully complex! Your workmanship is marvelous-how well I know it." God will use you to work through you to do great things, not because of who you are, but because of who God is!

But you've got to pray for it. You've got to believe it. You've got to reach for it, and you've got to ask for help.

I read about this little boy and a big bully who lived down the street and always bothered him. He was trying to get his nerves up so he could stand up to him, but he was just too afraid. He didn't have the confidence. And one day, his father bought him a new telescope. He was in the front yard, playing with it, but he was looking through the wrong end. He was looking through the big side. His mom said, "No, son, you're doing it backward. If you turn it around, it will amplify everything, as originally intended to do…" He said, "Mom, I know that. But right now, I'm looking at this bully. And looking at him this way makes him so small that I'm not afraid of him anymore."[5]

Maybe you need to turn the telescope around.

Faith is a telescope.

It allows us to see how our lives could be through God's eyes, not just how they are!

Before you give up, can you see the problem through God's eyes?

You've magnified that problem long enough. You've talked about how impossible it is and how it will never work out. But if you turn the telescope around, you'll see it from the proper perspective. You'll realize it's nothing for our God—a true story in the papers (remember newspapers) and online. You can Google this story—it's amazing. This seven-year-old girl named Jamie lived on a farm with her family, and they had a cow about to give birth. Her father had already told the family they wouldn't keep more cows. Every time one was born, they'd either sell it or give it away. But for some reason, little Jamie wanted to keep this cow, a desire of her heart. She started pleading and begging her father. "Daddy, please let me keep it. Daddy, please make an exception." After a couple of weeks, she wore her father down. He said, "Jamie, I'll make a deal with you. If the calf is born black, you can keep it, like the rest of our cattle. If not, we'll give him away." She agreed. Well, little Jamie didn't know any better. She started praying and praying every night before going to bed, "God, I'm asking that this cow be born black." Most of us adults would never pray anything like that. That's far out. That's kind of radical. But you know what I've learned? Radical faith gets radical results. A couple of weeks later, the little calf was born. It was solid black, but right between its eyes, there was a big J in white! Her name was Jamie. It's like God stamped it, J. He said, "I'm going to make sure everybody knows this cow belongs to little Jamie."[6]

What am I saying? When you pray God-sized prayers, God will show up in a big way. He'll give you the desires of your heart. Are there dreams you've talked yourself out of or problems you're convinced you'll never overcome? Why don't you do like little Jamie? Take the limits off God. Sin limits! God is without boundaries. What if it's not happening simply because you're not asking? Are we too "busy" with our lives that we are too busy to ask God to help us?

Here's the truth about me. I need help. It's a deep truth, and I'll tell you a little secret about you. You need help. Amazingly enough, from a human perspective, the whole story of the people of God and their great adventure together begins with a single word: Help. We're told this about the Israelites when slavery oppressed them in Egypt: "The

---

5 Harrington, D. J. (2022, July 26). *D.J. Harrington*. Recyclers Powersource. https://www.rpowersource.com/2022/07/is-your-telescope-set-right/

6 Published by: Captain Quote (2017, January 17). *Girl gets answer to her prayer with Baby Cow (true story-report)*. ...Ofthestory. https://ofthestory.wordpress.com/2017/01/17/girl-gets-answer-to-her-prayer-with-baby-cow-true-story-report/

Israelites groaned because of their slavery and they cried out. The cry of their bondage rose up to God. God heard their cry…" (Exodus 2:23-24, NCB).

God did not say, "Hey! Get organized! Hey! Show some initiative! Hey! Put your shoulder to the wheel. I'll help people who help themselves."

God just helped.

Who does God help?

God helps people who ask for help.

God helps needy people.

God helps weak people.

God helps scared people.

God helps people who are way over their heads.

God helps people who can't help themselves.

God helps people who are about to give up!

Now, to be clear, God helps other people too.

God loves to help so much that sometimes He shows up and gives help for no reason.

Jesus said one of the signature characteristics of his Father is that he makes the sun shine on both good and bad people. He sends the rain to fall for both the just and the unjust. One of the favorite hymns Christians sing to describe God is help. "O God, our help in ages past, our hope for years to come…"[7]

Mostly…mostly…being the kind of person God will help means being a person who is willing to pray and who is devoted to prayer.

What is prayer if it's not the belief that *it doesn't have to be this way*?

God helps those who pray because they are asking for help, looking for help, and hoping for help.

God helps all those who call upon His name, not just the highly motivated.

But God will not do what we can do for ourselves.

If God constantly worked to solve all our problems for us, we would remain forever emotionally and spiritually immature. Have you got a problem? Here's the answer: Pray and work. God likes us to pray, but he also likes people of action.

Pray and work. Don't attempt one without the other.

Dwight L. Moody was one of the world's great evangelists. He was on a ship that was crossing the Atlantic. The ship caught fire. The crew and the passengers formed a bucket

7 *Hymn #100: O God Our Help In Ages Past.* Semicolon. (2011, September 13). https://www.semicolonblog.com/?p=5299

brigade to transport water to the fire. One man turned and said, "Mr. Moody, don't you think we should retire from the line and go down and pray?" "You can go pray if you want to," Moody replied, "but I'm going to pray while I pass the buckets."[8] We have a phrase that's not heard much anymore. Have you ever heard someone say, "He worked like the dickens?" The *dickens* is another name for Satan. Someone may say, "He worked like the devil to get it done."

The implication is that the devil is always busy seeking to achieve his wicked ends. He never misses an opportunity to tempt, to discourage, to embitter. Well, there's a little truth in that. If you hit a rough patch in the road and sit around feeling sorry for yourself, the tempter will move in quickly and work like the dickens to cause you to quit trying. God helps all those who call upon His name, not just the highly motivated. But God will not do what we can do for ourselves.

I love the mantra: Pray as if everything depends upon God and work as if everything depends upon you. It's a combo deal; you pray while you pass the buckets! You pray, and you work. But it's not just self-help. We are called to prayer—a life of prayer, a heart of prayer, and an attitude of dependence! Wait, wait, before you close the book; I don't know where you are on the prayer deal. Maybe you have been disappointed by prayer. You cried out to God for something that mattered, and nothing happened, or perhaps you feel guilty about worship. Many people put prayer in this category as one of those things I know I ought to do more of, but I don't do enough of it, and I don't seem to find the time, and I feel guilty. Some people feel like you've got to have an English accent when you pray and talk like you wrote the King James Bible: "O, Thou, Great Jehovah from on High, I Beseech to endow us with thine intrepid love and Bestow upon thine pitiful soul…"

Like what? Huh?

Prayer is a conversation with God, as with your best friend.

We avoid it because we don't think we know the hocus pocus formula or magic words or can't get that English accent down, and it gets worse. Maybe you feel confused about prayer. You hear other people tell stories about amazing answers to prayer or feeling deep intimacy with God, but when you pray, your mind wanders. Soon, you're thinking about grocery shopping or your Amazon account.

How many of your minds are wandering right now?

Maybe, if you're honest about it, and this is a good place, you don't believe in prayer. Perhaps talking to an invisible, supernatural being doesn't make sense to you, or you think prayer doesn't really change anything (God already knows what he's going to do), or maybe prayer is the great joy of your heart. What if I told you that you were praying while reading this book?

---

8 Toler, S. (2009). *God has never failed me, but he's sure scared me to death a few times*. David C. Cook.

Prayer involves your hands and feet.

You pray the most with how you live your life.

You pray with what you attempt to do with your life. Maybe you have known secret moments of peace in times of trouble, courage in situations that would produce great fear, strength, and control in situations where you usually would make terrible choices, and you can't even express your gratitude for those moments of prayer. Wherever you are on the prayer deal, there is a story in the Old Testament of one of the first times God taught his people about the power of prayer, so I want to look at that:

God delivered Israel from the Egyptians after they first cried out for help. They were in the desert. They were on their way to the Promised Land. Then, we're told quite out of the blue, a group of people attacked them called the Amalekites. Their whole existence, their calling not just as a nation, but as a people blessed to be a blessing for the entire world…They had a mission. All of that is in peril, and they don't know why. Moses calls his number-two man, Joshua, in for a strategy session. We are told that Moses was the one man in all of Israel raised in Pharaoh's courts, implying that he would have received military training.

He would have been schooled in military strategy so that Joshua would wait for some great battle plan, but we're not told anything like that. Moses told Joshua, "Choose some of our men and go out to fight the Amalekites. Tomorrow, I will stand on top of the hill with the staff of God in my hands" (Exodus 17:9, NIV). We are not told what Joshua thought of this plan. If I were Joshua and I went to a strategy session like that, I would have expected more strategy. I might have expected that our leader, Moses, would be right down there with us in the middle of the fight, but he had another plan. The morning dawns, and Moses climbs up this hill. He goes there with his brother and another man named Hur. Hur was the son of a leader called Caleb. It is thought that the name Hur means liberty, which would be very relevant to this story of formerly enslaved people, but when I first read it, his name sounded to me like something out of Abbott and Costello's "Who's on first?" routine.

"Aaron, get Hur to come with."

"You want her? I thought you wanted him?"

"I do want him."

"Who is him?"

"I just told you. Hur."

Moses needs Aaron and Hur for an important reason. Moses goes up on the hill. He raises his arms toward heaven and God. It's pretty incredible. The text doesn't tell us a single word he prayed. The text does not even have the word prayer in it. Remember, back in those days, there were no books written about prayer.

The first books of the Bible (Genesis, Exodus, and so on) had not been written. Maybe Moses, like many people, felt reluctant to pray in public out loud. Earlier, Moses said he was slow in his speech and tongue, so maybe no audible words came out of him. Maybe Moses felt awkward, silly, or useless with all these men fighting, but prayer is not about coming up with impressive-sounding words; it's about the heart.

It's primarily about the one we pray to.

What we pray matters much less than who we pray to.

This is a single act of the will expressed by his body. "Help!"

The most amazing thing happened.

Help came.

Power came.

Power from God, power for the battle on earth. It was like an electric current flowing in and beyond him, and the men fought like men inspired. They can't be stopped. They can't be defeated. A bunch of ex-slaves… It's amazing! Then, Moses grows weary, and his arms are tired, and he can't keep holding them up, but when they come down, something happens to the spirit of the soldiers on the field, and they begin to lose the battle, so Moses raises his hands back up, and the tide turns yet again. Israel starts to prevail again, and it dawns on Moses and maybe on Aaron, Hur, and Joshua; when Moses reaches up to the heavens in prayer, power is released, and the battle is no longer merely a matter of flesh and blood. There is another power. There is another force. There is another kingdom at work. There is an unseen reality in the battle!

God gives his people a picture of a much deeper spiritual reality.

We are not made to live on our power.

You and I are not made to live that way.

Your life may not be as it could be because you are too busy to depend on others for help or power.

We are made to live in dependence on God.

Over time, this discovery deepens and is elaborated over and over in the Bible, supremely through Jesus, and it spreads to people and continues. An alcoholic named Bill W. lives in stubborn pride year after year after year, and his battle is with the bottle, and the enemy is killing him. Finally, he hits bottom. He realizes he is hopeless, and he lifts his arms toward heaven and prays that single word, "Help," and the battle for sobriety that he could never win begins to turn as long as he and millions of others live one day at a time with hands lifted, saying, "Help me, God! Please help me! I can't do this! My life is unmanageable. I have an enemy I'll never beat. God, help me! Please help me! Help me!"

Through that surrender comes victory. Through asking for help and raising hands in surrender comes victory in your life. What looks like defeat ends in victory. Be still and know that I am God, says the Bible, but God can't fight your battles if you are too busy fighting them.

Friends, this book is an invitation for you today: In your work, in your home, in your relationship, in your addiction, or your confusion, or with your diagnosis, or in your loss, or your fear, there is a battle going on. Everyone you see is facing a fight. We're not meant to battle alone.

Now, what will keep me from asking for help beyond busyness generally is pride and self-sufficiency.

When Renee and I married, one of us was way more emotionally immature and relationally challenged than he knew, and worse, was too proud and stubborn to admit he needed help, and worse, this person was (you guessed it) me. Ironically, I was getting a master's in divinity and psychology because I believe people need help. All people need help. But not me. The first step toward healing was very, very humbling for me. It was to admit I need help. I do not have this intimacy thing, this marriage thing or this love thing figured out.

I don't know what to do. I can't help myself. I withhold. I withdraw. I yell and scream and act like a gorilla. My temper gets the best of me. And I say things like, "You make me so mad, and I can't help myself."

I went to a human counselor, and I went to a divine counselor. (Of course, all counselors are human; I mean a counselor specializing in human relationships.)

Very often, God chooses human means to give us divine help.

I had to learn to lift my hands and ask for help, and I'm still learning this. Two great truths stand out, and if I can embed them in my mind, they'll help me raise my hands more often in prayer.

I associate them with two arms going up.

The first great truth is that God is able.

Our God is able. How able is God?

Well, according to the Bible, he is exceedingly able. He can speak the universe into being by saying, "Let there be light," and there is light. He can bring plagues that will change the heart of a pharaoh. When the Red Sea needed to be parted for Israel to walk through, God had the power to part it. When manna was required to feed the people, God was able to bring it. When a storm threatened his disciples' lives, God could calm them. God rescued Daniel from a lion's den, delivered three young men from a fiery furnace, and helped them escape the fire without smelling like smoke! God was able to take five loaves and two fish and feed a crowd of thousands of people, able to make a priest silent, able to make a donkey speak (proof that if God can speak through an ass, he can talk through me…)! God could make the lame walk, the blind see, the leper clean, and a dead man live!

How able is God? He is very able. He is exceedingly able, and his arms have not lost their strength. He has not lost his capacity to speak and have it be so.

God is able, and I have to trust that, at least enough, to turn to him and ask for help.

My faith life's basis and walk have been built on one factor: If Jesus's heart quit beating on Friday and never beat again, believe your lies. Play the short game. Keep trying for those "microwave" fixes. But if Jesus's heart began to beat on Sunday morning, if that happened, you realize *whatever* is dead in your life can have life again. Whatever is dead. Whatever—including your heart, your life, your health, your relationships, your very soul.

Here is the foundation of my entire faith walk:

If God can raise Jesus from the dead, God can do anything in your life. "To accomplish abundantly far more than all we can ask or imagine" (Ephesians 3:20, NCB).

Can you believe that truth louder than the lie of "I yam what I yam?"

Are you ready to surrender to a truth and power more significant than your lies?

Second great truth: **God is willing.**

God could be a powerful being, but if God does not have a caring heart and a listening ear, I don't want to hold my hands up to heaven all day. God is willing. He's not just able; He's willing to hear, notice, love, and act.

God is willing to join you and help you.

Why?

Because God looked in the tomb on Saturday and said, "It doesn't have to be this way!"

Have you ever looked on your "Saturdays" when all seemed dead and given up hope?

Are you in that place now? Before You give up, remember God is a God of resurrections!

God is willing to help you.

How willing? *Very* willing. The writers of Scripture say he's willing enough to count the hairs on your head and keep every one of your tears in a bottle, willing to hear the groans of his people and the blood that cries out from the ground of every single victim, willing to suffer like a lovesick father waiting for his prodigal child to come home, and willing enough to become like one of us. All this is to say that *it doesn't have to be this way*.

This is the doctrine of incarnation that in Jesus, God became flesh, and part of what that means is that God learned firsthand what it is like to need help. God learned that. Jesus would say this word to Mary when he was a little boy. "Help! Help me, Mommy!" It's one of the first words a child learns. "Help me get dressed. Help me eat my food." How amazing that God humbled himself in Jesus (the universe maker, asking for help to tie the laces of his sandals)!

When my mother was battling ovarian cancer—the cancer caused her to have two strokes that took much of her vision away. This loss of vision, as it turned out, was one of the worst parts of her cancer. She struggled to see the piano keys and read the lines of music. A month before she died, she said to me: "The worst part of my cancer is not that I am dying. It's that I can't play anymore." My mom lived to play and worship God! It came home to me the last time I was home. My mom, family and I were eating a meal, and she couldn't see her rice and beans on the plate. She was taking the fork and missing the food. She didn't want to ask for help, but I could see her frustration. I quietly dipped her spoon into her beans and nodded at her. No one in my family saw this, and I didn't want anyone to see it. I didn't just eat a meal with my family; I helped my mom find her food and fed her. I still cry when I think of this memory, and I curse cancer; it is the great thief stealing people and their time away from us! It was humbling to feed the woman who once fed me!

This thought struck me—If a parent lives long enough, the roles get reversed. Things change, and they end up asking their children for help. "Help me get dressed. Help me eat my food."

We are born needing help, and we die needing help, and in between, we can fool ourselves into thinking we don't need help. Still, all it takes is a little age, a little health problem, a little blood vessel that doesn't work just right, or a little email from work saying that job is no longer ours, and we remember that word: "Help!"

The deep truth about you is that if you want to change your life, you will need help!

In the end, Jesus (God in the flesh) could not even carry his cross by himself, and a man named Simon from Cyrene had to carry it for him. The story of Jesus ends as it begins with a God who somehow knows what it is to be weak and small and unable and need help. That's our God. He is so willing. He has such a generous heart. God is not frustrated or impatient. God is not weak or disinterested.

God is waiting right now, so where do you most need help from God? "God, give me the strength to face this crisis. God, give me the wisdom to know how to parent. God, give me peace amid this storm. God, give me the ability to overcome my anger, resentment, and bitterness. God, take away my fear. It's killing me, and I can't make it go away. God, give me your help to cope at work. God, I need your patience to dwell on this problem. God, I haven't lived in joy for a long time."

God is able, God is willing, and God helps people who can't help themselves.

Now, maybe like Moses, you need help from somebody else. Maybe your arms are getting pretty tired.

There have been times in my life when I have felt so profoundly burdened that I've had to say to a friend, "I don't even know how to pray right now. I feel like my heart is so downcast I don't know what to say. I don't know what to do. Would you pray for me? Would you stand in that gap for me?" and they have said, "Yeah, I will do that." Then, they are like Aaron for me. They are like Hur for me. Those are sacred moments; we get to do that for each other. It's a fantastic picture. This story shows us life in the Kingdom of God, where God hears and cares. God is able and willing, and he sends his power. There's a battle that looks like it is being carried on in human flesh, but the real battle is not down on the field.

The real battle is up on the mountain with a man named Moses, but Moses gets too tired. Moses gets too weary, so he has a couple of friends who come alongside him, and they hold up the hands that don't have the strength to hold themselves up. Somehow, amid that weakness, brokenness, and neediness, the power of God gets unleashed that never would through human self-sufficiency, strength, and ego alone. That's us. That's the reality in which we live. That is life in the Kingdom of God.

Maybe you need to ask somebody, "Would you be my Aaron? Would you be my Hur? Would you hold up my hands because they're tired right now? Would you support me in prayer because my heart is breaking right now?"

Now, when I tell people this, they will usually say, "Okay, you are right, but I am just so busy, busy, busy…"

With what? Your eternal destiny is at stake. Your abundant life on this earth and this side of heaven are at stake. Jesus told a similar story one time. The king invited all his friends to a party, and at first, they all said yes, but then, when the party was about to happen, they came up with excuses. One guy had just bought some land, one had just bought some Ford 150 Trucks, and one had just married. And none of them could come to the party, to the banquet. None of them were willing to come to the Kingdom of God. Why? It's not that they were terrible people; they were not selling drugs and getting drunk; they were doing good things.

So, God says, would you spend your life walking with me? Would you let me be your shepherd? Will you come to the party? People say, yes, I'm there. I'm there. What happens then?

Earth gets in the way of heaven.

Busyness gets in the way of *purpose*.

Jesus invites us into a relationship with God, and earth, life, and busyness get in the way. We get stuck praying ordinary get-me-by prayers. We think we can do it alone, and our lives are put on permanent pause because we refuse to ask for HELP!

We don't realize our time is running out; it's later than we think, and we need a shepherd! It's later than you think. Not one of these guys who gave excuses was shooting heroin. None of these guys had to do a robbery, a burglary quickly, and a B and E. Not one of them was ever kept away from heaven by bad things. Land, belongings, and a new bride are all good things.

But good things become bad when they keep us from the best things.

True story: A guy goes to the house where he grew up and knocks on the door. He became sentimental because he hadn't been there for twenty years. He asks the owners if he can walk through the house, and they let him. While in the attic, he finds an old jacket. He puts it on, reaches into the pocket, and pulls out a stub. It's a receipt from a shoe repair shop. He realizes he had taken a pair of shoes there twenty years before and had never picked them up amid the move. On a whim, he decides to go to the shoe repair shop. To be funny, he hands the receipt to the guy behind the desk, saying, "Are my shoes ready?" The guy goes back to the workroom for a minute, comes back to the counter, and says, "Come back a week from Thursday." That's the mind of the busy person today. They're always saying, "A week from Thursday." In my own life, I don't tell myself, "Never." I tell myself, "A week from Thursday." The danger is not that I say, "Never," it is that I say, "A week from Thursday." Words like *someday* are the favorite words of a busy person and phrases like *a week from Thursday* permit me to avoid doing what God is calling me to do today.

What do you do?

If you're willing to say, "I have a vineyard where there are some weeds," if you are willing to say, "There are some things in my life that are not buckled in…"

God has some advice: "Go to the ant, you sluggard; consider its ways and be wise" (Proverbs 6:6, NIV).

There are two lessons we can learn from the ant.

First, the ant knows that you should work hard in the summer of your life for the winter of your life.

Also, the ant does not require external motivation—no commander, overseer, or ruler applies the whip.

You have to want to change your life. No one else can do it for you. God cannot save you against your will!

The ant knows that if you're waiting for somebody else to get your life into shape—if you expect your boss, parents, teachers, spouse, or friends to make you do the right thing—you're in serious trouble. Ants take care of the vineyard.

My life is my responsibility. I'm responsible for my life, my vineyard.

No one else is responsible for the wine you produce but you.

Why are you blaming other people for your bitter wine?

Second, the ant understands the law of opportunity.

Even in the summer, the ant stores its provisions. Maybe I wish it wasn't summer. Maybe I'm tired and wish the kids weren't so young and demanding. But they'll only be this age one time.

Whatever season you are in is reality; it's your vineyard.

The writer of Proverbs says the ants understand time better than we do. We have this one life that goes so fast that we're surprised by it. We must go to the ant and learn to understand time because we have this one vineyard to take care of.

Here's the good news: though we can never overcome busyness and hurrying on our own—because it's too much for us—it's not too much for God. We can never self-help our way out of the way our lives are. But we can ask for help! We can surrender; while surrender looks like defeat, it's the first step toward healing!

The good news is that Jesus says, "Just ask me, and I'll help you with it."

This is the strangest thing about busyness or the unexamined life: it has power but is weak. If you answer the wake-up calls, trust God, and take one tiny step of faith in your vineyard, God will help you in such a way that you will think, you know what? This isn't nearly as overwhelming as I thought. If God will help me—if I trust him and take one step of action—busyness is not as formidable an opponent as I thought it was.

It begins with this question:

Are you living a life by design, or are you living a life by default?

Are you just letting the weeds grow and choke out what matters?

Are you willing to ask: Is what my life buckled into going to hold when I take a sharp left turn and hit the gas?

Design or Default?

Have you ever had this happen?

You never manage your money, you have no savings account, you don't keep track of your spending, you have no budget, and you never pay off your credit card debt, but you wake up one morning and discover you're a millionaire.

Or you never work out, eat whatever you feel like, have no exercise program, and spend the night in America's number one selling piece of furniture, the La-Z-Boy chair, watching TV, but one day you discover you can run a marathon!

Just like that—*poof*! Twenty-six miles is a breeze for you.

Or you're single, you never bathe, you never deodorize, you never brush your teeth, you never wash your clothes, you play video games fourteen hours a day and don't have a job, and you come to church one day. The most beautiful, attractive person you've ever seen says, "Come sit next to me! You smell fantastic! I want to spend the rest of my life with you!"

You can live by design or default, but you can't be the head or the tail. You have to pick one!

BY DESIGN

If I live by design, I will be intentional about my life. I will be willing to look at my vineyard. I will be willing to pray God-sized prayers. I will be willing to ask for help. I will be willing to find people who will hold up my arms. I have a purpose greater than myself, and I pursue it vigorously. I look for friends who will hold me accountable for my values. I examine my life regularly. I live with a strong sense of determination. I answer life's wake-up calls. A classic picture of this in the Bible is Jesus. When he was twelve, his mom scolded him for staying behind in Jerusalem at the temple. Jesus asked, "Why did you have to look for me? You should have known that I must be where my Father's work is" (Luke 2:49, ICB). Jesus had a fantastic sense of purpose, and we see it through his determination at the end of his life. The Bible tells us as the right time approached for Jesus to be taken up to heaven: "He steadfastly set his face to go to Jerusalem" (Luke 9:51, KJ21). That's an old translation I love: "Set his face." The Greek word is *stērizō*. It means not just to decide something but to be resolute, to be fixed in purpose, to make it so that you will not be turned back—life by design.

I can live by design with my only life God gives me, or I can live by default.

BY DEFAULT?

Now, this looks very different. To live by default means I follow the path of least resistance. I just kind of drift. I know something is wrong. I'm stressed, or I'm tired, or my marriage is stagnant, or I have bad habits, or I'm not connected with God in the way I would want to be. I'm not becoming the person or living the life I want to, but I don't have the energy or commitment to do what's right. People at work have a terrible attitude. I do too. That's where we end up by drifting. I get ingratitude by default if I don't choose gratitude by design. I get isolation by default if I don't select community by design. I get resentment by default if I don't choose joy by design. To live by default is never checking to see what the seat belt is fastened to! To live by design does not mean you have to be hyper-organized or a list-maker or something like that. It just means embracing the life God has for you and living by your values.

It means asking what the vineyard of my life looks like if I tend it and care for it.

What does the vineyard of my relationships look like? Do I have deep, meaningful, life-changing friendships? What does the vineyard of my finances look like? What does the vineyard of my soul look like? What vineyard will my kids describe when they gather one day at my funeral when my 3,910 weeks of life are used up when I have clocked out? Wake up. It's later than you think. Chances are your vineyard has some weeds that need to be pulled! Your life doesn't have to be this way; it won't always be this way.

The deep truth about you and me is we need help.

The deep truth about us is that God wants to help us and can help everyone!

This is your wake-up call.

Quit living an ordinary life with ordinary prayers. Start asking for help.

CHAPTER TWO

DING! YOU ARE NOW FREE TO UNBUCKLE YOUR SEATBELT!

It is only with the heart that one can see rightly:
what is essential is invisible to the eye.

—Antoine de Saint-Exupéry

I AM SITTING IN THE AIRPLANE wondering how long I can hold it—ever been there? Seriously, it's getting urgent with one more bump and one more drop! Once I turned fifty, it seemed that I had the bladder of a small mouse, a church mouse, and a holy mouse, no doubt! I pray for the seat belt light to "ding!" and let me know I am free. Please, dear Lord, set me free! I am flying back from Corpus from a speaking engagement in San Diego, California. It's a three-and-half-hour-long flight. I had to have that Starbucks Vanilla Latte before I got on the plane, along with the lousy hotel coffee on the Uber ride to the airport and the coffee I had just downed from the flight attendant! I am three coffee cups deep in urgency. Don't judge me. I will drink lousy coffee on the way to good coffee. I am a chain-smoking coffee drinker! About thirty minutes in, the sense of urgency hit me just as the lightning, rain, and thunderstorm hit the plane. The newbies on the flight are getting nervous. There's a lot of nervous peering out the windows. I always watch the flight attendants. If they are calm, I am good. If I see a flight attendant grab their rosary and start reciting, I might lift a prayer!

Have I mentioned in the last sentence or two that I must pee? Is that bad? Whatever you do, don't think of running water, Niagara Falls, or the water rolling down the little plastic window you are staring out of! My life needs to be modified, but the forecast for change does not look good. We are up and down. Turbulence has become the norm, and we are stuck in some broken elevator! I folded up my laptop and, like a little kid squirming in my seat, began to do the "potty dance" while sitting down. I know that the look of dismay is fixed upon my face. I no longer have time for small talk with the person beside me. No, I don't need restoration. I needed relief. I needed to go. It was not helping that the plane was in and out of these free falls. When would we level out and get to calmer airspace where we would be free to roam about the cabin? Was I worried about my ultimate safety? Like the plane crashing? No.

Why?

I thought it would be a relief if we hit a mountain right about now because then I wouldn't have to pee!

Speaking of hitting a mountain in planes, friends always sit in the back. Why? The first class is overrated. You never hear about a plane backing into a mountain, do you? Finally, we leveled out of the storm, and things were calm. Still, the problem was everyone had already consumed their complimentary free caffeinated drink, so when the pilot hit the switch, ding, "You are now free to move about the cabin," all you heard was the sound of those metal seat belts, click, click, click! A few other folks on our full flight also had a sense of urgent fullness in their lives. There we all were, in that polite way, getting out of the way and racing to get in line for the bathroom. I ended up third, although I had to push a couple of kids and one frumpy older gentleman out of the way. It was a good thing I did because the first person got in, and I found my way to the little aisle where the flight attendants were; of course, they came out and told everyone behind me to go back to their seats because "we can't have you blocking that aisle!" I was pleased to be third in line because the hope for change was only two people away!

Hope always needs a goal. Every great leader is a hope dealer.

I began to do what most people do, chat it up with the flight attendant. "Where are you headed to? Where are you based? How long have you been doing this?" Then she asked, "What do you do besides the potty dance?" It's always enjoyable as a pastor when people ask, "What do you do?" Before I respond, I ask myself, *Do I want this conversation to be long or short?* If I say preacher, it usually cuts the conversation way down. No more fun dirty jokes or dumb comments they've been lobbing my way since we first met. No more *double entendres* like you grew up with watching *Three's Company*! Usually, on the plane ride, once they know they are in the presence of a "holy one," folks put down their drink and apologize for their last comment, "No offense, Pastor." Then the plane ride gets quiet. People often feel judged if I tell them I am a pastor, as if I have been keeping a cosmic score for the Big Guy upstairs. "I am sorry for my potty mouth, Pastor." Unfortunately, Christians, historically, have tended to come off as black holes of joylessness, judgmentalism, and hate. Just imagine our reputation before we met Jesus! (smile) We've got an image problem, which always lands on me when I say, "I am a pastor." Jesus had the biggest problem with the judgmental religious folks in his day, not the average sinner.

I prefer to tell people I am a full-time hope dealer, and that always gets a look of curiosity.

If I want the conversation to be longer, I will say, I am a writer! Despite my urgent situation, I went with "I am a writer" to the flight attendant. Next question, "What do you write?" to which, I replied, "Books, daily inspirational devotionals." She replied, "Wait, what do you write about? Like, what's the book you are currently writing about, sir?"

"Plane rides and having challenges with going to the bathroom," I joked. "Seriously, it's about how changing your life is like falling off a bicycle."

"Huh?"

Lisa, on Southwest Airlines, this chapter is for you.

Southwest Airlines had an excellent ad for many years. Ding. "You are now free to move about the country." I loved how the advertisement implied that we needed a bell or some signal, ding, to know it was time to change the status quo.

How many times has God tried to get your attention? How many times has God given you a shoulder tap, and you failed to turn around? How many times has God given you a wink, and you missed it? Looking back, you swore you heard the ding, you felt that tap, you remember that wink, but at the moment, you were aloof, obtuse, or just too self-absorbed to see the Creator of the Cosmos in your midst! Sometimes things like the Almighty's presence are hidden in plain sight.

Ding! "It's time to live your life." Ding! "It's time to get moving."

Someone your age dies. Ding! "It's later than you think."

I love this question; I get it weekly. "Are we living in the end days, Pastor?"

Well, yes, I certainly am. As I figure it out, I only have about 7,665 days left on this side of heaven if I live to the average age a man lives in America. Yes, these are the end days for sure. Last time I checked, no one gets unlimited days on this side of heaven. I only get so many Christmas Eves to celebrate, and I have fewer of them ahead than I do behind me. End days, why yes, indeed. Jesus is coming, so look busy! Ding! "This is not your practice life." Ding! "You only get to do this once." Ding! "Wake me up. Quit sleepwalking through life." Ding! "You *have* to break some eggs to make an omelet." Ding! "Change happens when the pain of staying the same is greater than the pain of change."[9]

Ding! Your girlfriend of eight years breaks up with you the summer before you get married. There's nothing like the wake-up of a breakup! Ding! "You are reading this book right now. Is God trying to get your attention?" Surely, God can speak through a book, right? Get busy living or get busy dying![10]

Do you feel stuck? Like an observer in your own life? Do you feel like you can't do this anymore? You can't go to work every day, hoping something will change. Can you even

9   Thank you to Tony Robbins for that gem.

10 Remember that famous line from *The Shawshank Redemption*?

remember the last time you were lying on the grass, looking up at the sky, and dreaming about your life and what you could do? Are you ready to dream again? Are you prepared to say, "Never in My Wildest Dreams?"

Congratulations!

Instead of giving up, you have looked up and changed your future.

You are on the path to change, to rebooting your life.

You've fallen off your bike, the one you ride daily as you go through the same tedious motions. It's time to draw a line in the sand, hit the reboot button, and start over. Change will not be easy.

It will require discipline, and by that, I mean how Abraham Lincoln defined discipline: "Discipline is choosing between what you want now and what you want most."[11]

Changing your life is like falling off a bicycle because, first, it's embarrassing; asking for help is embarrassing. I remember thinking as a kid that adults live how they want to. They are free to tell anyone how to live, so they choose how they live. Ha! I can't wait to shave. I can't wait till I can stay up all night. I can't wait to grow up. In the meantime, everyone asks you: What do you want to be when you grow up? A policeman? A doctor? A teacher? Now that I am "all grown up," what do I want to be? How about younger? I want to be younger when I grow up!

So many adults are not living the life they dreamed of as a child. Most, I would say. Why? We vastly underestimated the power of destructive habits and destructive thoughts. We went with the flow instead of designing a flow. We surrendered to a line of thinking: "It is what it is!" We believed everyone else except God when they told us, "You can't change!" Changing your life is like falling off a bike, and the last time I fell off my bike, I broke my collarbone, but my main concern was someone going viral with the video of me falling! Yes, yes, I am vain, so what?

But here's the point: You can't be great if you're unwilling to fall! God can't steer a parked car. You have to get moving to move anything. You have to do something new in your life to change your life. I bought a mountain bike two years ago and began riding with "mountain bike riders." There are no mountains, but we do ride on trails and rough sidewalks. (smile) Corpus roads also qualify as a rough trail. Trust me on this one. I could have fallen less when I first began mountain biking with folks. I could have gone slower and more cautious. I could have taken fewer risks. I pass those people on the trail all the time. They're having fun, but they're not killing it. And that's okay. Everyone chooses their priorities. But to be great, you must constantly find the edge of your limits, which means you will sometimes go over the edge.

---

11 *Top 500 Abraham Lincoln quotes (2024 update)*. Quotefancy. (n.d.).
https://quotefancy.com/abraham-lincoln-quotes

The same is true with changing your life. There's going to be some falls along the way. You are not going to change in a straight line. Progress is always non-linear. Sometimes you look like the "Before" picture, longer than you want. But getting to the "after" picture will involve some change, which always feels like letting go of control. It's risky, like falling into the loving arms of your Father.

But you can only change one moment at a time, one habit at a time, one day at a time.

This means you learn to focus not on the mountains before you but just the next ten feet. Give us this day, our daily bread. You can only eat today's daily bread.

There's a hill; for Corpus, it's a hill. I wouldn't say I like it every time because it never ends. When I look at it, I don't want to bike ride. I want to get off and walk. One of the strategies I use to make it through a soul-crushing grind is to shorten my view to just a few feet ahead. Don't look at the massive hill that looms ahead; look at the next ten feet. Pick a rock, a rise in the trail ahead, or that next stop sign on the road, and make it that far. Then, pick the next objective and bootstrap your way up the hill. It's a mental game of chunking the challenge into smaller pieces you can handle. The same is valid with life change. Forty percent of your life is your habits. If you change one or two habits, you can significantly change your life. What if you focused on changing three habits every month for the next year? By the end of one year, you would have changed thirty-six habits and a great deal of your life. But focus on the next ten feet, not the next ten years. Think long-term, yes, but focus short-term.

But remember, **focus on the who before the do!**

Always build the **who of your life before you create the do of your life!**

Who do you want to become more than what you want to do? You can get paid to do anything, but who matters? That is why I say I am a full-time hope dealer. It's what I do whether I get paid or not; I give people hope. I can't ever take off the name tag of Hope. It's who I am. I get so tired of parents saying to their kids: You can be anything you want to be. No, that's just not true. It's well-meaning but a lie. I can't be all I ever wanted to be. I can't even be six foot one! But I can be all God intended for me to be, but that means I have to ask, "Who did God make me to be?" Not what job does God want me to get paid doing? What gifts and graces come naturally to me?

It's not always who I am, but rather *whose* am I?

Does God have a claim on my life? Everyone answers this question with how they live. Once I know who God made me to become, I get busy becoming, which means I am constantly growing and changing. Sanctification is lifelong. No one ever gets to a point where they go: Finally, I am all God intended me to be. At least anyone honest. But that doesn't mean you quit training and arranging your life in a way that Jesus would live if he were you. I pray with my feet, hearing the "dings" and cues that things must change. It takes twenty years to make an overnight success. After twenty-nine years of ministry,

I feel compelled to write down what God has been speaking into my life beyond the first introductory book. Helen Rowland said this: A bride in her second marriage does not wear a veil.[12] She wants to see what she is getting. I love that. Welcome to life, for better or worse. It's your life, in sickness and in health. It's your life to have, hold, nurture, and live. It's your life. You have reached the height of the airplane ride, where you are ready to say goodbye to naivete, self-pity, and "blindness that comes from wearing a veil!" You have lived long enough to know it's tough to change someone else and even harder to change yourself. Quit trying to change your spouse. They will hate you for it. If you want to change your marriage, change the one you can.

Ding! Welcome to the reality of marriage. Do you want to know what marriage is? Stand in front of the mirror, raise one hand, then raise the other; what does that look like? Surrender.

Ding! Welcome to marriage. Welcome to the fact that no one else can make you happy. It's an inside job. Of course, Helen Rowland was not always big on guys. She also said, "There are only two kinds of men: the dead and the deadly."[13] I thought that was funny. If you are still reading this book, Ding! Welcome the cue from God that some areas of your life need to be changed! You can get up and move around your life and change them. Welcome to the "second marriage."

Finally, relief comes at 35,000 feet in the glorious and unroomy bathroom of the 747, and I head back to my seat. When I got on the plane, I hoped to sit beside a "sleeper." A sleeper is my idea of a great traveling companion on an airplane, one who goes to sleep so that I can get some writing done. The person sitting next to me wasn't a sleeper, he was a walker, which is even better. Once I told him I was a pastor, he got up, left, and never returned.

Don't believe me? Tell a group of strangers you are a pastor and see what happens!

I have this empty seat next to me. The talker was in the row in front of me. Now, I am not an eavesdropper, and I can't even hear all that well anymore, but when you are packed into the coach, sometimes ding, you can't help but hear the conversation of those people sitting around you. The talker started immediately, getting acquainted with the man beside her. They decided to get comfortable and put their seats in the reclining position. If you have ever flown, I know you are thinking about how that looked. Let me say it this way. If I had been a dentist, I would have been ready to work. So here they are in my lap. I don't know the woman's name. I don't think she ever said it, not that I don't recall it, although I think I know everything else about her. As I write this chapter, I think of a few names, such as Motormouth, but that's a judgmental name coming from a guy who talks a lot! Ok, I think I will settle on Mrs. Garrulous. I chose that name after

12 *Helen Rowland - a bride at her second marriage does not...* Brainy Quote. (n.d.). https://www.brainyquote.com/quotes/helen_rowland_385987

13 *Helen Rowland - there are only two kinds of men; the dead...* Brainy Quote. (n.d.). https://www.brainyquote.com/quotes/helen_rowland_147607

looking it up on Google. *Garrulous* means *to chatter.* It also means *to talk ceaselessly about unimportant things.*

Do you have any conversational people in your life?

I challenge you to start using the word garrulous in your everyday life!

About an hour and a half into the flight, as I am gulping down yet another bad airline coffee, I think I might need to change her name to Fortissima!

I had to take Latin at SMU, so I like to incorporate Latin into my writings and sermons.

This is the worthless trivia you get from being a well-read soul.

Fortissimo is Latin and means very loud.

I liked what I named her: *Fortissima Garrulous.*

Everyone sitting in coach within twenty feet knew about her life. She was going to Corpus to buy a house. She and her husband were moving to Corpus from California, cashing out her 1980s home that had just been sold for 2.5 million to buy her house cash in Corpus. She could buy quite a few houses for that kind of windfall. Her husband had gotten a new job in Corpus. She was concerned because he was a job hopper in California and she wanted him to be more steady, Eddy! But on the flip side, he lands nicely and is always going to new jobs, always moving up. Who needs to have a boss with two-and-a-half million in the bank?

They have two children: six and four, a boy and a girl. They are into everything: soccer, dance. The boy is taking Karate to build his self-confidence. Six years old, and he needs self-confidence? Fortissima taught herself decorating. She is a decorator now. She's "into" decorating; that is how she put it. She used to be a cheerleader. She used to teach cheerleading. But now she is into decorating with her sister. She has three sisters. After a while, it was like watching Charlie Brown when the teacher spoke, but the teacher's voice was all I could hear: "Wah, Wah, Wah, Wah" and on and on. I thought to myself: Is that how people feel when I preach? Do you know about minute forty-two in the sermon? Don't answer that.

I was trying to write this amazing chapter, looking for material and tuning in and out of her voice like the old boom box I had in the eighties, trying to get Casey Casum's top forty countdown. But then I started listening to her chatter, Fortissma Garrulous talking, and I started hearing some DINGs!

Ding! There was sadness in what she was saying.

Ding! It wasn't idle chatter. It was more like a confession, a plea out of desperation. The deep truth about her was she needed some help! Fortissma Garrulous wants to change her life, and she's hoping a change in geography will change it. The only problem is, guess who goes with her everywhere she goes? Everywhere you go…guess who goes with you? You. Sometimes people focus on changing the outsides of their world, rather than the insides of their world.

She was screaming that she wanted a life of success and significance, and she felt like maybe moving to Corpus would do it for her. If you are unhappy without the two-and-a-half million, you will not be satisfied with the two-and-a-half million, for money makes you want more. They once asked John D. Rockefeller, the world's first billionaire, "How much is enough?" He said, "Just a little bit more."[14] When do we ever ask ourselves: How much is enough?

Ding! You have to change more than geography to change your life.

Ding! Fortissma Garrulous feels that her life is insignificant!

I realized God wanted me to write this chapter about her, you, me, and our struggle to change our lives. More than 200 years ago, Isaac Watts described in Horace Paraphrased

> "There are a number of us who creep - Into the world to eat and sleep;
>
> And know no reason why we are born,
>
> But only to consume the corn,
>
> Devour the cattle, fowl, and fish,
>
> And leave behind an empty dish."[15]

Admitting my life is a train wreck without the train is the beginning of change. Admitting my life is a mess, and I am often powerless to change it without God, is the beginning of change. It's step one in every twelve-step program. It's the deep truth we don't like to admit to ourselves, others, and God. I woke up the other morning and looked at how I woke up. It was not pretty. Shower, blow dryer, deodorant, cologne—I called in all available resources to change me. Beyoncé sings, "I woke up like this," and she has a picture of her beauty. Ha! She and thirty other hairstylists and makeup artists helped her to look like this. When women wake up, they can look in the mirror with hope. They have options for upgrades, cover-all, makeup, and hide-the-wrinkle cream.

When men look in the mirror, we say, "This is as good as it gets." When it comes to change, we often say, "Well, this is as good as it gets." Ding! I am not the end of any-thing when I think about myself. Ding! But I can be the beginning of many things in God's hands!

See, you are by yourself, and you probably are not much. But you, in God's hands, can be anything God wants you to be. But you still must place yourself in God's hands. You must leave the comfort of your seatbelt that you love to wear in life and start walking around the cabin. Sometimes it's dark, and you can't see around the cabin! But you will

14 Sherman, S. (2020, November 25). *How Much Is Enough?* Mindful. https://www.mindful.org

15 Watts, I. (n.d.). *Poets' Corner*. Poets' Corner - Isaac Watts - Selected Works. https://www.theotherpages.org/poems/watts01.html

most likely see the light when it's the darkest. People ask me: "Which is better, Pastor, to do funerals or weddings?" I used to say weddings. Now I say funerals. Why? Because people are listening at a funeral. People are open to seeing and hearing from God at a funeral. When I do weddings, the couple is not listening. They are all gaga with lust and kissy-kissy. But at funerals, people are quiet; their hearts are open and broken with grief, well, most funerals anyway. Pastor, pastor I am just not sure my loved one lying in the casket was saved.

Where are they? When my mom died, I tried to warn people in the wake. Don't repeat dumb clichés to my dad because he had lost his filter. You know, that is the age when people say what they want because they are retired, and they don't care anymore. So, this well-meaning guy says to my dad, "Jim, she's in a better place." My dad says, "Really, I don't know. She's lying over there in a box about to be put into the ground, and that doesn't seem like a better place to me." Ouch!

But what does it mean to be saved?

Does Fortissima Garrulous need salvation? When a preacher says she needs help, is it just the afterworld I am discussing here?

No, not at all. That ticket has already been purchased. It's the abundant life she's not living. Jesus's number one subject was how to make up their come down here, thy Kingdom of God, not how to get into heaven.

Four well-meaning Baptists knocked on my door the other day, having no idea I was a preacher. They knocked and said, "Sir, have you been saved?"

I thought, *This is going to be good. They have no earthly clue about who I am.* I said, "Saved from what?"

"Well, sir, from eternal hell and damnation?"

"Well, how do you know I am headed there? Presumptuous of you to knock on my door and tell a stranger I am bound for endless torture for all eternity."

"Sir, you will go to hell if you don't say this prayer."

I love religious people; they always know where everyone is headed! I say, "I am? Are you all on the heaven and hell committee? Was there a nomination process or email that I missed? How does one land on that committee?"

I Thought All I Had to Do Was Say "The Prayer"

One of the other popular misconceptions about salvation is that all you have to do is recite the Sinner's Prayer, and you will be saved. One problem with this idea is that "The prayer" doesn't appear anywhere in the Bible. Trust me, I've checked. Another issue is that many people don't feel the dramatic inner change they expected to experience after praying the magic prayer. They wonder if they did it right. Then they pray the prayer again the next night, the next week, forty more times in church! They're deeply troubled that perhaps they're not really "in." The problem is not that they said the prayer incorrectly. The problem is that their definition of salvation is too small. They think Jesus defined salvation merely as a ticket to heaven; you will be ok in the next by and by! They're defining salvation as having their entrance application to heaven accepted rather than receiving abundant life from Jesus every waking moment. Salvation for Jesus was always twofold: Eternal life, which we should not worry about, and abundant life here and now, which we are invited to right now!

After explaining all this, I knew from the looks on their faces that they regretted knocking on my door. I think I have a little bit of my old man in me, willing to challenge these dumb religious clichés.

I continued, "Well, I don't know about that speculative future stuff you are talking about, but if hell existed, why is it not mentioned in the Old Testament? And when Jesus mentioned it, he's referring to the trash dump?"

"Sir, what do you do for a living?"

"I am a writer," I yell out with enthusiasm.

"Sir, you need to say this prayer immediately!"

"What about right now? Can you say a prayer to help my marriage, my drinking problem, my temper, or my relationship with my kids? No doubt I need salvation, but it's mostly being saved from a barren, busy, empty life of working to pay my mortgage."

Most of us have plenty of hell to deal with on this side of heaven!

As a leader of religious people, I have some problems with spiritual people.

Do you want to knock on doors and ask people if they are saved? I think a better question is this one:

Sir, if you don't die tonight, how are you going to live tomorrow? Abundantly? As you dreamed? How do you live an abundant life that God wants to give us?

The problem with religious people is that they are so focused on the next world that they forget the importance of this world. Don't become so focused on what you can't see; you forget to deal with what you can see.

God sent His Son.

Why?

It was more than just getting you a ticket to heaven.

Jesus said not to worry about the next life. Instead, Jesus's number one subject was the Kingdom of God—making up there come down here, God's will be done on earth as it is in heaven! That's the meaning of the Kingdom of God. It's abolishing slavery, racism, sexism, and all the "isms!" It's seeing everyone as a child of God, not the pigment of their skin or orientation! Read the New Testament sometimes. Count how many times Jesus referred to the Kingdom of God. If you take Matthew, Mark, and Luke, Jesus refers to the Kingdom of God 111 times. If you talk about something 111 times, it's probably essential.

Jesus's primary mission was Not only to get us into heaven but to get heaven into us.

Quit worrying about heaven in the next life! Start focusing on bringing heaven here!

Knock on doors and invite people into making this world a better place, making up there come down here! That's an invite I will accept! The disciples asked Jesus, how do we pray? They could have asked, "Jesus, teach us how to love, how to forgive, how to heal," but it was to pray. What was Jesus's response? Again, it was about the Kingdom of God. He told them that when they pray, with their words and actions, they should make sure it's about making up there and coming down here. God's will be done on earth as it is in heaven.

After all this rant, they stood there looking at me dumbfounded and unsure whether to walk off or keep arguing with me. Amid this whole scene, I began to recall a sad pastoral moment. I will never forget it. I was burying Wilfred Ott's second son! I had already buried his older one three years ago; he died in a car accident! This son, the younger one I am getting ready to bury, died a slower death, but also from an accident. He got injured in a factory and couldn't use his dominant right hand. They gave him a little money, and he drank to forget. He wanted to forget too much, and liver failure followed.

On the day of the funeral for the second son, who was all of fifty-one, Wilfred looked at me and said this, "Pastor, I don't want to hear anything about hell today in your eulogy. Don't tell me that there's a hell waiting for me when I die because I am already in hell. No Dad wants to bury both his sons."

You never know the level of pain in someone else's heart. I didn't argue or disagree with him. His losses were heartaches, not hassles. Sometimes people find themselves trapped in hell right here on this side of heaven. He wept, I did too, and so did Jesus. Sometimes all we can do is cry and give it to God. But we can also get stuck in grief, and that is a hell in and of itself. You want to move from grief to gratitude. "Don't cry because it's over; smile because it happened." Dr. Suess said that.

From my well-meaning Baptists, salvation was more expansive than Jesus taught; salvation was always twofold: Eternal life in the next life and abundant life in this one. Both are important.

Salvation is forgiveness for your past, purpose in this moment, and eternal hope for your future. Salvation is saying yes to the abundant life that Jesus offers you now, today, and forever. What a gift: It's free. Salvation is free to you but cost Jesus everything. When my dad was the Vice President of USAA, he received courtside tickets to the San Antonio Spurs game during the NBA finals. These seats were expensive, worth thousands, but they cost us nothing more than a trip to the Will Call Office, show our IDs, and give us an envelope with the seats on them. Likewise, Jesus died an expensive death. It cost him everything to provide you with salvation, life abundantly, life eternally. But you must still go to Will Call and pick up the tickets. There is a plane called Salvation that will take off. You have a reserved seat on the plane, but you have to choose to say yes and put your butt in the seat.

Ding! Your tickets to a better life await you. Eddie Money had a great song, "Two Tickets to Paradise." He sang, "Won't you pack your bags and leave tonight?" There's a sense of urgency when someone invites you to paradise. Your ticket is waiting. You can't wait to catch that plane! You have to lay claim to that which Jesus gave up his claim! That usually means losing the safety of your devices, ways, and plans to change life. It involves surrendering and taking off the seat belt of security. Ding! It's time to explore outdoors, leave the comfort of the great indoors, unlock your door and the safety of your lair and camera doorbell, and go outside. Maybe it's not safety first, but safety second and Jesus first.

Don't worry about losing it! Salvation: You can't lose it. How can you lose what you never earned? You have to receive it. You can't lose it, but you can reject it. You can say no to God, and God will honor that freedom! Salvation is inviting God into your heart to change your current life. The only concern for the next life you should have is like the leading real estate concern: location, location, location.

But that's also been decided. My Jewish friend, Rabbi Joseph, said it best: "It won't be heaven unless everyone is there." What if I told you the whole world is my parish? God tells us as much: It's Good News for the World…it's Joy to the World…Remember, according to the last book of the Bible it tells us that the Gates of Heaven are never shut. In fact, it says, The sun never sets in heaven! Have you never read Revelation 21:25 (NIV)? No locked pearly gates and no setting sun, for there is no night-time in heaven. The sun always shines. God's gates, like the arms of Jesus on the cross, are wide open, waiting for you to be welcomed home!

I am a hope dealer and a hopeful Universalist. I am here to tell you that God's Good Book says this about your loved one: whether they believed in God or not, God believed in them. If you are alive and have a heartbeat, it's from God, and God believes in you. If you have ever had a heartbeat, God believes in you.

What's More Important: You believing in God or the Almighty believing in You?

My money is on God every time. Chances are, like one hundred percent, you and your loved ones will walk right into their loving Father's arms, not because of anything you have done but because of what Jesus has done. Historically, the church has not wanted to celebrate or discuss this because it cuts down on the offering. But if you don't claim the ticket now, you are missing out on the abundant life you can have today. Don't look surprised when you see people you didn't like on Earth in heaven! I think the first five minutes might be a lot of shocked faces. What are you doing here? But heaven is not going to be a potluck! You aren't going there because you are bringing the best bean casserole ever tasted. You are going there based only on what Jesus has done for you, despite you. Others, well, will be just as surprised to see you there. But it's not because of what you have done or what they did; it's just because you all picked up your tickets.

I said to the four well-meaning Baptists, "What about saving my life right now? I got some chains and seat belts around things I want to be free of?"

"Sir, what is wrong with you?" one brave lady inquired.

Well, a lot. A lot is wrong with me, but a lot is right with and within me. Do you know what I say when people ask me what's wrong with the world? *Me.* I am what's wrong with this world. I need to get busy changing myself, which will change the world.

Salvation? What is that?

Ding! For me, it's refusing to live a life less than what my mom prayed over me when I was born. Prayers don't have expiration dates. Salvation is about making up there come down here. It's about making God's will be done on earth as much as in heaven. Salvation is just as much about having abundant life today as it is about having eternal life tomorrow.

Salvation says I don't have to be resentful; I can be forgiving. I don't have to be hateful; I can be loving. I don't have to be greedy; I can be generous. I don't have to live in guilt; I can live in freedom. Salvation says I don't always have to feel shame; I can feel forgiveness and have a new life. Salvation is about saying I once was a caterpillar, but now I am a butterfly. Think about it: no one ever sees a butterfly and says, hey, look at this converted worm, it's a converted caterpillar. Salvation is about becoming the me God intended me to be. Living free of the guilt and shame cycles we get stuck in. Salvation is about saying shame off you. What Jesus was trying to say to us is simply this: "Salvation is at hand, like the Kingdom of God; it's within you, take it, choose it or not! If you invite me into your heart and life, streams of living water will flow within you!"

Jesus was sent to help me from me, save me from me, and bring me peace so that I might live at peace with myself, God, and others.

I never said their four-part prayer and have not heard another knock on my door.

As I was sitting on the plane, working on this chapter, I started having more "DINGs" go off in my head. I remembered Saint Exupery, who wrote *The Little Prince.* He also wrote about flying. True story: Saint Exupery was one of the first aviators. He flew the mail in North Africa and South America at the beginning of this century. He wrote beautiful books about flying. In his book, *Wind, Sand, and Stars,* he wrote about an experience on a plane that was much worse than having to go the bathroom or listen to a talkative, desperate soul. He wrote that on one flight, his plane crashed in the North African desert. He barely survived the ordeal, and like all people who look Mr. Death in the face and live to tell about it, he lived differently from then on. Ding! He came out of it with a heightened expectation of what life can be, what we are capable of, what heights we can achieve as human beings, and what little time we have to achieve it.

After the crash, he returned to France. He took a train from Marseilles to Paris. He wrote about the faces of the people on the train. I am writing right now about the faces on this flight. He wrote: "All I can see in these faces is the silent misery of wasted lives." He described a man on the train called "The Bourgeois of Toulouse." "Why didn't somebody shake this man early in his life before this clay hardened and get him to live the kind of life he can? And now that musician, that poet, that artist, that craftsman under this man is gone, and it will never happen."[16]

When Michelangelo carved the famous statue of David, he was asked how he knew what David looked like. How did you know where to put the chisel and hammer to? He replied, "I just removed everything from the block of marble that was not David!" Have you given God the chisel? When you do, that's salvation.

Ding! "Why didn't somebody shake him to get him to live all the life he is capable of?"

When did you quit living and start existing?

I thought of that passage as I listened to the woman talk incessantly, especially when she said, "You know, I asked my husband if we could settle down now, not move anymore. We have enough. We ought to spend more time with our children before they go wrong. But he told me that he doesn't have enough. He wants more." You won't be enough with millions if you are insufficient without millions.

Saint Exupery was appalled when he returned from the desert experience and saw what he described as how the "machine stamped out these every day, joyless lives, all of them looking alike." I am not sure much has changed. Do you feel like the machine has stamped on your life? Artificial intelligence is here, and I fear it might start stamping. Are you just a social security number?

Because Saint Exupery had almost lost his life, future self, and what he could become, he valued life more than those without that experience.

"Lord teach us to number our days" (Psalm 90:12, NIV). This is the value of knowing that you are in the "last days"—yours anyway. Most of us only get 27,375 days this side of heaven—3,910 weeks of life. Three thousand nine hundred ten weeks of living with the fact that you are hurtling at lightning speed toward your death means you make this day and everyday count. Don't waste a breath, a heartbeat, a moment. You only get to do this once. Live with urgency.

---

16 Saint-Exupéry, A. de, Galantière, L., & Cosgrave, J. O. (1939). *Wind, sand and stars*. Reynal & Hitchcock.

Saint Exupery's life took a dramatic turn when he experienced a life-altering incident. In that plane crash, his old, stagnant self-perished, making way for a new, vibrant life that was born out of the wreckage. He was reborn! This transformative experience led him to pen these profound words:

"It is only with the heart that one can see rightly: what is essential is invisible to the eye."[17]

Salvation, the Kingdom of God, is often invisible to the eye. It's not something we can see with our physical senses. It's love, friendship, forgiveness, and restored relationships. These are the most significant things; we can only perceive them with our hearts, not our eyes. It's ironic that right after Jesus is in the desert, he returns, perhaps having witnessed people living dull, joyless lives, and he says to them (you and me): "I have come so that they may have life and have it in abundance" (John 10:10, CSB).

Today, abundant life is in this moment, not just in the next life.

Today, you can be alive and fulfill your purposes! You don't have to fidget your life away, wondering why you are here!

Your life is now!

Jesus says what every good hope dealer says: "You can let your hopes, not your past hurts, shape your future." At least in my mind, this is what I hear.

What does he then say? Follow me.

Following is our job. Changing us, much of it, is God's job. But it's still a partnership.

But the change can't happen unless we follow. He says, "Follow Me," and it's in that following God does some of the changing. Our job is to follow; God's job is to help with the change, but we must follow. We must follow Jesus into loving indiscriminately as he did, choosing forgiveness as he did, and it's our choice. Do you want to know God's will and where Jesus is at? Do the things Jesus did: Feed the hungry, have a water ministry (cup of cold water), visit the sick, love your neighbor, whoever that may be!

We choose to love our neighbor, whoever that is, with as much love as we do ourselves. This is following Jesus. When we take those steps, we can't help but be changed. When driving down the road, you can't take two exits at once; you must choose the road and the exit you will take in life. One leads to abundance, and one leads to hell, right here on earth.

You don't have to die to live an abundant life. You don't have to die to live in hell. I have seen people in both camps. I didn't use to think it could be that simple, but now I think it is. I think you get to an age where you realize this is like the second marriage. I am not entering into my new life with a veil on; I am tired of being tired, I am tired of being bored looking at my belly button, and I can't buy anything in this world that will

17 Ellams, I., & Saint-Exupéry, A. de. (2020). *The Little Prince*. Oberon Books.

fill me up. When you realize you have less than 7,665 days left, you become one who has gained enough wisdom to know that making it big isn't as important as making your life count.

As you follow Jesus, you become one who sees that life itself is a gift given to us with infinite potential but with a limited time to experience it.

Jesus knew his days were numbered here on the cross. The Bible says he was always walking. Walking where? Toward the cross! It's that simple for those who have discovered that the fullness of life can be found only when we give ourselves to something greater than ourselves, like the Kingdom of God, up there coming down here, God's will being done. Nothing is better than having a day when you rip a corner of heaven's glory and bring it to earth! One of my church members, sarcastic, funny, outspoken Dick Hamilton, heard God speak to him in a very imperfect sermon on a quiet Sunday morning. Ding! In a sermon, on a Sunday. Jesus said to Dick, "Follow Me to forgiving those who have hurt you, crucified you." He was a longtime church member, and I preached on forgiveness and how we must forgive everyone; God has forgiven us of everything. We don't want to put ourselves above God, do we? Usually a boisterous and talkative guy, I remember watching him cry the entire sermon. I knew he had heard the ding!

He called me later that afternoon and said he had called his brother, whom he had not spoken to in seventeen years, and made amends. His brother flew out the following week and sat by him in church. Do you know how powerful it was to watch Dick introduce his once bad-mouthed brother to the entire church and tell everyone he had finally picked up his ticket? Salvation had arrived: forgiveness.

They had a year together of reconciliation and love. Then, tragically, his brother passed suddenly from a heart attack. But I will never forget standing at that grave and Dick saying, "I am so glad I decided to follow Jesus in forgiving him and reconciling. I am so sorry I wasted seventeen years holding onto bitterness instead of forgiveness. But I can now go to my grave knowing that we didn't waste our last 365 days holding onto pettiness but holding onto each other!"

It's not hard to hear that ding!

Now, it's not easy, and it's scary swallowing your pride and following Jesus down the road of forgiveness, but it will take you from pettiness alley and bitterness road to an abundant life. He had heard God's celestial Ding in his life, calling to take off the seat belt of comfort and truly live his life as it was meant to be.

Have you heard God's Ding in your life?

Didn't Jesus die so you could truly live—not in the cocoon of security all the time, not in the cocoon of safety and a fat 401 K? Not in the safety of having a bunch of temporary dust-collecting stuff that will not go with you to heaven.

But to save the you—that makes you—you!

To save your soul. To give you abundant life today! The only thing going to heaven is your soul. Eternity is already in session. You are already a part of it. Jesus said to the disciples and said to you, "Follow me." He never once said to become a Christian. He never once said go around and tell people about burning in hell. He did say, "Follow me! Follow me. I've got something for you to do. I will help you lead others to a life of significance." Jesus didn't say, "Follow me, and I will take you to a spiritual life retreat." Jesus said, "Follow me, and I will take you into the world to change the world."

What a flight I am on....

I named my son Jacob because God told me to. I also called him Jacob because Jacob's story is the story of many of us. We all start cocky, thinking we are going to grab the world by the tail and stuff it in our pocket. (Think about how dumb your parents were at sixteen.) I knew it all; they could tell me nothing. Those same parents got bright again, somehow, when I was twenty-four. Jacob's entire life had been a struggle. From the very beginning, he struggled with his twin brother, Esau. Jacob was his mother's favorite. If you need to watch Jerry Springer reruns or Dr. Phil to see dysfunctional families, just read the Bible's first book, Genesis.

Jacob knew that his brother Esau was his father Isaac's favorite. It was a classic sibling rivalry that resulted in heartache consequences. Jacob conspired to steal Esau's birthright and blessing. In fear of his life, he ran away from home. He went to a faraway land and fell in love. He agreed to work for seven years in return for Rachel's hand in marriage. But, his future father-in-law, Laban, was as much of a scoundrel as Jacob. Laban substituted his older daughter, Leah, for Rachel on the wedding night. How drunk do you have to be on your wedding night to consummate the marriage with a completely different woman? That's a lot of Bud Lite! Jacob had to work for seven more years for Rachel, whom he loved. Love, as always, was expensive! Then Jacob and Laban got into a dispute over possessions. First, Laban cheated Jacob, and then Jacob cheated Laban. Their family reunions and Thanksgiving dinners were worse than yours! The point is that Jacob was always wrestling with the need to change things in his life and battling: It is what it is, I am who I am…

Much of his struggle, he brought on himself. Sound familiar?

He needed salvation mostly from his ways, from himself. From the very beginning, Jacob was a man of deceit and cunning. Even in the womb, the story says, he grabbed Esau's heel, trying to keep him from being born first. His name, Jacob, means "supplanter" or "grabber." He grabbed his brother's heel. He grabbed his brother's birthright. He grabbed some property from Laban. He grabbed at whatever he wanted! You don't have to teach a two-year-old to say mine or no! Early in his life, he was not a very lovely person. Not the sort of person you would want for a neighbor, and not for a brother, for that matter. But something happened to him that night in the wilderness.

He needed help from God, and he was determined to wrestle that help out of God's hands.

He had an all-night wrestling match with God and came away from that encounter with a new man. Amid the wrestling, Jacob said, "…I will not let you go unless you bless me" (Genesis 32:26, NIV). So, God blessed him.

Have you ever wrestled with God over changing your life? If you do, God will bless you.

Jacob wrestled the angel, and the angel was overcome.

When you encounter the living God, it constantly changes your life.

It's like growing in love with your spouse. Love does not always change the one you love but constantly changes you.

And God changed his name from Jacob to "Israel," meaning "one who strives with God."

Gone was his old life, like his old name. Now, he lived a new life, differently, with a limp.

The limp was evidence that now he would follow and walk differently than ever.

He would walk with wisdom. He would walk with an awareness of God's presence. He would walk with forgiveness. He would walk in the abundant life. **When you wrestle with God, it doesn't just change your today; it changes your forever.**

Jacob's sons were the founders of the tribes of Israel. Since his time, all the people of Israel have traced their ancestry back to him. They say proudly, "We are the descendants of Abraham, Isaac, and Jacob." One of life's most significant questions you will wrestle with is this: What will you do with this difficulty that comes to us all? When Jacob was in his wilderness, he encountered God. And the two of them went at it. Out of it, Jacob received a blessing.

One reason struggles often lead to blessings is that we recognize our limitations and weaknesses and reach for resources beyond ourselves.

Just as Paul said, "For when I am weak, then I am strong" (2 Corinthians 12:10, NIV). When we think we are strong, we have only our strength and resources; in the face of life's difficulties, that is weakness. When we realize our limitations, we open ourselves to God and all the resources of faith, and then we can become intense.

Salvation has come to this house. Zacchaeus would change his daily life and how he lived. Isn't that salvation? He would begin to make up and come down here, God's will being done!

Legend has it that Zacchaeus, the tax collector in his later years, rose early every morning and left his house. His wife, curious, followed him one morning. At the town well, he filled a bucket and walked until he came to a sycamore tree. There, setting down the bucket, he began to clean away the stones, the branches, and the rubbish from around the base of the tree. Having done that, he poured water on the roots and stood there in silence, gently caressing the trunk with both hands. When his amazed wife came out of hiding and asked what he was doing, Zacchaeus replied, "This is where I found Christ! This is where Jesus saved me!"

I can imagine that for the rest of their lives, that woman who touched the hem of Jesus's robe that day on the street and the daughter of Jairus who was raised in that room in her home continually brought people back to those sacred spots and said, "This is where I found Christ!"

Ding! "This is where Christ loved me into life!"

You must undo the seat belt to find a sacred spot like that!

God is not interested in parts of you, for having a part will never change the whole.

God doesn't promise destinations. He promises Himself.

"I will be with you always, even until the end of the world" (Matthew 28:20, CEV).

Salvation is salvation from yourself, your shadow self, your selfish self, the lesser self that always wants to take the easy way out.

Elijah hides in a cave, running away from Jezebel, the wicked queen. He is feeling sorry for himself. God comes to Elijah and speaks to him. Only the text says that God does not talk through "earthquake, wind, and fire," which was the expected way. It was expected that God would speak through nature. I Kings 19:11-13 (CEV) says, "But the Lord was not in the wind. Next, there was an earthquake, but the Lord was not in the earthquake. Then there was a fire, but the Lord was not in the fire." But ding, God spoke in a gentle whisper, in a still, small voice.

God's voice says to Elijah, "Get out of here. I've got something for you to do. I've got a mission for you to perform, so stop moping, meditating, or whatever you are doing up here in this cave and get to work! Take off that which is binding you and live!"

The Bible is not a book of nature.

It is a book of history. It is a book about how God has helped us and promises to help us always.

The Bible claims that the God of Abraham, Isaac, Jacob, and the God of Jesus speaks to us in historical events, like flying on a plane at 35,000 feet, even right now, through a book. I like what Schweitzer said about following Jesus as he discussed people who had tried to write about the "historical Jesus."

Schweitzer concluded that you cannot write a historical biography of Jesus. Anyone who writes a biography of Jesus, he said, is writing about himself. History is like a deep well. As you look down the shaft of the well, through two thousand years of history, you see your reflection in the pool at the bottom. But, he said, Jesus is not discovered through biography anyway. He used the scene at the end of the Gospel of John to illustrate this. The Gospel of John is at the end, after the Resurrection. The disciples think that Jesus is dead, so they return to Galilee and take up their old fishing business. Jesus appears to them just as he did at the beginning of his ministry.

In the beginning, he says: "Follow Me!"

Now, he comes to them in their despair after the Resurrection.

This time he says: "Feed my sheep."

But it is the same thing. It is a call to discipleship. It's the call to surrender your lesser self so your greater self can live now and forever.

Schweitzer says that is what we should expect in this post-resurrection era.

We live in the time after the Resurrection, so we should expect Jesus to be with us and still call us.

These are Schweitzer's famous words. "He comes to us as one unknown. As of old by the lakeside, he came to those men who knew him not and spoke to us the same words, 'Follow thou me,' and set us on the tasks that he has to fulfill in our time."[18]

That's the clue.

God calls us to fulfill the tasks he has for our time, and time is limited. You don't have to survive the plane crashes of life to realize this.

Salvation means God has raised Jesus from the dead to say to anything in your life, "It doesn't have to be this way!"

The Resurrection means that Jesus is not some figure who lived in the past and is now gone. Jesus is someone who lives with us now. He speaks to us in our conscience or on sunsets. Sometimes he says to us on plane rides with other people, "Ding! The plane just landed, and a captain is flying the plane of your life." He has just told us, "You are now free to unbuckle that which restrains you!"

When was the last time you heard the ding?

Before you give up, will you listen for it?

---

18 Schweitzer, A. (2005). *The Quest of the Historical Jesus*. Dover Publications.

CHAPTER THREE

THE WAYS YOU LET IN BECOME THE WAYS YOU GET SET IN!

All life is an experiment. The more experiments you make, the better.

—Ralph Waldo Emerson

WE ALL HAVE WAYS; YOU have your ways, and I have my ways. Our ways are how we choose to react. Our ways are the way we choose to speak. Our ways are when we choose to insert ourselves and when we choose not to! When we accept and when we decline! When we stay and when we go. To ask for help or not is your way. To number your days or not is your way. Who you let into or kick out of your castle is your way. Your passions speak of your ways. How you spend money is your way. Your boundaries are your ways. Your text message history speaks of your ways. It's just the way I am… we say.

Many of our ways were modeled by our parents. We adopted our ways because that's how Mom handled conflict: Mine with a tennis racket, shoe, or whatever nearby became the weapon of choice. That's how Dad spent money. He had his ways, and some of those ways became your ways.

Two sons: One alcoholic father. One son's way was to adopt the father's ways. The other son's way was to reject his father's ways. Both sons were asked, "Why are you the way you are?" Both said, "My father was a drunk!"

Your kids have their ways.

My oldest son, Jacob, told me about a test he had last year at Texas A&M. This is a major professor at a major university, Texas A&M in College Station, one of the largest universities in the country. He was in a Mechanical Engineering class, and the professor was about to pass out the final exam, the most important test of the year. Before he did, he told his students how proud he was of them, and because they had worked so hard, he made them a special offer. He said, "Anyone that would like an automatic C on this test, just raise your hand, and I'll give you a C. You won't even have to take the test." One hand slowly went up, then another, and another until about half of the students opted out of taking the test. They walked out of the room, so relieved, so happy. The professor passed out the test to the rest of the students, placed it face down on the desk, and asked them not to turn it over until he instructed them to. For the next few minutes, he encouraged them about how they would do great things in life and how they should always strive to do their best. Then he said turning the test over and getting started was okay. The test only had two sentences. "Congratulations! You just made an A."

Some people's ways are easy, and some people's ways are more complex. We often settle for a C without realizing that God has an A in our future.

"I don't think I'll ever get over this sickness. I'm just learning to live with it."

That's taking a C! Be careful because the way you let in, you will get set in.

The thoughts you allow to enter your mind shape the life you lead. They can transform your reality, turning a C into an A. It's all about the mindset you choose to adopt.

To change your ways, you have to change your thoughts.

Wrong ways of thinking don't lead to the right ways of living.

Think wrong, live wrong. Think right, live right.

It's impossible to think wrong and live right.

Here's the empowering truth: you, and only you, hold the reins to your "thought life." If you shift your thinking, you can transform your life. "God is restoring health unto me. I will live and not die. I'm getting stronger, healthier, better." That's aiming for the A. "Well, I'm getting up there in years. You know how your health starts to go downhill." That's settling for a C. How about: "I am going to age with awesomeness" as my life coach and good friend Dane Boyle says?

"I'll never break this addiction. I've had it since high school."—another C.

"This guy I'm dating, I know he's not good for me. He doesn't treat me right, but I may never meet anybody else." That's not a C, that's a D, that's an F.

God has an "A," but you'll never see it if you keep taking the Cs. Yes, the Cs are more accessible. You don't have to stretch. You don't have to get out of your comfort zone. You don't have to take the test, but did God make you a C? I can't think of much that would be sadder than to come to the end of life and have to wonder,

"What could I have become if I didn't settle for good enough?"

What could I have been if I hadn't taken so many Cs; instead, I pressed forward, striving to be my very best. I know some of you are thinking, *Well, I married a C!* Well, you stick with him and help make him into an A. Don't look at your husband now; that's the wrong time. Eyes straight ahead. When God breathed his life into you, he put a part of himself in you. You have the DNA of Almighty God. You were never created to be average, barely get by, always struggle, and have to take the leftovers. I can blame you for my ways, or I can redefine them.

Through Facebook and Instagram, we learn from others' perspectives. However, you have your ways of seeing, thinking, and speaking about things.

Just because you were raised in specific ways doesn't mean you must continue living in those ways.

Just because you grew up that way doesn't mean you must stay that way.

I don't expect my neighbor to mow my lawn, although he is invited to do so anytime. Likewise, I don't expect my neighbor to define the boundaries of my castle. It's my castle. I decide who to let in my castle and who cannot come across the moat. Why do you keep giving the controls to your drawbridge to others? Is it their castle? I am responsible for my heart, my ways, and my attitude. Whether you think you can or can't—you are…right! Is it your way to go with the flow? Is your way one of design or one of default?

What if I told you that one of the reasons Hitler lost World War II was because of his ways?

I know you are like, wait, what, Hitler? How is he bringing up Hitler in a book like this? Well, because sometimes you can get a wake-up call from the past. Everyone has ways, right or wrong, evil or good. We all have our ways!

June 6, 1944, in the heat of summer, was D-Day, the most decisive event in World War II. It was the battle, the invasion, that turned the tide. D-Day is incredible for many reasons: It was the largest amphibious assault in history. It was the largest deceit, most incredible deceit since the Trojan Horse. One hundred sixty thousand troops came into France to take it out from under Nazi-controlled forces, which was just astounding. They managed to completely deceive the whole Axis army about where the landing was to take place. Now they knew when it was coming. You don't get to mobilize that many people without them knowing it's going down. So Eisenhower, the supreme commander, knew that the Nazis knew when they were going to be coming. But they didn't know where. You see, there was this whole Atlantic Wall that Hitler thought was impenetrable that ran from the Arctic down to basically Spain. And he felt that with this massive stretch of defenses, as he made sure there were guns, pillboxes, and barbed wire, he would watch it all. The Allied forces tried to trick Hitler into thinking they would land in the South of France because it was the closest to the nation of England, just across the channel, at the shallowest depth. They did some incredible things to make them think that was where the invasion would take place. On the morning of D-Day, they rained out paratroopers who were mannequins all over the South of France. And some of these mannequins were rigged with explosives, so as they landed, there would be bombs going off. They covered the area adjacent to where they were trying to make Hitler think they were going to land with inflatable tanks so they would feel that they were amassing a massive force. In aerial reconnaissance photos, it looked like there were so many tanks in southern France, but they were just dummy balloon tanks.

Meanwhile, of course, the invasion happened at the five beaches of Normandy in central France, where 5,000 ships would quickly come across these artificial ports that created harbors. And they were going to storm the beaches there, and they had hoped all the gun stations had been taken out. Of course, the Omaha ones weren't taken out, which is why it was so bloody and devastating at Omaha. And this whole thing worked. One of the big reasons that this massive turn-the-tide event happened in this war was because Hitler was not a morning person.

His ways were sleepy. You see, he liked to sleep in, sometimes as late as noon.

On D-Day, when this was happening—and remember, Hitler knew when it was happening—he was so confident that even that morning, he slept in. And his men were so afraid—all of his generals were so afraid of waking him up, that even once they figured out that it was raining mannequins in the South of France, and when they finally figured out it was happening in Normandy, they needed his permission to move the elite SS panzer divisions of tanks!

Hitler had to personally approve rerouting all tanks from the South of France to Normandy. The speed of reinforcements was everything in battle, is everything in battle. It could have changed the outcome of the D-Day invasion in favor of the Nazis. But because he had to give permission himself, and because he was asleep when the battle took place, when he finally woke up at 11:00 or 12:00, it was too late, and they already got a foothold on the beaches of Normandy that led to them taking France back. This was the event that turned the tide in World War II.[19]

I'm not saying that if you're a night owl, you should change your ways and become an early bird.

I am saying that you can't win a war while you're sleeping!

Romans 13:11 (TPT) says, "To live like this is all the more urgent, for time is running out, and you know it is a strategic hour in human history. It is time for us to wake up, for our full salvation is nearer now than when we first believed."

Opportunities can't be taken if you are sleeping.

Sunrises can't be seen if you are sleeping.

Winning a war doesn't happen if you are sleeping.

19 Riis, D. (2019, March 18). *What Hitler got wrong about D-day*. History.com. https://www.history.com/news/d-day-hitler-germany-defenses-miscalculations

This is your wake-up call.

Your ways are brief and few; you will only be here temporarily. Live in urgent, not wasteful ways, and you won't waste your days. One of my ways is to fan the flames of the love of my life and to keep dating my wife. If I don't date my wife, someone else will. If you don't date your spouse, someone else will. If you don't take your spouse to bed, someone else will. Fan the flames so you have a flame to fan. So, there we are: Baby Doll and I are out on another date night. It's chips and queso night. I have never been unhappy with my wife or my life, with chips and queso in front of me. Chips and queso are faith food. It helps you believe that God loves and wants us to be happy. (smile)

Every couple has ways. Every marriage has its ways. Some marriage ways work, and some don't. One of our marriage ways is weekly check-ins. We ask each other questions once a week, such as: What's it like to live on the other side of me? How can I be a better husband? What can I do more of in the marriage? What can I do less of in the marriage? I ask questions and then listen, listen, hear, and change so I can love her better. But we are intentional about our marriage; no marriage is excellent by accident. Here's the rule: Sometimes you must be utterly inaccessible to others to be accessible to your spouse. How can your spouse reach you if you always reach for your phone? Research says you touch your phone 2,500 times daily. You do it wrong if you feel, scroll, interact, and laugh with your phone more than your spouse.

What did the Bible say, "It's the little foxes that spoil the vineyards" of our love (Song of Solomon 2:15, ESV).

Little things like cell phones can become big things in our lives! Being utterly inaccessible to everyone else, so we can only be accessible to each other, is a priority. If your marriage is a priority, have a weekly date night and check-in. It has revolutionized our marriage. Have some designated times in your relationships when you put the phone down. Face time is best, and it is best done in person. This way, being inaccessible to all but one communicates: "You are a priority!" Some of you are too available to everyone else and not available enough to the ones you committed your lives to.

The same is true with God. How can God reach me while everyone else can get me? Weekly, go where no one else can reach you so God can reach you. Jesus practiced this. Why do you think you don't need to? Some of my ways are alone and time with God, myself, and my spouse.

Why don't we do this? We think we can microwave our relationships so they taste good. Have you ever seen a restaurant advertise that they have the best microwaved food in town? No one wants that—soggy bread, limp fries, and a dirty microwave. Nothing good in life comes fast; not construction projects, not healthy babies, not good scotch or whiskey, not marriage, not your relationship with God, not food, not your dreams, not a meaningful life, not weight loss. Nothing good comes in a hurry. I want a marriage in the oak barrels of love, not in the lustful honeymoon stage full of the feels! What if one of your ways was always playing chess instead of checkers? God and true love roll with a crock-pot. God is not found at the drive-through but in the sit-down meal.

Have you ever tried to love someone and grieve with someone in a hurry? Yes, I know you lost your loved one, but can we hurry all this crying up?

Have you ever tried to put hope on a quick deadline? It just doesn't work.

Love always means unhurried time together—with your spouse or God. Love and hurry are incompatible with one another. It's why you keep dating and keep checking in. It would be best if you put the time in. Make it a rule: Spend unhurried time with the ones you love. Crock-pot your time with your loved ones; schedule it because good relationships are like falling asleep. I can't force it. I can't make falling asleep happen, but I can turn off the lights, crawl into bed, put my head on the pillow, and trust God for all my troubles. I can set the table for love to happen, but it doesn't happen at the drive-through. I can arrange my life so that deep, meaningful love is possible or not.

What if the only thing we were ever in a hurry to do was to love one another?

What if every time you walked in the door, you greeted your partner with a hug and a kiss and said it's good to see you, regardless of what happened that day? Try it for a week and tell me things have not changed.

I know. I know. It's dangerous to ask your wife: What's it like to live on the other side of me? How do I come off? What are my blind spots? What do you need more of or less of in the marriage? Sometimes I wish my wife was a better liar. One night, I came home from work set in tired, grumpy, irritable ways. I asked: What's it like to live on the other side of me? She says: Everyone at work gets the best of you. I get the worst of you. Everyone at work gets Pastor John. I got Jerk John. Ouch. Her ways are sometimes too honest for my ways! Instead of getting defensive, I made some adjustments. It was true for her if she felt that way, and I needed to adjust. I now drive into my garage and say a little prayer. "Lord, help me leave work at work, and when I walk through this door, be who my wife wanted me to be on our wedding day, but even better." That prayer has changed my marriage because it changed me.

But there we were on Friday night date night. After twenty-seven years, we still long to gaze "lovingly and longingly" into each other's eyes and get some "relief" from the week! It was chips and queso night at On the Border. It was on this night when, out of the corner of my eye, I saw this "couple that didn't couple well."

Have you ever seen two people and thought: How did these two end up together? Did someone win the lottery? That was my thought and more, as in walked the most gorgeous woman I think heaven could allow. She was striking in every way. You might even argue that God spent some extra time on her. Right next to her, practically attached to her, was a dopey, nerdy, lumpy, dumpy sort of guy. Have you ever seen the play

Beauty and The Beast? She looked like a thirty-five-year-old who just jumped off the cover of Glamour Magazine. He looked like a fifty-year-old who had just climbed out of his parents' basement.

On the surface, at least, his and her ways were divergent!

Yet, despite his obvious outer, limiting shell, the two were obviously in love, as they giggled and strolled into their love booth, complete with their relief in two frozen 'ritas! They sat, not across from each other but right next to each other. Shockingly, they were talking to each other and not scrolling on their phones. I turned to my wife of twenty-seven years, a beautiful baby doll, and said, "Wow! What's an amazingly gorgeous young woman like that doing with a leafy-dopey, pudgy, middle-aged guy like him?" Baby doll quipped back, "You think people say that about us?" *Well played, wifey. More chips, please!* Renee's ways may be tiny, but she is small and mighty, like the hummingbird.

The ways he let in, he had become set in. His ways were not the typical ways. A guy like that would often ask himself: How do I overcome what I can't fix? I will not be on the morally depraved TV show, *The Bachelor.* Although now they have *The Golden Bachelor* for the older gents, sponsored by Viagra, right? He knew he would not be voted Most Handsome by GQ magazine! You might as well get used to being lonely.

I am who I am.

You can't fix your face, can you?

He didn't believe those lies.

How do I know? I asked him. We met up in the restroom. Do you know that awkward point when you wait to wash your hands as he washes his hands because only one soap dispenser is working? I don't just people watch; I people ask. I am always curious about how people think because how you feel is how you live. I asked him about his ways. "No offense, brother, but I couldn't help but notice that you outkicked your coverage and, like me, ended up with all that heaven would allow in your wife! How did you do it? How did you land such a hot wife?" He looks at me and says the most excellent quote:

"I've always been a sort of what-if kind of guy."

Did you hear it? He said he always was that way. It's his way; he was already set in, and asking her out was natural. I gave him a fist bump and went back to my booth with a smile on my face. I knew what had happened. This man, who had no business on the outside, at least, had what it took where it mattered most, on the inside, to dare to dream, to say—What if? What if I ask her out, and she says yes? He realized a significant relationship with another means looking beyond the flowers and grass of a person's outside and looking at what lies under the hood! Instead of catastrophizing his world and forecasting doom and gloom and cloudy skies, which only becomes a self-fulfilling prophecy of self-pity—he was willing to ask a more giving question:

What's the best thing that can happen? What if the Sun shines brightly on my life today? What then? Opportunity dances with those on the dance floor, not on the sidelines. His way was to be on the dance floor. He was willing to go for the A when the world told him to take a C!

Haven't you spent enough time asking: What if this goes wrong? What if that goes south? Haven't you spent too many of your 27,375 days asking: What's the worst thing that could happen? The fear and that answer have kept you stuck. You are believing the lie that luck, fate, or life has dealt you a poor hand, and you cannot fold up and refuse to take a bet.

You are the result of your decisions, not fate.

All that your life holds right now, the cup will never get bigger! That's a lie.

This is as good as it gets. That's another lie.

You're out of luck. Your back is against the wall. That's a lie.

How long will you believe and listen to the evil one whose nickname is Father of Lies?

The evil one impregnates people with lies, helps lies be born, lies that keep us from living the whole life God intended when he breathed His breath into our lungs. Let's roll it out anyway, even if we go negative here: "What if I ask her out and she says no?" Well, you will be in the same place you are now. Alone. Maybe a bit more of a bruised ego, but still in the same place, alone.

If we flip it: What if she says yes? What if I can show her the best side of me? What if she discovers the most beautiful part of anyone, their soul, heart, the inside? Talent and beauty may get you the job, but character keeps you in the job. Competency may get in the room; character keeps you in the room. Beauty fades, but who you are on the inside—that's forever. She did say yes—four kids, and twenty years later, there he is, having chips and queso on a Friday night date night, cashing in on the results of asking the right question.

You can't live a proper life by asking the wrong questions.

What-if questions were part of his way. If it's not part of yours, maybe you should quit saying, "I can't change my ways." Start admitting that you won't change your ways! Is your "I can't" really a "I won't?" Living proof, he was, sitting in the booth next to me, growing deeper in love with a woman that most people would never put together. Don't be most people. What if your life is only one decision away from getting better?

What if your life is only two words away from getting bigger, richer, and more meaningful? What if?

I got this text as I sat back in the booth after the restroom chat. It made me quit reaching for the chips. It was a text from a dead man:

"I just refused the ventilator again. The doctors tell me I will die now. They tell me I am dying. I feel pretty good about dying, but I have never died before. I know I should say more. I love you all. Goodbye."

That text was from my dad, a dead man, according to those who were treating him. I got it that night, and for him, on day ninety-five in the hospital, battling for his life fighting off the "Rona" or COVID-19, at eighty-two years old!

The ways you let in become the ways you are set in, as there was no doubt that text was from my old man. Sarcastic till the end, that is my intrepid father. My favorite line, and the one who told me it was my old man: "I feel pretty good for dying, but then again, I have never died before." That's a sense of humor, even with Mr. Death knocking on your door.

If you are the third born out of four, how do you answer that text from your old man? What were my ways in that moment? I thought I would first let my oldest sister answer and follow her lead. I texted her, "Sherri, what will you say to Dad first? You are the oldest!"

Have you ever thought life would never be the same? That is true. It will never be the same. Your next moment will not be exactly like your last one; it might be even more prosperous. Life often changes without consulting us first, but we get to return to life once it lets us know.

I share this story because I know what you are thinking. You are saying, wait, wait: You can't control some things. Some things hit you that you never saw coming. No one saw COVID-19 coming. No one saw the death and destruction it would cause so many.

How could we respond?

The way of faith!

What is faith in this situation? It's like jumping off a cliff and assembling an airplane on the way down. What does that look like? It looks like my dad's response. He refused certain death. Statistically, he had about a 10 percent chance of coming off a vent alive at the advanced age of eighty-two. He had about the same chance of living if he did nothing. Faith says: They are telling me I am going to die. Ok, I am ready. I've picked out my gravesite at the Fort Sam Veterans Cemetery. Lots of people die at 82. No one will say, "He was so young…"

The way of faith says: I know that death is not the end. It is the doorway as we move from life to life. You don't have to get ready to die if you live prepared to die.

Don't live your life fearing what is certain, your death. You and I will die, no doubt. That's certain. Fear what is uncertain: You are NOT living your best life! Fear spending your life refusing to ask: What if? Fear dying when you are fifty, and your funeral service happens when you are seventy-six.

Fear being stuck in ways that don't lead to life.

Fear dying on the inside yesterday and going through the wrong motions for the next twenty years, dead to what could be!

How do we handle things like COVID-19? How do we react to what we can't change? How do you say, "*It doesn't have to be this way!*" to something that has to be this way? *With faith.*

What does faith look like? Like this: You are someone who knows you can't always control what happens to you, but you can always control how you respond to what happens to you! You didn't choose illness; you didn't choose cancer. You didn't choose COVID-19. You didn't choose this day to get told this news. Bad news never has good timing.

No one ever chooses hardship, but you must decide how to respond.

How do we do that? Get set in the way of faith now, today.

Build your life on the foundation of God's love.

Don't let hardship or trauma become your template. Let God's love be your template.

Know who you are beyond all the name tags you wear: a child of God. Build your life on that. And know that you are headed for hardship. You say that's not a positive way, Pastor. No, I am pretty positive you are headed for hardship. Because you and the ones you love will sometimes get sick and not get better. You and your loved ones will face death. I am optimistic about that. What is death but hardship? Not only that, but you will face difficulties related to all sorts of things in life. Everyone is either coming out of a problem, headed into a problem, or has a problem, which means hardship.

Get set in the way of faith today while the sun shines before the rains.

Crisis doesn't build character; it reveals it. The rain, the storms, and the wind don't always make your roof more robust; it shows if your roof is strong. COVID-19 revealed the ways my dad was set in. They were the right ways. Haven't you lived with the wrong ways long enough? Are you ready to reset? The way of faith is the only way to live. Everyone has faith. It's not a matter of whether or not you will worship but what you will worship. There is no such thing as an atheist. Everyone worships someone or something; everyone has a master passion that drives their life. There is nothing wrong with being driven; it's just who or what is driving.

Jesus lived by faith. He could not always control what the disciples or what people did, but He could always control how he responded with indiscriminate love. When you have nothing but love in your heart, that's all that will come out. This is why Jesus prayed for forgiveness for the men "squeezing him" or crucifying him. He only had love in his heart, so when his heart was squeezed, love was the only thing that could come out.

It's not what squeezes the tube of toothpaste that matters; it is what is inside that matters because it's what always comes out.

Something is always going to squeeze you in life. What comes out is what matters.

Jesus lived a life of faith—a life surrendered to God's will for his life. That involved the cross and being slaughtered for our sins. He could not control that; he surrendered to it. He could not control the hate and vitriol of those who crucified him, cursed, and spit on him as they drove nails into his hands and feet. He experienced something much worse than hardship. The only thing he could control he did control, which was his response on the cross, which was love and forgiveness. "Father, forgive them, for they don't know what they are doing." (Luke 23:34, NLT) Did you give the real F word? Forgiveness?

What do you say to those who crucify you? When you have nothing but love in your heart, that's all that will come out. Faith is not: Tell me how you feel! Faith is: Tell me what you are going to do about how you feel. It's always easier to act your way into a feeling than wait until you feel like doing it. It will never happen if I wait until I feel like working out at the gym again. But dopamine is released once I work out at the gym, and I am happy. I have acted my way right into the feeling. The same rule applies to intimacy in relationships. It's easier to feel love for your spouse when you act that way, even if you are acting. The feelings will follow. If you don't feel loving toward your spouse, start acting in loving ways.

I am the son of a strong man! I am not the son of a weak man. My dad's life was two bookends of crap he never wanted to have to deal with. At six, he overcame being paralyzed for over a year with polio, recovering so well to get a football scholarship with the US Naval Academy. Then, at eighty-two, he was hospitalized with COVID for 132 days. Two worldwide pandemics, and he is still going strong without a walker and oxygen at eighty-five. Why?

The ways he let in, he became set in. He let Faith in; he lived Faith out.

He said to the doctors if I go on that vent, I will surely die. If I lay here on this bed, I might live. What if, what if I try to live? What's the best thing that could happen? I live. I live so my son can write about this in a book one day! What is your will to live today, not just on the day you might die?

What if I say *it doesn't have to be this way* to people who say it does? Why pray "If it is what it is?" Such fatalism does not lead to new life.

God has His ways. His ways are not your ways; his thoughts are not our thoughts. God's ways are weird. His ways are to forget our sinful ways. His way is to turn the other cheek. His ways are to bless those who curse him! What if my ways became weird ways, like God's ways? His ways are to "forgive and forget!" He can do what we try to do. Scripture says he remembers our mistakes no more. God's ways are supernatural. Here's the good news: You can become weird. Everyone is normal till you get to know them. Why be normal? Why not be the salt of the earth? Why not have the ways of a light on a hill? You can join God in changing your ways. It's up to you: Your ways, your responsibility. If you believe the lie that you can't change your life, you will be right. If you think that change is possible, you will be right. Be careful about what you believe about yourself, because it will all come true. Like a wheel inside a wheel, it will turn on you, and turn true.

There are two types of people in this world: Those who complain about the world and those who seek to change the world. Those who make your life easier and those who make it more complicated. Those who lift you and those who tear you down. Those concerned about doing the work—and those concerned about getting the credit. Those who leave you feeling up—and those who leave you feeling down.

But when it came to my dad, there were these two types of people: Those who agreed with him and those who hadn't yet agreed with him! I learned to decide quickly in life.

So, how do I respond to a text I'm afraid I have to disagree with? Dying? Refusing the vent? Goodbye? This is how the story ends for him: lying in a hospital bed alone? No family allowed in the room to say what we need to say, touch his hand, kiss his forehead, and receive the final "I am proud of you, a blessing?" It was a hopeless text to a man who hands out hope like candy. It took away all my words. Usually, I am a man of many, many words. I mean, I get paid to speak and type words. But I couldn't find anything that seemed right at that moment. Frankly, I always loved what Mark Twain said about speakers like me: "There are two types of speakers: those that are nervous and those that are liars."[20] It's why I am nervous as I type this book.

Are you going through the motions in your way? Are you one to phone it in? Another day, another dollar. Keep your head down, and don't make too much noise. Are you not putting your heart into your ways? Do you know anyone who has lazy days and lazy ways? Going through the motions is only a problem if you go through the wrong motions. Getting stuck in your ways can be the best or worst, but there is no neutral. Your ways lead to life or death. But remember, it's later than you think. Time is not on your side. Time is not your friend. My dad went through the motions of his usual ways, and those who said it was his last day were dead wrong. At the time of this writing, he is three years down the road, off the walker and oxygen he went on home.

God's Word says: "But make sure that you don't get so absorbed and exhausted in taking care of all your day-by-day obligations that you lose track of time and doze off,

---

20 *Mark Twain quote*. AZ Quotes. (n.d.).
https://www.azquotes.com/quote/812796

oblivious to God. The hour has come for you to wake up from your slumber. The night is about over; dawn is about to break" (Romans 13:11-14, MSG).

Do you hear God say to your ways today: "Get dressed, be about—your dawn IS breaking! Today is your day!" Today is the best day of your life. Not because it's perfect. Not because you finally have enough money or because your family is healthy. No. Because today, this moment is all you have. What makes today great is not because you are on vacation or chunking your cell phone into the ocean and cracking open a Corona while you sit on the beach, like in the commercial. That's a great vacation and commercial, but it is a train wreck if it's your whole life. No one should vacation their life away. You are wasting your vineyard. Fruit can spoil, and so can we if we don't share our fruit and gifts with others.

Today is the best day of your life because it's all you have. You don't have yesterday. You don't have tomorrow. You have right now, this moment, today.

It's the best day of your life.

Your life and your ways seem so real right now. Your way is to be out buying things. Your way is to drive around in your F-150. Your ways are double-clicking stuff on Amazon. But before you know it, your ways will be no more. Your ways will not be on this earth anymore. Your ways today are in the prime ways of your life. But you are going to blink, and it's going to be decades later. The longer you live, the faster it goes. Time is not on the side of your way. One day, your ways will become good old ways. Aristotle said, "We should measure time in heart throbs," meaning that every time your heart beats, it's a gift. You are not guaranteed that the gift will happen again. One day, the gift of your heartbeat runs out. You only get so many beats on this side of heaven. Six days, six months, and six years from now, some of you reading this today might be on the ground! Who knows—I could be?

Let's not fill this moment with worrying ways about our future days. Let's not let our ways become one of anxiety and fear about the past days. Let's not wish away today but look forward to another day. Your dawn IS breaking. This moment is your best moment, not because it's pain-free, you can read, or you have money in the bank because it's all you have.

Sunrises and opportunities only last so long. Right now, choose these ways: The way of faith in the face of hardship. Choose the ways of Happiness. It's an inside job and an inside choice. Choose the eternal ways in life. Choose the long game. Choose the way of chess, not checkers. Choose the crock-pot, not the microwave. Choose the ways so that something will outlive you. Have ways to get pregnant with God's work. Have a way to have the baby, even if you are not ready. You will never be prepared! Let in forgiving ways: Forgive everyone of everything today. Let in loving ways: Love fully and completely now! Quit skimming the surface of your relationships. Take your spouse and partner into your hands, look them in the eyes, and tell them how much they mean to you today, *and do it every day!*

Let in generous ways: Give generously today. You can't take it with you. Invest in your kids. Plant a tree from which you will never eat fruit. Provide shade for the next generation today. Someone is sitting under a shade tree today because someone planted that tree twenty-five years ago today. Plant a tree today. Don't put this book down like you picked it up. Ask God to help you change your ways! Take responsibility for your ways. Quit blaming your father, your mother, or some dead person in your life. They are dead.

I don't wish you to be better. Choose to be better. Don't just choose to be grateful, express gratitude. Unexpressed gratitude is un-gratefulness.

Today is the best day of your life because today is the day you will choose faith.

Today is the best day of your life, because it's all you have.

Today is the day you will ask: What if?

Your dawn is breaking. You get to choose what you do with this day.

It's the best day of your life because it doesn't have to be how it has been!

Can you believe it?

CHAPTER FOUR

THINK ABOUT WHAT YOU THINK ABOUT

Learn from the mistakes of others. You can't live long enough to make them all yourself!

—Eleanor Roosevelt

I AM CALLED TO HATCH THEM (baptism), match them (marriage), and dispatch them (funerals), but I am also called to listen, coach, *and lead.* I have learned from the mistakes and the faith of my church members. Like a person's mistakes, you can tell a lot about a person by their handshake. You can tell if a man works outside or, like me, inside, in the comfort of air conditioning, as God intended! When my well-lotioned soft hands met Jose's hands, I immediately knew he had lived a hard life. He had the hands of a welder, a plumber, a carpenter. It was like shaking hands with a brick.

Jose was a "first-time church guest" who wanted to meet with me immediately after church. Usually, this means people want money, but in Jose's case, he wanted something deeper than relief: restoration. Jose stood about five foot eight, weighed 160 pounds, and was covered with colorful ink and language. I mean covered in ink. I know what you are thinking. I am judging him by his outer cover, and look, no one judges better than Christians, especially a pastor, right? There is no judgment here. Frankly, I was glad he was willing to endure a sermon! I strive to love as Jesus did, with indiscriminate love. He came to church in shorts, a t-shirt, and flip-flops. Corpus Christi was casual, yet he abided by our strict dress code at the church: Put Something On. Anything. That's our dress code. Just don't show up naked. Please, that's a nightmare for all of us.

Yet, he showed up emotionally and spiritually naked, and that's where the lesson came in. "I grew up in a rough neighborhood, Pastor, the Westside, Molina." Broken homes often produce broken children, hearts, and lives, but what happens after that is up to Jose. Despite his parents telling him to leave at sixteen, he was the first in his family to graduate from high school and to "actually make something out of the raw materials God gave him!" He learned to work with his hands more than his mind and became a woodworker and carpenter, making bar stools, tables, benches, and chairs. His wood shop was his safe space, the creating place where Jose could breathe. I told Jose that meeting him was like meeting a unicorn. Who "makes" anything in America anymore? You can't buy what he's selling at Plastic Mart or Wally World.

Jose told me how he grew up as an "angry kid." Those were his ways, taught to him by his father's ways! His father was more spewer than stewer and lashed out at others. His father taught him how to think, but not well. His father taught that it was always someone else's fault if something went wrong. He grew up and lived on the porch, blaming everyone else. In addition to his high school diploma, he received a complacency certificate! He didn't use that language, but it was close! Have you received yours? You know the one that says: You must learn to live with what you can't rise above. The one that says: Your life as it stands today will never change, at least not for the better. Why bother trying to change anything? Nothing you tried in the past worked! That fatalistic phrase I can't stand: "It is what it is!" Sometimes we receive certificates of complacency in our marriages, relationship with our kids, relationship with God, and relationship with our health. We learn to live with a limp all our lives. **Maybe we need to raise our expectations first of what could be, rather than settling for what is? Of course, the certificate of complacency will tell you it's all their fault, those people. Have you ever heard of those people? If everyone else is to blame for your problems. You are not likely to be changing anything.**

The certificate of complacency is the quickest to make you the victim.

When you play the victim, you remain the victim.

It's like going to your mailbox, taking your bills out, and putting them in someone else's box, hoping they will pay for them. After all, it's their fault you are in debt. It's their fault you were trying to keep up with the Jones. If everyone else is to blame, it sure prevents you from looking at your heart and your responsibility for changing where you are in life. When did you last pay someone else's mortgage or electric bill? You might think it's ridiculous I wrote that. But in twenty-nine years of ministry, there has not been a month of my life where someone in or outside the church asks me to "pay their bills."

One hallmark of spiritual maturity is taking responsibility for one's current and future state in life.

It's never their fault that they can't afford their bills. It's the bank's, wife's, or kid's fault. (hmm…they may be right there—kids are expensive) So, this was Jose's worldview growing up. He didn't own a mirror called self-responsibility.

Jose came to tell me his story, and as he told me about the battles he faced and the mountains he climbed, I recognized he had faced both hassles and heartaches! Whenever someone comes to me for counseling and they present that he had faced both hassles and heartaches! Whenever someone comes to me for counseling and presents the issue, and we get to the real issue underneath the problem, you know, the thing under the thing, that's when this distinction becomes very helpful for me.

A Hassle or a Heartache?

Before you give up ask yourself this question: Is what you are dealing with a hassle or a heartache?

Let's ensure we don't make all our hassles into heartaches because life becomes unbearable and unsolvable. I also call this the 95-5 rule of life.

Ninety-five percent of your problems in life are hassles, not heartaches.

- Hassles are fixable.
- Hassles can be solved.
- Hassles are transitory.
- The hassle is the car breaks down.
- The hassle is getting a letter from the IRS wanting more tax money.
- The hassle is your property taxes go up because the value of your house goes up.
- The hassle is that there is not enough money, and it will take too many months!
- The hassle is you lost your job.
- The hassle is your boss is a jerk.
- The hassle is your kids not listening to you.

Hassles are something you can overcome. You can get another job. You can get another boss. You can get another car. You can always have more kids. (smile) I mean, learn to work it out with your kids.

Heartache:

- Five percent of life is a heartache.
- Heartaches are unfixable.
- Heartaches are terminal cancer.
- Heartaches are when your child dies.
- Heartaches are when your loved one is six feet in the ground.

As you face your challenges in life, begin to ask yourself: Is this a hassle, or is this a heartache? How might I invite God or others to help me in this situation? I know I need help, but what do I need help with? Define it. You can't fix or give it to God if you don't define it. The biggest mistake we make is when we turn, in our minds, a hassle into a heartache because we don't think about the problem. Or when we take the sum of our hassles and let them build into a singular heartache! How many hassles does it take before we feel they become one big old heartache?

If it's a hassle, we can get busy working toward fixing it.

If it's a heartache, I will cry with you. I will pray with you, and in the end, I will do what you can do—give it to God.

How do we give it to God? With faith. Let's say you lose a loved one. Well, that's a heartache. It's unfixable. We grieve and know that it's going to hurt. We don't run from our grief. We don't suppress it. We lean into it. Stuffing feelings, repressing feelings, and not leaning into grief will work temporarily. But the problem is, those repressed feelings tend to have resurrections at the wrong times. We get ambushed by grief when we hear a song, see a face that looks like our loved one, smell the perfume, or see an old photo. We want to lean into our grief and let our hearts grieve. When we do that, we focus on grief being a journey, not a destination. We journey through sadness toward gratitude. We know that we will never "get over it!" No one gets over losing their spouse, their mom, or their child. *Get over it?* That's something dumb that people who have never lost loved ones say. We don't judge them for it. They are well-meaning, but you don't get over it.

You learn to live in a new way.

You learn to live in a new reality.

You recognize grief is the price tag of love, and you never get done paying this side of heaven. **Most importantly, you learn that you can hurt and hope simultaneously. You hurt because they are gone, but you hope because you will see them again in heaven.** We hurt, and it sucks, but you also know that the intensity of this feeling will wane. The intensity of grief will wane, and you will learn to live into a new normal, but you will always grieve heartache. Let's make sure when we are struggling with an issue, we clearly define what it is. But don't underestimate the possibility of a hassle, if left unchecked, turning into a heartache. Does your marriage need some healing? That is a hassle. Did your marriage end in divorce because you never dealt with all those hassles?

When you neglect to tend to your vineyard, the challenges in your marriage can escalate from mere hassles to profound heartache. Excessive hassles are like unchecked weeds; they can hinder the growth of your vines, preventing them from bearing grapes and producing wine. This unfortunate outcome results in a life marked by enduring heartache. Jose told me how his initial marital hassles evolved into a profound and lasting heartache.

Running To Something or From Something?

True story: Georgene Johnson lived in Cleveland, Ohio. She was forty-two years old. She woke up one day, looked in the mirror at her body, and was unhappy. But she also said, "It doesn't have to be this way." Her lazy ways had become the ways she was set in. She said, "I will start today and make some new ways." She strived to improve her life by adding one good habit: a daily run. She said, "I am going to look like a good forty-two." You know you are getting old if people add a little phrase to your age. You look good for your age. It's never you look good in absolute terms. It's always in comparison to others your age! Compared to the flabbiness and deterioration that everyone else your age is showing, you look good! She did well in her running. She was running farther every day. She thought she would try a little competition and entered a 10k race. That's about six miles. Nervous about her first race, she got up early and arrived at the start of the race. To her surprise, many people were milling around, stretching, getting ready. Suddenly, a voice on the microphone said, "Move to the starting line." This is it. Just like that, ready or not, here it comes, and a gun sounded, and they were off, like a massive wave of hundreds of runners sweeping her up.

She was in the race.

After about four miles, she realized they should turn around and head back to the finish line. She wondered why they didn't turn around. She stopped and asked an official, "How come the course isn't turning around?" He said, "Ma'am, you are running the Cleveland Marathon—Twenty-six miles." Her event, the 10k, was to start a half hour after the marathon.

How many of us would have stopped there and said, "That's it, I'm going home."

Would you?

Would you have settled for a C or gone for an A?

Would you have settled for your certificate of complacency? You have done enough.

To her credit, she kept going right and finished the race. She said, "This is not the race I trained for. This is not the race I entered. But for better or worse, this is the race that I am in."[21]

Now she's ready for the certificate of victory from running the race life put before her! That's the way it happens. Life has a way of doing that to us, picking us up and putting us into situations we didn't train for, volunteer for, or want. How many of us have ever woke up and said, "This is not the life I asked for!"

But the day you were born, you got married to your life, so, for better or worse, this is the situation you find yourself in. Divorce does that. We never dreamed of divorce when we got married, but there we are, running the race of divorce. Sickness and the debilitation of old age and disease do it. We are healthy until we are not. We never thought this would happen to us. What do you mean I have to run through this season? Is it called disappointment? Life has not gone the way I planned! I thought my life was going to be different. Welcome to the club called Reality. Where's the signup sheet for the good

21 Ritter, W. (2020, April 20). The Race That Is Set Before Us. *RitterWrites*.
https://www.ritterwrites.com/writings/2020/4/22/the-race-that-is-set-before-us

life? What is a good life, and how did I end up on the wrong path? You can scream and shout that life is not fair and it's not, and life won't care! Or you can use the same energy to get busy running.

Growing up, my sister would get a bigger piece of the apple pie.

"It's not fair."

My dad always said, "Life's not fair; deal with it, son."

I love that response now. I didn't love it then. Spiritual maturity is learning to quit and expecting life to be fair. People don't always get what they deserve. Sometimes they get way worse than that! You can complain about your vineyard and how someone else's vineyard is bigger, more fertile, and has better grapes. But at some point, you spend energy complaining or tending your vineyard!

Embrace Your Response Ability

Anyone reading this grow up with brothers and sisters? I have two older sisters. I called Jungle Jane and the other "the Sarge." Which one do you think bossed me around a bit? Sherri, "the Sarge," got sea monkeys! Does anyone here remember sea monkeys? You can still order these tiny brine shrimp today! She got them, and my parents said I was not old enough to care for sea monkeys. What? You add water and a bit of food to a plastic bowl. So I said, and say it with me now, "That's Not Fair!"

They gave in, and I got sea monkeys. My sister, "the Sarge," didn't like that, so she started a Sea Monkey Club! She was the only one in the club, but I also wanted to be there. Have you ever joined a country club? There are dues to pay, and likewise with the Sea Monkey Club. I had to give her my weekly allowance to be in the Sea Monkey Club. I gave her my quarter a week. That was my allowance. That's how old I am!

Think back to your childhood, to something you said, to something we all said at one point or another: "That's not fair!" The truth is that life isn't fair, yet there's something in all of us that wants life to be fair sometimes. I'll confess that I'm primarily concerned about fairness when my piece of the pie is the smallest. I can care less about what's fair when I get the larger pie. When I get the large piece of pie, I say, "God is so great." I don't think about those who got the smaller piece who are out there thinking: My life is so unfair. I prayed. I work hard. When we say life isn't fair, what we're saying is life isn't even. While I think life should be even, we can all see that that would be impossible. There is no way for things to be even.

Here's why this is important for us to look at: the unfairness of life, the unevenness of life, can quickly become an excuse for our irresponsibility:

"If I don't get a big piece of the pie, can you expect me to be responsible? Why try? Why go the extra mile if I don't get the benefits? I have every right to walk away from my responsibilities because someone else got my fair share."

Let me tell those who lean in that direction: Don't do that! Irresponsibility eats a hole in your soul, and you begin to spiral. You're the one whose irresponsibility will most negatively impact you, and you'll never be happy. Irresponsible people aren't ultimately happy because irresponsibility creates conflict with others and within yourself. Benjamin Franklin said, "He that is good at making excuses is seldom good at anything else."[22] He's describing that downward spiral of irresponsibility that comes when we view our lives as unfair!

Learning to blame everyone else means you blame God too, right? I mean, this was all His idea, right? God, it's got to be his fault. God, it's not fair they got a better start in life than me. God, it's not fair she got a better preaching voice than me. God, they married someone with money. What happened to my spouse? It seems God gave people around me better looks, pedigree, more money, better backgrounds, etc. And again, it's not fair.

Jesus even told a parable about this: A master went on a long trip and decided to give three of his servants different amounts of gold (or talent levels) to manage his money until he returned and settled accounts with him. One person got five bags of gold, another person got two bags of gold, and the third person got one bag of gold. What mattered was not that they got different amounts but that each person was responsible for what they had received. It's just like in this race we call life. Everybody gets an uneven amount of opportunity and is held accountable for what they do with it.

Everybody has the privilege and the responsibility to somehow, someday, give an account for what they did with their uneven amount of opportunity. The issue isn't how to make life fair. The real problem is what we will do with the hand we were dealt. What are we going to do with the lives God has given us? The more you focus on the unfairness and unevenness of life, the more you will be tempted to excuse irresponsibility because of what someone else has or hasn't done. We are all one-bag, two-bag, or five-bag people. We all know some five-bag people. They get into the right schools. They marry the right people. They have talent that gets recognized in the public sphere. They make a lot of money. They're beautiful. We hate those people! Everything seems to have come naturally to them! But if these five-bag people aren't careful, they will take what they've been given for granted—because it's just that easy. Then some people had to work their way through school, whose parents divorced when they were young, who aren't all that attractive, who don't have good communication skills—life is tough for them. These people know when they look around them: I don't have much going for me, especially compared to others. And then there are most of us—somewhere in the middle. And the question for us is this, What will we do with what we have? The tendency is to look at everybody else—what they have or don't have—and make excuses for what we will or won't do. This parable teaches us to look at our bag and decide how to leverage it

22 Brooks, J. (2018, January 20). You Can't Go Wrong With Ben Franklin's Wisdom. *Dayton Daily News*. Retrieved from
https://www.daytondailynews.com/news/opinion/commentary-you-can-wrong-with-ben-franklin-wisdom

fully. As the Capital One commercial says, "So what's in your wallet—or bag?" What if instead of saying it's not my fault that immigration is a problem, it's my time to do something about it? What if, instead of saying it's not my fault, 3,800 children will die today due to unclean drinking water? But I can do one thing about it: save one's life. What if we moved to say: It's not my fault, but it is my time. I have been blessed with amazing things like wealth, time, and opportunity; I could share some of what I have to change someone else's world!

I remember one time Zachary, at age fifteen, was complaining to me and his mother. He was angry at life and life's terms, and he said, "Dad, I never asked to be born."

I said, "Neither did I, but here we are."

No one gets to decide to be born into this world, the year you were born, or the time and space in history in which you were born, but here you are.

You didn't get to decide your parents and how they raised you, but here you are.

You didn't get to decide the color of your skin and the benefits or minuses that might come with that, but here you are.

You didn't get to decide your socioeconomic background and the perks or minuses of that, but here you are.

You didn't choose your siblings, the house you grew up in, or if you had a house to grow up in, but here you are.

You don't get to decide how you start, but you do get to choose how to live today and how you will finish.

That is your superpower!

You didn't decide to be born, but you can choose *how* and *if* you will truly live!

You didn't decide the beginning, but you can determine the middle and the end!

In thirty years of ministry, I have done over a thousand funerals. Every time I look into the casket, do you know who I see? Me. My death. I get so tired of people saying: "Boy, he looks good!" I always want to say, "No, he looks dead, quite dead!"

What do you want people to say at your funeral? You can have that phrase: "He looks good." I want them to say, "Look, he's moving…" (smile) Because when the body moves, the funeral is over. When you move, life is happening.

I have lived with my impending death for a long time, so much so I don't fear death, but I do fear not living all my years.

You want some fears: Fear settling. Fear complacency. Fear complaining about how it's unfair. Fear death before death. Fear the second death, the death of being forgotten. Fear settling for a C when an A awaits you. Fear settling for second best. Fear settling for the certificate of complacency rather than victory. Fear surrendering to your circumstances rather than overcoming them. I have buried people at 85 who died at 65. They quit thriving and merely survived for another twenty years. Don't be one of them. Don't fear the mountains in life. Fear not grabbing your shovel!

Jose ran a race in life he never wanted to run.

It wasn't fair: his parents, his background, his lack of money, love, and care. He learned to distrust people. This distrust resulted in anger and alienation and lashing out at the world. The race he ran as an adult got harder, and he didn't want to run it anymore! He says, "I got broken by my broken parents, hurt by my hurt parents, broken by my broken neighborhoods, broken teachers, and ultimately, I got broken by myself." Like unchecked weeds, his hassles had overtaken his vineyard, and his heart was broken.

He says to me, in between sips of water as he sits on my couch, staring down at the floor:

"I woke up one morning, looked in the mirror, and felt I was too broken to be fixed."

"Ever felt like that, Pastor? Like you are just damaged goods, too far gone for anyone to save?"

His life, like his heart, was in pieces. Failed marriages and four kids who don't know Jose as a dad. He realized he had repeated the ways of his parents. The sins of the parents are visited upon children and their children.

Here he was a carpenter, and there was not enough wood glue, nails, or screws to keep himself together and in one piece. He was Humpty Dumpty, and no one could ever put all the pieces back together again. Ever felt so broken to be fixed that even a carpenter can't put you back together again? He felt depressed. He felt unloved. He felt unwanted.

He felt.

You can feel heartache, and you can feel hassled. Are feelings more heartache or hassle? I would say hassles, but left unchecked, they had grown into heartache and depression.

Now, feelings are important, but they often get confused with facts. Never confuse your feelings with facts. Just because you feel something is true doesn't mean it is true. I feel like I should be the best-looking man in the world. Please quit laughing. But, ahem, it's not a fact. Not even close.

You may feel unlovable because someone did not reciprocate your love, but that does not mean it's true.

You may feel you can never overcome, but that does not mean it's true.

Feelings are the warning light on the dashboard of your life. Your tire pressure is low. Your battery needs changing, but they should never tell you to throw the car in the junkyard!

Feelings are not always a trustworthy guide to reality.

Feelings are a guide to how you think about reality.

Feelings are beautiful indicators that something can be right or wrong, happiness or madness! But feelings make for terrible dictators. Why would you let something temporary, a hassle, and something that will pass into permanent heartache?

Why would you let your feelings of being mad dictate your behavior and turn into a gorilla around your spouse? Even if a family of gorillas raised you?

Feelings pass, and facts remain.

Feelings are like the weather; if you don't like it, wait, it will change! Facts are like the sunrise and sunset; it's going to happen. You may not always see it. Some clouds of feelings may block it, but the sunrise and the sunset will occur. A man who was more than a little intoxicated got on a bus late one night, staggered up the aisle, and sat next to an older woman who was clutching a Bible. She looked at the wayward drunk up one side and down the other and said with conviction, "I've got news for you, Mister. You're going straight to hell!" The man jumped out of his seat and shouted, "Oh, man, I'm on the wrong bus again!" Well, he was on the wrong bus. People make that mistake from time to time. Is there any hope for them unless somebody confronts them and helps turn them around? I got a text the other day from someone on the wrong bus. It said, "Pastor, He makes me so angry, I don't think he will ever change."

Wrong bus.

I replied, "No one makes you anything. No one can make you mad! You choose to get mad. What if you reacted differently this time and didn't let him get your goat?" Oh, Pastor, they always get my goat! Maybe it's time to tie up your goat somewhere else! Who's in charge of your goat? No one gets to make you happy; you choose to be satisfied!

Happiness, "Madness," and sadness are all inside jobs.

"But, Pastor, you don't understand; this situation will never change."

Perhaps that is true. That makes it a heartache. But when a circumstance does not change, you can still change who you are and how you react. It's the greatest freedom you have always had, and it's how to respond and play the cards life deals you.

You can get on another bus besides the *let's get all angry* bus!

You can't change the direction of the wind, but you can adjust your sails. But you must ensure your feelings stay as indicators, not rule your life like dictators. If you let your feelings become dictators, then your "madness" will take over your life, and you will become an angry person! If you allow anger in, anger will become your way. But you can change your ways. Anger used to be my way.

Do you want people to say of you: "He is always angry!"

"She is always upset about something!"

"He has a short temper!"

Anger is not a sin. It's what you do with it that is either sinful or not.

Being unable to process your anger healthily will lead you to an unhealthy life.

Make sure you get angry about the right things in life. Even God gets angry, but He is slow to do it. I first realized feelings could be managed when I lied to my mom. She was distraught with me for lying. I remember she was yelling and yelling and spanking and spanking, and then, mercifully, the phone rang. She went from:

"You little #$%# to Hello, this is Mrs. Roberts, why yes Father Rafferty. I will be glad to stay late with the choir and teach them the notes of Handel's Messiah."

When she picked up the phone, she went from John McEnroe to Mother Teresa in a second. She controlled her anger, wrapped it up, and put it on hold! I remember looking at her as she switched into Mother Teresa mode, and I thought, "Ok, this is her way; you can turn this on or off."

You manage your feelings, or they will manage you.

You control your feelings, or they will control you. You are always the one responsible for your feelings. No one else can "make you" feel anything.

Jose continues talking about his ways, mindset, and thinking at that time. He said, "Finally, Pastor, you ask yourself the question: Why are so many people out to get me?" The only logical answer for Jose was, "Even God hates you!" After all, isn't God in charge in this race we call life?"

Jose said, "My feelings that God hated me grew as the years passed, and I perceived each setback as further evidence that my belief was correct." One thing that gave Jose life meaning was his job building custom furniture in a wood shop. One day, Jose spotted a man walking down the street carrying an elegant Queen Anne chair. He instantly recognized it as a valuable antique and asked the man if he could have it. It only had a broken rung, and Jose knew he could fix it. The man said, "No." He was going to throw it away. Jose asked him: "If you're going to throw that away, may I have it?" The man said no, throwing the chair into a dumpster, permanently breaking its frame and ruining it. This moment reinforced Jose's feelings that people are no good and that God doesn't care about him. A year later, Jose's feelings of anger, sadness, and all his life's hassles left unchecked and untended to finally drive him to burn out.

Depression, left unmitigated, always turns inwards.

That's what depression is: Anger turned inwards.

Depression is anger at yourself. Depression is: "I am running the wrong race in life; I didn't sign up for this race, and I can't enter another one." Depression is: "I am on the wrong bus, and the bus driver won't slow down and let me off." Depression is: "There is a black cloud following my life, and I will never see the sun again." Depression lets hassles mount up and up until they turn into heartache. Depression is awarding yourself the certificate of complacency. It says: "I don't like my life, myself, my ways, and unlike the weather, my life will never change." Eventually, depression turns to self-hatred and loathing of oneself, hating the very gift of life that God gave you.

Depression is: "I don't like my belly button. It's ugly, and it will always be ugly. I wanted an innie, and I got an outie."

This is why the very first effective treatment for depression was given by Maslow, who told depressed persons to quit looking inward and start looking outward. Quit staring at your belly button (I don't like mine either after double hernia surgery) and start looking at how you can help someone else's belly button. He told a depressed person to go out and do nine nice things for nine people who can never repay you. When people do that, they get less depressed. It's amazing. They get a *helper's high*. God has wired us scientifically to get a rush of endorphins when we help other people, so much so that we can feel "high!"

The most selfish thing you can do is to help someone else!

Before you give up, will you try and help someone else's life become better and then see how you think and how you feel?

Do you want happiness? Quit chasing it. Stop. Happiness moves. Happiness changes addresses. We think we will be happy when we make this much money, get this job, or have sex with this person. It's true that those things when we achieve them, give us a tiny burst of happiness, but they recede. People don't believe the address for happiness moves, but it does. You reach that benchmark you set and wonder why you are only happier for a while, and then your average baseline returns. So, what do you do? Again, studies show that if you chase happiness, it's elusive, and that's why the Bible says it's like grasping oil. But studies also show that if you chase meaning, significance, and blessing other people's belly buttons and not your own, guess what gets thrown in? Happiness.

Come on, the most selfish thing you can do is find someone who can never repay you and take meaningful action for them.

But Jose had to learn this hard, which almost cost him his vineyard.

Jose says: "Often, Pastor, I would go out on my little boat, right here in Baffin Bay or the Laguna Madre, I would go out alone and have a pity party, a life's not fair party." Pretty soon, these feelings would lead to some depression-laced fantasies of just throwing himself out in the water and ending his life!

REV. JOHN W. ROBERTS

Slowly, his hassles began to feel like heartaches. Nothing changes if nothing changes. It is what it is, he thought! The temporary feelings of depression were about to make a permanent life-ending decision. The temporary feelings were about to distort the fact that he mattered to God. His life was precious, not something one throws away.

Never make a permanent decision based on your feelings. The same is true sexually. I always tell young people: Never let your physical commitment exceed your spiritual commitment to another person.

Why would you drop your pants if you are unwilling to give them your heart?

Because it feels good?

What happens when the feelings run out?

Jose made up his mind that he would do it. His hassles had become a heartache, and the dark cloud of depression made him feel like he would never see the sunshine again.

He didn't buy any bait, and he bought enough gas to get himself out to where he would drown. He journeyed into the water, shut off his boat, and stood on the edge of his ship in liminal space, of life and death. He tried to be prepared for his final moments on this side of heaven. He stood on the edge of his boat, trying to get the final bit of courage to end it all. But as he stood on the edge of that boat, he suddenly recalled the angry man who had thrown the Queen Anne chair into the dumpster. And in the middle of that quiet moment on the water, with not another soul in a two-mile radius, he heard a stranger's voice say to him:

"If you're just going to throw that away, may I have it?"

God said, "If you are going to throw your life away, may I have it?" Jose says he knew it was the voice of God. He had never heard the voice of God, but he knew it was the voice of one who loved him. That was a fact that outweighed all his feelings. There was no one else within visible sight of his boat. He fell to his knees, inside the safety of the boat, as his soul finally fell into the safety of His Father's loving embrace.

The love of God overcame his feelings of self-hate.

God reminded Jose that he was, is, and always will be a child of God. He will always have refrigerator rights. He can go to God at 2 a.m. and ask for something from the fridge, and the King won't be upset. The King will be able to deliver it. The King is willing and wants to help!

God's love was a fact that overcame all those ugly temporary feelings.

He had come home. Jose finally quit chasing relief and surrendered to restoration.

He would let THE Carpenter and THE cross bring him not just forgiveness for yesterday but purpose for today and hope for tomorrow.

Jose had a moment, and this moment was the start of healing a lifetime of anger!

Some of you reading this book might want to stop and listen and hear God say over you:

If you are going to just give up on your life, can I have it?

If you are going to give up on your marriage, can I have it?

If you are going to give up solving your problems, can I have them?

If you are going to give up having a loving, forgiving heart, can I have your resentful heart?

It's this paradoxical thing, but with God, surrendering your life leads to finding true life. This is the beginning of salvation: allowing your shadow self to perish, letting the lesser self fade away so your God-given self can thrive. You can't sit on both chairs; you have to choose one. It's not death to self, but death to the lesser self, your shadow self, so that the greatest self can truly live.

In the Bible, we read about a young man, not called Jose but called the Prodigal Son, who was on the wrong bus. He was tired of living by his old man's rules and regulations. He went off to truly live in the "far-off country" and finally be happy alone.

Self-discovery, he thought. I got to be me. I got to do me. I got to be me. I can't be me, living under my father's roof and my father's rules. If he could backpack across Europe, he could find himself.

I can relate.

When my senior year in high school rolled around, I could not wait to go to the "far-off country" called college! Finally, to be free of my old man's rules and regulations. See, in high school, I didn't care about grades. In that order, I cared about athletics, girls, and athletic girls. My report cards reflected my priorities. My only A in high school was in PE. The rest were Cs and Ds and an occasional B! Two days before I went to college, my Air Force full Colonel dad said to me, "Son, if you don't do well at Southwest Texas State University, you will be going to community college, living under my roof, and my rules!"

It was not a threat. My dad didn't threaten. He promised and delivered.

That was all this prodigal needed to hear. I studied every day, five hours a day, whether it was Sabbath or not! I came home for Christmas break in my first semester and handed my report card to my old man. Miraculously, it read: "Straight As. Dean List!" How did someone in the slow Math class get an A in college Algebra? How did someone in the caterpillar class, not rockets, finally grow his wings? I remember being put in the caterpillar group in Math, and I said, "Hello, I get the insult here. I am decent in English and vocabulary…"

What had happened? Had I suddenly become bright and intelligent? Ha. Nope. One Word:

Motivated.

I didn't want the pain to remain. I wanted freedom. I was willing to pay the price of liberty- studying. Motivation and habits can change the course of your life.

I will never forget seeing my dad's shocked look, watching him go into his bedroom, and I heard him call the school registrar, "Yeah, I just want to confirm that my son's report card was not forged."

True story.

I still laugh about this. I don't blame him! I would have called too! My dad comes back and says: "What gives? Why the good grades?" I said, "Oh, Dad, I don't want to live under your roof and your regulations." I was on the Dean's list for the rest of my college career, which landed me a scholarship to graduate school at SMU. They thought I was smart; I was just motivated.

Lazy ways had become studying ways. My grades didn't always have to be a certain way. I didn't care if the teacher had deemed me in the slow class; that was years ago. I am not going to let her forecast determine my day. Under fear and love for the far-off country, I could apply myself and change my future instead of surrendering to the ways of my past.

Yet, in the Biblical story, the discussion is not on grades but money. As a young man, he asks his dad for his inheritance. This is a risky proposition, isn't it, parents? Suppose your eighteen-year-old son comes to you and says: "Mom and Dad, I know you're going to leave me an estate worth a half-million dollars someday. I want to get it now." After you pick yourself up off the floor, how are you going to respond? Some parents can start their children off quite substantially, and that's fine. But I wonder how often it works out well for these kids. My dad used to say to me, "If I give you everything, you may never realize the value of working for everything."

Truth—I bought my first car at twenty-four, a used Ford Escort with, as it turned out, rolled back miles on it; a shady dealership! It took me three years to pay it off, and trust me, I learned the value of a dollar by doing so. My dad would have never cashed out assets early and given me my inheritance, but some would have. I would not have had the maturity to handle any inheritance or sizable sum at eighteen. Some eighteen-year-olds would have the maturity to handle a half million dollars quite responsibly. But I guess that most of us who are put in that situation at that stage in our lives would do just what the young man in Luke's Gospel did. He squanders his inheritance: It's party, party, party. All the drinks are on me, and don't you know everyone is your friend when they are on your dime? But the friends ran out when the money did. Soon, the bank is calling. The accounts are overdrawn, and the money is gone.

Now, you and I might not be party animals at our ages. My idea of a wild night is a heating pad in bed by about 8:30 with a good book. Most of us are not party animals.

That's not to say we would not have wasted the money. We might find other ways to go through the funds. A BMW convertible, a shopping spree at the mall, and a European trip would be nice. I have yet to outgrow spending money. He spent his fortune, ran up his credit cards, burned up his allowance in record time, and now he has hit rock bottom. Can you see him lying in his dorm room? I'm sorry. I know the scripture doesn't say a dorm room, but it does mention a pig pen, and I just naturally made the association. He's wondering what in the world he's going to do.

The Bible tells us, "But when he came to himself…" (Luke 15:17, NRSV). Those are some of the most important words in Scripture. Are your ways to come to yourself? "When he came to himself." He realized he was on the wrong bus and his life was heading in the wrong direction! Suddenly, this young man knew it was time for him to take charge of his life. It was time to get off that bus of victimhood and get on the bus of victory. He realized he had signed up for this race, but there was another race he could be running! You only get one shot at your vineyard. What he learned is that God is the God of the fatted calf. God always adds an extra leaf to the table, and there is a chair with your name on it, a robe, and a family ring waiting for you.

But he had to come to his senses. We all do as we grow up.

Likewise, the people of Israel have been wandering in the wilderness for forty long years. What should have been an 11-day walk turned into a forty-year trek! God fed them with manna from heaven when they were in the wilderness. Finally, they enter the Promised Land. Here is what the writer of Joshua says at that critical point in Israel's history:

"The manna ceased on the day they ate the produce of the land, and the Israelites no longer had manna; they ate the crops of the land of Canaan that year" (Joshua 5:12, NRSV).

God was saying, "Come to your senses!"

Do you get the picture?

For forty years of wilderness wandering, God provided the children of Israel with manna from the skies to meet their physical needs.

Don't you imagine they got tired of eating the same thing every day? They passed a recipe book, *101 Ways to Serve Manna.*

Can't you hear the grumbling? "Oh, man, not manna again."

Forty years.

That's the Bible's way of saying a long time.

Forty years is a long time to live with things the way things are, especially when they are not good.

I'm sure God made it appetizing for them. Even more important, it kept them going. It met their needs. God promised them that they would be provided for, and they were. But the manna stopped on the day they could provide for themselves.

God is saying to them. "From here on, it's up to you. I gave you everything you needed to survive in the wilderness, but it's time for you to take responsibility for yourselves." This is the practical truth about life that everyone has to realize sooner or later. God will not provide for us what we can provide for ourselves. God expects us to take charge of our lives. Pray as if everything depends upon God. Work as if everything depends upon you! I wonder if God doesn't get tired of listening to the prayers of some people:

"Lord, help me do well on that test." God asks, "Did you study?"

"Lord, help me get that promotion." God asks, "Have you done your part?"

"Lord, help me get down to a size ten." God asks, "Have you put down the chips and queso?"

Do we think God will do what we refuse to do for ourselves?

Can you understand what God can and will do for you as you run the unfair race of life? This is not to say God won't help us. He will, but if we can do it, God lets us do it. This means we must always attempt things we can't do alone. We must attempt great things to see the greatness of God. We must leave room for God to show up in our church budgets and our relationships so that we will see God show up.

Don't just do what you know you can, but do what you can, and leave room for God to show up as you attempt more!

Jose had been restored. Jose and I went out for lunch. We began to talk about what he thought about.

Think about what you think about.

Are you willing to give up your old way of thinking that led you to giving up?

If you want to change your life, you must change your thoughts. Think about what you think about. If we are all addicted to anything in life, it's our thoughts. You cannot change anything if you cannot change your thinking.

When I do counseling, it used to be the first question out of the gate, "Let me know how you are feeling. How are you?"

I don't ask that anymore. Now I say, "How are you thinking?"

Why? You can't live well if you are thinking poorly!

Start asking the people in your life not how you are but how you think about yourself. Your life is always moving in the direction of your strongest thoughts.

There's only one thing I remember my driving instructor telling me, and it's also an excellent rule for life. You tend to steer at whatever you stare at! You tend to steer at whatever you look at on the road. As you run the race of life, you tend to steer toward what you focus on! If you focus on worries, you will become a worrier. If you focus on fear, you will become fearful. If you focus on faith, you will become faithful.

Your life is always moving in the direction of your strongest thoughts. Now that you know that, do you like the direction of your strongest thoughts?

Most people never think about what they think about. They just let any old thought land in their head, like any old bird land on a tree. Yet, who is responsible for your thought department? You! Only you. Why would you leave your mind open to any old thought? Do you leave your front door wide open when you sleep at night? No.

What's your first thought when you wake up? Is it to reach for your phone, like about 89 percent of Americans do? Do you start scrolling and complaining about how unfair your day will be? It would help if you ran a marathon and signed up for a 5k. Is it to check your calendar? Is it to start thinking about how many mountains you must climb that day and how you will ever have the energy, the strength, and the resources to do it? What if you put your phone in the other room and didn't charge it near your bed? What if you set an alarm clock to remind you to wake up not with anxiety but with gratitude for the gift of today? What if your first thought was the God who made everything has promised to be with you today? What if you made it a habit to wake up and record four things you are grateful for every day? Guess what that habit will do for you? It helps you find and grasp happiness because it's impossible to be thankful and unhappy simultaneously.

What if you let that eternal FACT that there is nothing you can do to make God love you more or less determine your outlook?

What if you let that fact override your temporary feelings? What if your entire identity was framed by God loving you and thinking you are a gift to this world? What if that was your most vital thought? Guess what happens? You become a gift to this world. What if your most critical thought every morning was: The same God who made the heavens and the earth, the billions of galaxies we can now see with the James Webb Telescope, the God who is taller than any mountain in my life, has promised He will guide me, strengthen me, and give me wisdom and discernment my whole life? What a life! I can turn to God for help today, and God will show up!

What if tomorrow you think this: You can rise and shine or increase and whine? It takes the same amount of energy to do either! It's always up to you which one you choose to do. Rise and shine or rise and whine. I don't think most people decide to become extraordinary. They decide to attempt, with God's help, incredible things. But it all starts on the inside. The exemplary life is found on the inside, its perspective. Every time I drive thirty-five North to San Antonio, a two-and-half-hour drive, I say to myself: "If you look for the flowers, you will find flowers. If you look for roadkill on the side of the road, you will find roadkill."

Again, if your life is always moving in the direction of your most robust thoughts, are you excited about the direction your thoughts are taking you?

I asked myself that very question several years ago.

And my answer was no.

If my thoughts were directing my life, and I looked specifically at my thoughts, I did not like the direction they were taking me in. They were consumed with negativity, fear, and self-doubt, and my inner dialogue was not good. I was letting any old thought called fear, shame, guilt, and you will never be good enough to take permanent residence in my head. In the last three years, and through the writing of this book, my number one top personal spiritual priority was to renew my mind with truth. I got consumed with it! The Bible says renewal of the mind, guarding your thoughts, is the way to "knowing" the will of God for your life.

"Do not conform to the pattern of this world but be transformed by the renewing of your mind. Then you will be able to test and approve what God's will is—his good, pleasing, and perfect will" (Romans 12:2, NIV).

If you want to renew your life, you need something to renew your mind and thoughts. If you drive a premium gas-powered car, chances are you don't put cheap fuel or diesel fuel in it and then expect it to run well. Likewise, why would you expect your life to run well if you keep filling it with cheap thoughts?

Think costly thoughts. Think expensive thoughts. Quit dwelling on cheap thoughts like it's unfair and quit looking for the dead stuff. Think good thoughts. Think flowers. Think love. Think about dealing with hope. Think about someone else's belly button more than your own. Watch how you think about your problems. Most are hassles; deal with them without letting them become heartache.

Think about God's power unleashing in your life. See yourself becoming a new person with new habits. You are not responsible for your first thought, but you are responsible if you think another thought on the first one. You are responsible for your second, third, and fourth thoughts. Think expensive thoughts, for this is what the Bible is saying when it says:

"Finally, brothers and sisters, whatever is true, whatever is noble, whatever is right, whatever is pure, whatever is lovely, whatever is admirable—if anything is excellent or praiseworthy—think about such things" (Philippians 4:8, NIV).

Most of my counseling is not about eliminating people's problems; it teaches them to think right about their problems, how to see them, how to deal with them, and how to increase their "spiritual containers and capacities"! Everyone has invisible spiritual containers and capacities for coping with challenges. The goal is to expand our containers and increase our capacities. The goal is to expand our thinking and let God help us with our problems, to trust more, and to try things in a new way. Quit the old Calgon prayer—"Oh, Calgon, take me away." Quit believing your life is like the Corona commercial where you can chunk your cell phone into the ocean and sit on the white sandy beach with your cold Corona forever.

Don't pray for less problems. Pray for greater strength.

Don't pray for external pressure to go away. It never will. Pray for internal pressure to be equal to the external pressure. Pray for internal strength to meet the challenge of external problems.

Why do they pressurize tennis balls?

Why does all that air come flying out when you open the can?

Because they know life's rackets will be swinging and striking them. Internal pressure means the tennis balls can bounce back when the rackets of life start knocking them around. You are no different. It would be best if you had internal pressure and internal strength. It begins in the mind.

If I squeeze an empty Coke can, I can crush it. Because I am strong? No.

Why does the can get crushed? There is no equalizing pressure inside of it.

But if I squeeze an unopened, carbonated, pressurized regular Coke can, I can't make it burst. Why? Because I am weak? No. It's not about external pressure or internal pressure. It's about how a Coke can have equal or greater internal pressure.

Life is not about choosing the race you run. Sometimes you get thrown into a race you would have never run. There will always be external pressure in your life. Quit trying to build a life free of pressure. It will never happen. Quit trying to manufacture life with circumstances that are free of pressure. No Calgon, soap, beer, food, or relationship will eliminate stress and pressure from your race of life. You can't drink it away, sex it away, or drug it away.

You want to train your soul and build up internal pressure to be greater than or at least equal to whatever squeezes you in life. It all starts with how you think.

If you believe you can, you are right.

If you believe you can't, you are right.

Jesus always prayed for internal strength to face the insults, the nakedness, the crown of thorns, the cross, the humiliating death, and the ability to forgive those who nailed him to a wooden cross. He said to God, if there is no other way, if the cross can't be moved, may I be strong enough to overcome the cross.

What if you prayed not for the strength for your crosses to go away but for the strength to embrace them, climb up on them, and surrender to the new life that waits on the other side?

You didn't choose to be born in these unfair circumstances. You didn't choose the beginning, but you can choose the middle and the end. You didn't decide how your life started, but you can choose how you finish!

Living life presents challenges. That's baked into our human experience. So, the goal in counseling isn't to make all the problems in your life go away. The goal is to help you recognize what a hassle and heartache are. The goal is to show you that if God can raise Jesus from the dead, anything is possible in your life, in and through God's help!

I can handle anything, thanks to the strength of God. When Moses was at the Red Sea, 1.3 million people were with him, enslaved people and not warriors; the most powerful man in the world, Pharoh, and his army came to crush them, to kill them in the desert. The people asked Moses, "Were there not enough graves in Egypt? You brought us out here to be slaughtered and to die?" It certainly looked that way. The people were trapped. They could not cross the Red Sea, and they could not go back toward the army that was rushing to them. At that moment, God said to Moses, "Here's a stick!"

A stick.

What is a stick going to do?

It wasn't a spear. It wasn't a knife. It was just a lousy stick.

Welcome to ministry—here's your stick. There's the mountain—here's your stick. There's your mountain—here's your shovel.

When Moses held up that stick and said to God, "Okay, God, work through what is weak and feeble, this stick, my life," and God showed up. Because it's not about the sticks or shovels God gives us. They are just sticks and shovels. It's about how God uses the weak things in life, like us, to overcome the mountains so that God, not the sticks, not us, gets the glory.

What's your stick? What's your shovel? What has God given you that you can hold up, dedicate, give back to God, and watch God work through?

For Jose, it was his woodwork. He now dedicates much of his money to people experiencing poverty, building them furniture they could never afford. Jose now also works with Habitat for Humanity three days a month! Come on, who does that? Only God.

He builds homes for others, from one carpenter in Jesus to another in Jose. When Moses held up that stick and dedicated it to God, God showed up and parted the Red Sea. God solved the problem, but Moses had to use his stick. God will move your mountains, but you must have enough faith and energy to lift your life and stick to prayer. You must do your part, and God will do his! The armies, the Red Seas, the crosses, the mountains will always be there. But so will God. And God always gives us a stick. It may not look like much, but with God, a stick, a shovel, it's all you need. It starts with how you think.

What is your stick?

How often do you surrender to the problem instead of to God?

Think about your faith thoughts.

What are your Default Thoughts?

The more often we think of a thought, the more connection there is, and it's easier to think of that thought again. Before long, whatever we have been thinking becomes our default thought.

Imagine this. Every day, I get up, walk out in my front yard, and walk across the lawn for one hundred days straight in the exact location and patch of grass.

If I walked across that patch, what would I do? I would create a path in my yard. If I think of a lie for one hundred days straight (let's say the lie is that I am a failure or will never be good enough), I start to believe the lie. I create a neural pathway through my brain.

What can I do? Walk a new path. Create a new path and stay off the old one. What we're going to do is renew our minds. We're going to keep off that old path. And if I stay off that path for one hundred days, what happens? The grass grows back. There's more resistance. It's not as easy to walk. And I forge a new pathway in my brain toward the truth, and the truth ultimately sets me free.

I don't know how this will play out in your life. But maybe your path is this: It's a frustrating day at work, and you come home, and it's been crazy at home because it's always wild when you have kids, and the house is a mess—and you walk in, and your old path says, yell at your spouse. And what you do is stay off that path. You capture that thought and might count to three, ten, or 110. And you say today I am going to walk a different road, and you come up and say, I'm sorry, it's been a difficult day. And you hug, and you change the tone by changing the path. What if the rule was every time you walk through the door, you greet your partner with a hug, a kiss, and a warm embrace before you had the contest about who had the most challenging day? How would your relationship be different if you acted your way into some new feelings and set the tone for the whole day with a loving embrace regardless of whether you "felt" like it?

You love them, even when you don't feel like loving them. The fact is God loves us, even when we are temporarily acting very unlovable. Facts always outweigh feelings. Maybe your path is you feel bad about yourself. So, when you feel bad about yourself, there's a straightforward path to the freezer. And you eat ice cream when you feel bad, and then you feel worse because you ate the whole thing. Now you have the shame cycle and feel a lousy loop looping in your mind. You know, the whole reliving of eating the entire box of thin mints, the whole bag of chips. Because you sought relief, but what you needed was restoration. What you're going to do is create a new path. Instead of walking to the freezer, you walk to the front yard, take a little walk and exercise. Walk the dog, even if you don't have a dog. Walk the dog every day for three miles. Do you know how many more days you will add to your life if you walk an hour daily? Google it. When you exercise, you get some dopamine and adrenaline, feel better about yourself, and create a new path. Exercise is a fact that changes how you think, not just physically but also in terms of how you feel about yourself!

When you're bored, what do you do? You pick up your phone, and you look at Instagram. You scroll through all your friends, and you hate them. Because their life seems better than yours, they are posting their highlights, which you are comparing to your everyday life, which seems like many low lights.

Why? Because social media is built on: Show the Best, Hide the Rest!

You're not there with them where they are right now online. Why weren't you there? And you feel like a loser. Why didn't they invite you? What you might do is create a new path. You open up a Kindle, read a book, and put something different in your brain that renews your mind. You start your day with the right thoughts and prayer and reach for your shovel, not your phone. To think differently, we will forge a new path in our brain because the more you walk that path, the easier it becomes to travel. The more you stay off the old one, the more it weakens, and it's harder to think those same thoughts again.

Can you even think about doing any of this?

If so, you are on your way in a new direction, and your life is always moving in the direction of your most powerful thoughts.

Your life can be different.

Your life can be better.

Your past can be forgiven.

You are who you are.

But that's not all you will be.

In God's hands, dead relationships can come back to life.

In God's hands, resurrections are everyday events.

In God's hands, used tombstones go on sale.

God can change anything in your life.

What did Jesus say? "…With men this is impossible, but with God all things are possible" (Matthew 19:26, KJB).

But you have to believe this and think these thoughts. Invite Jesus into the situation, and then take steps to make it so. Your race won't be fair. It might be more complex because your calling is more challenging, but it can improve. Tell your mountains about God. When you don't surrender to circumstances but surrender to God's will for your life, change and lasting change happen. Before you give up, I dare you to pray today and give all your problems to God, surrender them to God, and then say, "But I know God… whatever it is today I am facing, *it doesn't have to be this way.*"

CHAPTER FIVE

RE-STORY-ATION?

---

*No matter how you started, God can rewrite your story and
give you an ending you never thought possible.*

—Ngina Otiende

LEGEND HAS IT THAT THERE was a small jazz club in New Orleans. In the corner of that club sat an old, dilapidated piano. All of the jazz artists complained about this antiquated instrument. The piano players dreaded playing it. The vocalists dreaded singing with it. And all of the combos that played in the club wished that they could bring in their own "piano" just like they could a saxophone or a trumpet. Finally, after years of listening to these jazz musicians complain about his piano, the club owner decided to do something about it. He had the piano painted. How's that for restoration? Not very effective. Many people focus on the flowers and the grass and forget that the most important and truly beautiful part of a person is the part you can't see with your eyes but can see with your heart. The flowers fade, and the grass withers; charm is deceptive, and beauty fades, but the right heart lives forever! Quit focusing on your exterior. It will fade, so start focusing on what's forever—your interior.

Why do people even keep coming to church or reading books like this?

People keep coming to church because they trust that Christ has changed my life and can change their lives as well. Yet, from my thirty years of experience, I know that some congregation members nod in agreement but never allow God's love to penetrate their lives. They are there to tickle their ears and grab the "feels" from worship. They are satisfied simply by painting the old piano. They will never take the necessary steps to make the changes they need.

Don't be a person who is content to paint the old piano.

I am riding with my friend. He's mechanical, thank God. We were going to lunch this past week and saw a woman with her car hood up. My friend says, "Let me see if *I* can help this woman." He pulls over. We get out, and he offers to help. The woman says, "Thank God you two guys are here to help." I said, "Ma'am, I am only good to pray over you and your car." She looks at me funny. I begin to tell her I am a writer. (smile) She tells my friend, "I can't start it, but if you jiggle the wires on the battery, I think it will work." My friend and I peered into the hood. This is funny because I do not know what I am looking for. Ha! It's like peering into an abyss. I have no idea what I am looking for. God could provide an arrow pointing to the problem under the hood, turn the manual to the page where to fix it, and hand me the manual, and I would still be lost.

I get paid to pray, not play with cars. I will pray for your mechanic.

But my friend grabbed the positive battery cable, which came off in his hand. The cable was too loose. "The terminal needs to be tightened up," he told her. "I can fix it with a wrench." The woman replies, "My husband says to just jiggle the wire. It always works. Why don't you try that? Sorry, but I am in a hurry!"

My friend whispers, "I wonder why her husband doesn't ride around town with her so he can jiggle the wires when needed."

He says: "Ma'am, if I just jiggle these wires, next time you stop, you will need someone to do that again, and every time you shut the engine off. Give me a minute, and I will solve the problem, and you can forget about it."

How many times in my own life have I reached for the quick fix instead of the actual fix? Come on, God, microwave this situation, fix it for me. I am in a hurry here, God! Nothing good in life comes fast. Show me in the Bible where God says, jiggle the wires; I know you are always busy and in a hurry!

The work of restoration cannot begin until a problem is fully faced. Sometimes you must stop the car, take it to a mechanic, and let him work on it slowly.

Look, I am writing this book for myself. I am glad you are reading along.

I am so guilty of this prayer: "God, can you help me but make it look like I did it all myself? Jiggle the wires and hurry up, will you God?"

Every two years, I read the Big Book of AA. This week, I have been reviewing the Big Book of AA and thought I would skip to step 12. The Big Book says Step 12 is: "Having had a spiritual awakening as a result of these steps, we sought to carry this message to others and to practice these principles in all of our affairs."[23]

That leads to the great question of this chapter:

What message are you carrying?

---

23 *The twelve steps*. Alcoholics Anonymous. (n.d.).
https://www.aa.org/the-twelve-steps

Most people are like electric wires: What comes in is what goes out. Someone calls us a name, and we call them a name back. Someone says a hurtful word; and we say a hurtful word back. Most people pass on the same energy that is given to them.

Now compare an electric wire to those big, green transformers that you see. Dangerous current or voltage comes in, but something happens inside that green box, and what comes out is, in fact, now helpful and productive. That is precisely what Jesus did with pain: He did not return the negative energy directed at him. He held it inside and made it into something much better. That is how. "He took away the sins of the world." He refused to pass on hate, negativity, anger, resentment, hostility! Not to say he didn't receive the nails of hate; he just refused to nail anyone else with the nails from his hands. Jesus was a transformer.

There is no such thing as a neutral exchange between two people.

People either bring you up or down. They give you more joy, or they rob you of your happiness. I remember one time studying hard for a master's level counseling test, and when I got my paper back, I earned a 92. Woohoo, right? I was so excited; I went to lunch and told a group of my friends about my grade, and three of them gave me a high five. The fourth friend said, "Well, it must have been easy." Bam, I got hit by a *joy robber.* Every time you interact with someone, they either make a deposit or a withdrawal to your heart. They either fire bullets or plant seeds. Are you a farmer or a gunslinger? They either compliment you or remind you of your failures. Drug dealers deal drugs, and athletes deliver plays and memories, grocery stores sell groceries, referees deal judgment, Mother Teresa deals love: Everyone is dealing with something. Apple trees give apples; orange trees give oranges; hope dealers give hope. Every exchange you have with someone is an opportunity to give them hope, even if they are on their deathbed. Trust me, that's when we need the most hope! I am trying to live as a hope dealer.

What is hope?

Hope is reaching into the future to grasp something you don't have or can't even see with your eyes! Hope is the divine possibility. Hope says to someone: Your life doesn't have to be this way; it can be and will be better. Hope believes the best is yet to come, even if that means in the next life, because the best yet to come is Jesus.

I think of how Jesus always dealt with hope, even in death on the cross. What did he say to the thief who believed in him? Your future is secure. Though your life is ending this way, your future is secure. "You will be with me in paradise." He encouraged that thief to reach a future he could not see because of the veil of death.

Come on, everyone carries a message. What's yours?

My brother gave me a hilarious and influential book about one of my old favorite comedians, Rober Schimmel. He wrote a book called *Cancer on Five Dollars a Day*, as he was diagnosed with non-Hodgkin's lymphoma, which he overcame! He attributes a big part of his success to his outlook, which his doctor helped him with. His doctor offered him a powerful piece of advice about people who either accept this is the way it is or people who do more than paint the piano. The doctor said that cancer patients can be separated into two groups: *The transmitters and the transformers.* The transmitters hear the news, the dreaded C word, focus on unanswerable why-me questions, eventually become negative and bitter, and they spread that negativity to everyone around them. They are the electric wires; what comes in goes out.

On the other hand, the transformers look for positives in their situation. How can I overcome the C word? Is there a treasure in this darkness? They spread their good feelings to those around them. They might take in something negative but transform it, so what comes out of their mouths and actions is positive and loving! Though each person never chose cancer, they could choose to either be a transmitter or a transformer. "It's not the hand that you're dealt that matters; it's how you play the hand you're dealt!"

Whenever I preach a sermon, there are four sermons involved. There's the sermon I write, the sermon I mediate over in my mind, the sermon I preach on Sunday morning, and the sermon that's heard. Whenever someone says, "That was a good sermon," I always say in my head: "We'll see!" We'll see if this was merely a piano painting or if they will take the words and let God retune and rest the keys! The point is that our words or messages are not always the messages others receive. Likewise, the message we think we are carrying may not always be what we put out in a transforming way.

The point is to start thinking about what you are dealing with. Everyone deals with something. Are you more of a transmitter or transformer? Are you more of a thermometer or thermostat regarding your relationships?

I am not saying you should dim your light to please someone. Your light drew them to you; now they want you to "dim" it? Work on pleasing God and being what God made you to be! Yet, be conscious of how you are coming off. God reminds me of this every time I get up to speak to my congregation. It began years ago. God would say to me, and still does:

Never underestimate the pain in the room.

Everyone may look good, dressed in their Sunday best, showered up, teeth brushed, and shirts buttoned, but I know the truth. Everyone in the room has pain. Everyone has brokenness in their life. When I look at my church, you know what I see? *The Island of Misfit Toys.* Thanks to the *Rudolph the Red-Nosed Reindeer Special* for that image. But that's what the church is for. It's a hospital for sinners, not a museum of saints.

Do you need a refill?

When I meet someone, I know they are holding a cup. Everyone has a cup named Hope that they carry, but most of our cups have holes in them. Our hope leaks out as we encounter life's hassles and heartaches. Our hope has holes in it from people who have stabbed us in the back. Our cup of hope has leaked out, and we don't know where or who to turn to!

Everyone needs a refill of hope.

God reminds me of it every time I meet or interact with someone.

Never underestimate the pain in this person's heart.

Just try it.

Recognize that everyone has some battles, some things going on in their life that you don't know about, that maybe you would have never guessed would be going on in their lives, but it's there! Everyone has losses in life, everyone! There are those who are wounded and those who pretend they are not wounded. Effective pastors are nothing more than wounded healers. Folks who have been wounded, healed by God's grace and love, and now point the way to the grace from God's love!

The other day, I got a box from Amazon that had a label saying, Fragile, Handle with Care. If I can handle a box with care, I can handle other's hearts with care too. We are too rough with other's hearts because we underestimate the pain in someone's heart.

Likewise, we should never underestimate the power of God's love to restore us and others!

But it goes beyond jiggling the wires; this is a chronic condition for all of us to reach for the quick fix. It goes beyond painting the piano; it's a wrestling match between two important players, and trust me, I have wrestled with these two players.

While working on this chapter, I decided to sit on my back porch and watch the sunset. It's a warm summer evening with a cooling breeze. The beautiful sky is now turning that deep navy blue just before dark. I am trying to decompress. It's the beginning of a short weekend before I preach on Sunday. That's when the carnival started in my head!

Have you ever heard the carnival barker in your head, complete with music?

Hear ye, hear ye, step right up, don't be shy; I know just what you need, sir!

Some agitated place in me started clamoring for relief. Some wires need jiggling; I feel stuck: stuck in a habit, stuck in a mindset, stuck in a toxic relationship, stuck in a financial pattern where you can't seem to get ahead, stuck in the claws of an addiction, stuck in grief, stuck in unforgiveness, stuck in a job that feels like it's a dead end, stuck in bitterness or in progress toward some goal, whether it's getting healthy or getting your budget. It feels lousy to feel stuck, like you're not moving forward as a human being.

And I am looking at my life and how I am dealing with things, and the carnival barker is back, and he's taunting me with this phrase:

"How's that working out for you? How's that working out for you?"

I think that's a fundamental question to ask ourselves because we can get so trapped in what we're doing that we never stop to ask ourselves or consider: Am I doing something that's moving me to where I want to go?

Does everyone have a carnival barker in their head? I was trying to untangle my soul when the circus tents showed up. The carnival of desire started jockeying for my attention.

The carnival barker shouted to me: "Hear ye, hear ye: You know what you need. There's some ice cream in the freezer. Two of those Nestle vanilla cones with chocolate at the bottom. You know you want it; now go get it!" Renee (my wife) is not even home! "You can take two! She will never know! Throw the box in the trash can in the garage... so she doesn't see it all empty in the trash can like she saw last time."

The carnival offered relief, but it was not what I needed!

I needed restoration, not relief.

Relief is easy, quick, and fleeting.

Relief is so momentary.

Relief is numbing, sedating, self-medicating myself.

Scrolling on my phone is a relief.

Television is a relief.

Eating both sleeves of the Girl Scouts "Thin Mints" is a relief.

Tequila is a relief.

Chips and queso are a relief.

We reach for relief because it's easy, immediate, and within our grasp. Relief is just jiggling the wires.

Now, this is the part where I tell you how I told that carnival barker to go away and quit tempting me. Well, I would like to say that's how it happened. Do you think I would say I sat there and numbed myself with two ice cream cones?

Of course, I would.

There I am, wolfing down both ice cream cones. I would have eaten a third if three were in the box! They were as good as advertised. After five minutes with the wrappers shamefully crumpled in my hands, I immediately regretted coming to the carnival of relief.

Sweet is the sin, but bitter is the taste left in my mouth.

Relief is so fleeting, and all those problems I faced were still there. Despite the ice cream, my soul was still disjointed, a tangled web.

It seems that I am always either running to something or from something! Why? Why is it so hard to just be still? Why is it so hard to let God fight some of my battles? How can God fight my battles when I am always grabbing the sword?

Think of sitting on the beach watching the waves roll in at sunset and compare that with turning on the tube and vegging in front of *Stranger Things* or *The Walking Dead.* The experiences could not be farther apart. This is what David was trying to put words to when he reported finding God in green meadows and beside quiet waters, emerging with a refreshed soul. Or, as another translation says, "He renews my strength" (Psalm 23:3, NLT). We need the immersion David spoke of. We need the renewal, the restoration.

Relief is painting the piano. It's not tuning and replacing the strings.

What is the difference between relief and restoration in your life?

Relief is short-term. It lifts the pain or the pressure for a while. It doesn't last.

Restoration, however, gets to the heart of the matter. It fixes the core issues from which you feel the need for relief.

Restoration is the permanent solution, the final cure. It is making things right. Relief is just easing the pain while things aren't right.

I know a woman who leads a large firm but who struggles with what is called today "body image issues." She was the ugly duckling in high school and college, then she "sprouted." Her word, not mine. Though she became a "stunner" (her word, not mine), she always feared the return of the ugly duckling. So, today, she is addicted to exercise, and secretly, she purges and suffers from anorexia. All of her efforts to be "in shape" are relief. She needs restoration from the wounds she sustained when being rejected for being the ugly duckling. Those hurtful words that people said to her when she was young, she still lets them be her template. She has let hurtful words be her template for her life, and they have only led to her focusing on the exterior.

I know a CEO who is about 400 pounds. He's a fine man, but his eating is manic. He is digging his grave with his teeth. He has traded donuts for sex. Why? As I've gotten to know him, I've come to understand that he was abused as a boy. Rather than getting a restoration for his soul from all the abuse, he eats to find relief.

Consider this pattern in your own life. Do you have issues from which you seek short-term relief rather than the restoration you need?

The actual healing Jesus offers when we commit our lives to him; the actual healing is restoration. It's a changed life. Now, please don't misunderstand me. Relief in its proper form is great. No one enjoys a massage, a jacuzzi, that quiet glass of wine, or the peace while reading a good book by the sea more than I do. I love a good ice cream cone as much as anyone does.

Relief is part of life.

Enjoy it.

The problem comes, though, when we allow relief to replace restoration.

That's when deformity and addiction set in.

Here's the principle. Relief is for short-term issues—tired feet, a week of hard work, the bruising conversation, and the challenging few months.

Restoration is for the long-term issues—the childhood trauma, the bad stuff that has produced lousy fruit for years.

Be courageous enough to go after restoration.

Be courageous enough to do more than paint the piano.

Now, let's think about this regarding boundaries and other people! Because this is where these issues come alive. Remember, my rule on boundaries is simple: If you don't set limits for your life, other people will!

We all have that "Needy Ned" in our lives or that "Demanding Donna" that won't leave us alone. They are the joy robbers; they are the ones making withdrawals with no deposits.

Most of you, when you have Needy Ned come clamoring to you, you are good at giving them relief. Here's some wine. Here's some ice cream. Here are some chips and queso, so let's numb out! Here's some money, now go away.

But restoration, ugh. We're not so good at this. The reason we're not as good at this is because, honestly, it takes a lot of time and a lot of effort. It takes much longer to redo a piano's inside with new strings, tuning, and keys than to slap some paint on the outside.

Relief is telling someone to take a week of vacation.

Restoration – This is months, or maybe even years, of working with someone who has an addiction, and they're hooked. You hang in there with them, and you help them get to rehab, and then to a 12-step group, and you help them find accountability, and they go three months sober, and then they fall off the wagon. You help them pick up the pieces *again,* and kick their butt (with tough love), and you work with them a*gain*. After a long period with lots of ups and lots of downs and celebrations and tears, finally, by the power of God through His people, they become spotless, and you've helped them be restored to their God-given potential. They are ready to serve the coffee and lead the 12-step groups. Now, they are prepared to be leaders in the church.

Needy Ned?

This is the chronically insecure person – "Meet my needs, please. Will you love me? Will you value me? Will you make me feel special? I need a guy; I need a friend!" You take them into your life, do coffee, and pray with them, showing them who they are in Christ. And you help them get involved in the community. Over time, you teach them where their security comes from, not from other people but from whom God says they are. Over time, you help restore them to their God-given potential.

This is the person who never has money – They're always hurting. They're always broke, and you don't throw $500.00 at them to solve the problem. That's what they are always asking from you. Just help me pay for my car, Pastor; it's past due, and they will repo it. Please give me some paint for my piano. Just give me some relief. But guess what I have learned? When I give them 500 bucks *for just this one time*, they are back again next month for one more time and one more time.

They don't need relief. They need restoration.

You give them $500.00, and within a few days, they're in trouble again because that doesn't help solve the problem. They need a budget. They need a job. They must put the PlayStation down, shower, shave, and send a resume! They may need more income and fewer expenses. They've spent years getting into a financial hole, and it will take years to help them. So you work with them, teach them a new language and way to think; debt is bad, debt is stupid, we're paying cash, no credit cards. You sign them up for Dave Ramsey. One day, they're debt-free and generous, and God has used you, not for relief, but for restoration, and it takes time.

The challenge is that, by nature, most of us want to offer relief when, often, the right thing to offer is restoration.

Relief is: Give me one sentence from this book to change my life. Restoration is Knowing you have to read the whole book twice. Then pray, then work. Then, partner with someone else and God above, and the piano starts to get rebuilt. Restoration concerns the foundation of your life, not just the exterior walls of your life. But I get it; no one ever buys a house and says, well, I bought it because of the foundation; you should see it!

One of the biggest lessons I have learned in pastoring people is this:

People want you to jiggle the wires instead of helping them fix their lives.

There is a great Bible story about relief versus restoration that we can study to help bring people back to their God-given potential. If you want to join me as a hope dealer in bringing hope to people's lives, it's good to see how it has been done and how we might do it in the future.

Scripture says: "One day Peter and John were going up to the temple at the time of prayer—at three in the afternoon. Now a man who was lame from birth was being carried to the temple gate called Beautiful, where he was put every day to beg from those going into the temple courts. When he saw Peter and John about to enter, he asked them for money" (Acts 3:1–3, NIV).

This was a guy that was lame. He was born this way. For his whole life, he couldn't walk. He was disabled from birth.

Pause, what do we have here?

We have a guy in significant need, and people have offered him relief for his whole life. They carried him. He begged. They gave him money, and somebody carried him home.

This guy was brilliant because there were three familiar places to beg during this time in history. The three most popular places: one was what they would call the highways where there was a lot of traffic; they'd go out there and beg. Two, they were in front of the homes of wealthy people because they thought wealthy people would give more. But the most lucrative place to pray was in front of the temple because this is where everybody would go at one time of the day. Why not beg on the steps of the doorway to church? You got guilt. You got religious people. You have some high-explosive elements for giving!

Let's call it the way it was. The Pharisees, who were very self-righteous, loved to give publicly. "Hey, look, there's a coin! Hey, I gave you five dollars, and you only have one! I'm so spiritual!" And so, this guy was trained that people would meet his needs. Verse three, when this guy saw Peter and John about to enter…what did he ask for?

What do all the guys standing on our street corners ask for?

Money! He asked for money. Shocker, right? Wrong.

Most people think money is their greatest need. Please give me some money. Please give me some relief!

Here's what has been confirmed in my life. When I was broke, I had problems, but I just needed money, right? Then I got money, but I soon realized I still had issues that money couldn't fix! One of the ways I knew I needed God is because there are some things money can't fix, including the inside of you!

Peter looked straight at him, as did John, then said, "Look at us!" So the man gave them his attention.

What was the beggar expecting? This guy was expecting to get something from them.

Why? Because for his whole life, people had given him what he wanted. He wanted money, and they gave it. He wanted relief, and they gave him relief.

Relief is provision.

Restoration is peace.

Sometimes we pray for provision, when we need to be praying for peace. For without peace, we will not be able to enjoy the provision God provides.

In verse six, Peter changes things up and says, "Silver or gold I do not have… You want money, I don't have money…but what I have, I give you. In the name…" This name is above all names, in the name of. "…Jesus Christ of Nazareth…"

He said, "You're not getting money, I am giving you restoration. I'm telling you to walk."

Verse seven says, "Taking him by the right hand…"

What did Peter do?

The Bible says, "…he helped him up."

This is a classic example of not giving a handout but instead a hand-up. Instantly, the man's feet and ankles became strong. He jumped to his feet and began to walk. Then, he went with them into the temple courts, walking, jumping, and praising God.

What happened?

They helped bring restoration.

They worked with him!

We're not handing out money or relief. We are handing out restoration. You stand up. You believe God can do this. You take the step of faith. Talk about being a hope dealer; come on. This was no neutral exchange. This was a significant life-giving deposit of hope, helping this man reach a future he couldn't even see, one where he could walk!

This was a transmitter, a beggar, who met a transformer.

This was a painter who met the piano tuner.

When they worked with him, God restored him.

The problem for us is we typically don't work with people; we work for people because we wrongly believe that we are the necessary ingredient for them to get better.

I used to believe this about me. It's me. I am magic, and I can do it.

Ha! You can stop laughing now.

It didn't take too long to figure out that I was just a sign pointing to the real healer!

But we place ourselves in their lives in the role of a functional savior. You need me to save you! I have the answers. I am the solution! If I don't meet your needs, nobody will.

What happens? I tried, and you didn't like it. I pull back, and I feel guilty. Why? Because I thought it was necessary to make you better. We are not the ones who restore. God is the One who restores. He is the Power Source. We are the connector, and we need His wisdom; we need His help, or we will end up trying to help people in a way that doesn't help them, and in the end, it hurts us.

We want to do it God's way. There is a prayer I pray before I counsel anyone, before I meet with Needy Ned, or Demanding Donna. Right after I remember not to underestimate their pain. I say to God:

God, help me give people what they truly need, not just what they want.

Would you say that aloud?

God, help me give people what they truly need, not just what they want.

This is what Peter did. The lame guy said, "I want money!" He said, "I'm not giving you money. What I have, I give you in the name of Jesus, walk."

People are going to tell you what they think they need.

It's almost always relief-oriented!

They may say, "I need money, I need money! You have money, John. Give me your money!"

God may show you very clearly, "No! They need a job! That's what they need! And we're talking about a real job that's forty hours a week. Put the video games down and grow up and get a job, brush your teeth, put on some deodorant, and then the girlfriend comes." If you give them money again, they will stay on your couch because you offered relief when they needed restoration.

I don't mean to be hard; I am not underestimating the pain in their hearts, but you must encourage folks to let hope be their template.

"But I need $580.00 to make my car payment!" "No, no, no, no, no, no! You don't need a $50,000.00 car. You need a $2,500.00 car, and you need it now! You're in bondage to something that you cannot afford, and I'm not going to continue to give you something that's going to end up hurting you in the long haul."

"But I just need you to make me feel special! You're the only one! I texted you, and I saw the bubbles. You were going to reply. Why didn't you? I'm devastated you didn't call me for the last seven minutes! Why didn't you come over to my house today? I need you! I can't make it."

"No, no, no, no, no, no, no! I can't meet that need."

"You have a God-shaped spiritual void that only God can meet. I'm telling you, I want to love you, but I'm going to do it in a way that will help you."

God makes us restless till we find our rest and restoration in him!

God, help us to give people what they truly need, not just what they want.

I've got a buddy that I've known for years since college. I officiated his wedding to a great gal. And over the years, I watched their marriage deteriorate. He came to me ticked to high heavens and had good reason. He's like, "I'm so done, I'm out of here, I'm done! My wife's emotionally engaged with some other guy and maybe worse, and she's inattentive and…" on and on. And he said, "I'm out of here, I'm done, I'm gone." And I just looked at him and said, "No, you're not!" He's like, "Yes, I am!" And I said, "No, you're not!" And he said, "Yes, I am!" And it went on for a while. And I said, "You're right that she's being sinful, irresponsible, dishonoring, and on and on, and her list can go on and on and on. But I know your side of the story too, and I will tell you what you'll not like, but what you need to hear."

Because there are three sides to every story—yours, mine, and the truth!

I told him that most marriages that have some years to them come down to this: growing, not falling, in love, many times with the same person. Quit being selfish. Marriage is not meant to complete you but to make you a better person. So, you either grow up, or you grow apart.

Those are your options. In your marriage, you will either grow up and learn to be unselfish and think of the other person, or you will grow apart. Quit being part-time archaeologists and digging up the past on each other.

Do you want a long marriage? Have a short memory!

And I said as lovingly as possible, "You have worshipped the idol of materialism. You have worked and tried to communicate love by giving your family more, but giving them more is not love. You've neglected your kids. You're on the golf course and at a football game every weekend. Your family is not in church. You have not led them spiritually. What we're going to do is get you into counseling. I will get you a mentoring couple, and you'll go home and lead your family back!"

And he just puffed up and said, "I'm not doing it!" And I said, "Listen to me, I'm not backing down. That's what you need to do!"

So I said to him: "It would be best if you had restoration."

And after kind of a heated deal, he finally just broke down, and he said, "You're right; I've got to own up to my part of it." That's what he did. He did everything that I asked him to do. And here's what's amazing, it's amazing! Nine months later, and I'm talking for nine months, which isn't very long, he wrote me the best three-page email I've ever gotten! I don't take any credit for this besides that God gave me the words to say what he needed to hear, not what he wanted to hear!

God gives us the words people need, not those they want to hear!

There will be times when you're tempted to give them what they want! You are so right. She's a horrible wife, and I agree you should have an affair first and then get an attorney, and then end this thing in divorce. No, no, no, no! God, help me see past what they say and what they truly need. What's the thing under the thing that is causing the thing?

This is a prayer I always pray: "God, I pray that you would lead us to give people what they truly need, not just what they say they want."

Relief or restoration? If relief is not the long-term answer, and restoration is, it begs the question, Restoration to what?

Are you restoring me to my old self? No. Are you restoring me to selfishness? No. Are you restoring me to what?

What if I told you God wants to restore you to the masterpiece he originally made?

Ephesians 2:10 (NLT) says: "For we are God's masterpiece…" Do you feel like Picasso?

Ephesians 1:4 (TLB): "Long ago, even before he made the world, God chose us to be his very own through what Christ would do for us; he decided then to make us holy in his eyes, without a single fault—we who stand before him covered with his love."

In other words, God thought of you, you know the glowing, loving, forgiving, take the high road you can be, before the beginning of time. There are things and assignments we have in this moment of history that God has planned and equipped us for, but will we answer God's call?

Eternity is already in session, and you are a part of it.

What if the restoration God seeks in our lives allows us to become who God saw when he formed us, wonderfully and fearfully, with a sense of awesomeness and wonder in our mother's secret place? (See Psalm 139.)

William Shakespeare once said, "We know what we are, but not what we may be."[24]

But if we could know what we are in our identity, then we see what could be, might be, should be, and could grow into being!

What if God wants to restore us to our real identity, not our shadow self?

Much of the anxiety today revolves around identity confusion. Who am I? What is the correct behavior for who I am? What are my values? What points me true north? Why am I alive right now in this moment of time and history? What unique gifts do I have that no one else brings? If you can answer these questions without confusion, you are on your way to a successful life and a life of significance.

Identity determines activity. Knowing who you are determines how you live your life.

Again, being confused about identity is the source of much anxiety in the world.

You are not your job. You're not how much money you have in the bank. You are not the car you drive. You're not the contents of your wallet. You are not your khakis. You are

24 *William Shakespeare - we know what we are, but know not...* BrainyQuote. (n.d.).
https://www.brainyquote.com/quotes/william_shakespeare_164317

not your gender. You are not your orientation. You are not rich. You are not poor. You are not White, Black, Yellow, or Brown. There is no Jew or non-Jew. There is no *other*.

You are a child of God. That's it.

Intelligence, looks, jobs, gender, and orientation can all be decided upon and changed to varying degrees, and Father Time is undefeated at making sure your grass and flowers fade.

If you have a heartbeat, you are a child of God.

We are made in God's divine image.

God created everyone.

What if we saw ourselves as children of God and everyone else that way too?

Can you imagine that?

You will always be a child of God.

The world can never strip away this name tag.

You can't take away my medal because you didn't give me my medal.

God did.

Once you know this, you begin to live like a child of God, especially regarding restoration and relief.

Just as God said about Jesus on the day he was baptized, "This is my beloved Son," so on your baptism, God said over you,

> You are to be different.
> You are mine!
> You are a child of God.
> You are infinitely loved.
> You were bought with the blood of Jesus; you are not your own.
> You are not self-made! (No one made their kidneys in their garage.)
> Salt of the earth. Light on the hill. Yeast in the bread.
> *I planned for you before the beginning of time.*

Now that you know *who* you are, here's how you are to live:

> You are to love your enemies!
> You're to do good to those who hate you!
> Bless those who curse you!
> Pray for those who mistreat you!
> Turn the other cheek.

Give to everyone who asks of you.

You're to go the second mile.

You're to do unto others as you wish they would do to you.

You must be a hope dealer, life-giver, encourager, and restorer.

When Jesus talks about loving other people this way and seeing other people this way, it's *indiscriminate love.*

To love everyone with indiscriminate love takes new eyesight; the eyesight of the heart and soul that sees the most valuable thing about a person is what you can't see: Their God-given soul that God has placed eternity in.

It's no coincidence that before Saul became Paul, God blinded his physical eyesight to restore his spiritual eyesight.

You must have new eyes to see yourself and others as children of God. Otherwise, you get lost in the color of your skin, orientation, smoking or drinking, skinny or fat, Republican or Democrat, Jew or Muslim, etc.

I am so good at discriminatory love. I love those who love me, look like me, vote, think like me, and are just like me.

Jesus loved everyone as if they were the only person on this earth.

Jesus saw everyone as a child of God, regardless of gender, religion, culture, etc.

Jesus said in Luke 6:27–36 (NKJV): "But I say to you who hear: Love your enemies, do good to those who hate you, bless those who curse you, and pray for those who spitefully use you. To him who strikes you on the *one* cheek, offer the other also. And from him who takes away your cloak, do not withhold *your* tunic either. Give to everyone who asks of you. And from him who takes away your goods do not ask *them* back. And just as you want men to do to you, you also do to them likewise. But if you love those who love you, what credit is that to you? For even sinners love those who love them. And if you do good to those who do good to you, what credit is that to you? For even sinners do the same. And if you lend *to those* from whom you hope to receive back, what credit is that to you? For even sinners lend to sinners to receive as much back. But love your enemies, do good, and lend, hoping for nothing in return; and your reward will be great, and you will be sons of the Most High. For He is kind to the unthankful and evil. Therefore be merciful, just as your Father also is merciful."

Jesus has no word here for the victimizer, but he has a strong word for the victim. Jesus naturally assumes that behavior does not belong in the Kingdom of God, and a child of God does not practice that behavior.

But if you don't know you are a child of God, you might be tempted to act differently!

He doesn't address the victimizer but addresses those who are children of God who may be victims. He is saying that you can choose not to be a victim. You have the choice to determine ahead of time how you are going to respond when something happens to you. What if you had decided to love everyone? You have the ability and the power through Jesus our Lord not to respond in kind, and you have the power to take the first step and to respond in love. Just because someone sees you as an enemy doesn't mean you must see them similarly! You can decide not to reciprocate based on identity! We have the ability through Christ to take the initiative and respond in love, kindness, blessings, and prayer when abuse comes our way.

Restoring people can be challenging. Sometimes you only manage to provide relief. When that happens, take comfort in knowing that you acted like a child of God and loved indiscriminately. A month ago, a first-time guest approached me and asked me for one hundred dollars for a new tire. He even took me to the parking lot and showed me his balding tire. Of course, an astute mechanic like me knew the tire needed replacing. (smile) I said, "Okay, where are you buying the new tire from?" He says, "Discount Tire." Monday morning, I called Discount Tire, gave them his name, and put one hundred dollars on my debit card for him.

I was feeling pretty good about myself. Then I thought to myself, *He took you. You're a sucker, and you swallowed that bait hook, line, and sinker. He lied.* Then I thought, *So what if he lied? You just wasted one hundred bucks on someone else instead of you?* Then I thought I would call Discount Tire back and find out if he lied. Do you ever have conversations like this in your head? I couldn't help myself; the voice of doubt won. I called Discount Tire and spoke to the manager. I found out that he did lie. The manager said he had gotten all his tires replaced and his wife's tires replaced as well. He says, "Pastor, I think you bought his eighth new tire this month."

I hung up the phone feeling dumb. Don't let the noise of your weaker self drown out God's inner voice. I thought I heard God say, "Good Job!" I smiled the biggest smile I had all week. I am so glad he and his family will be safe on the road. There won't be a wreck due to a balding tire as he travels 75 mph down Highway 35. It is a good thing to help make sure our roads are safe. He can pass his vehicle inspection now. His kids and family have new tires. Thank you, God, for allowing my identity to determine my activity and even being happy about generosity in the face of disingenuous people. It's probably the best one hundred bucks I spent that week! Jesus says that if you perceive a need, respond with love and generosity. If the other person is lying, that's his problem. I am to treat people as I would like to be treated if I were in their situation. For once, just one time, I had finally loved indiscriminately. It didn't cost much, one hundred bucks. It didn't feel natural, but I will keep trusting and stepping into it. It's called being a child of God.

I am not trying to refute what I wrote earlier, but I am saying that we do it with indiscriminate love as we seek to restore people. I wanted to ensure I wasn't cheated by calling Discount Tire, but it didn't work. I can be more cautious in the future, but at the end of the day, I am responsible for my behavior, and if you err on the side of love, that's a good thing. That's what a child of God does. It's gray. It's not always so easy—this balance between relief and restoration. But the goal is for you to know your identity as a child of God. Claim it, live it, and understand that all activity follows identity.

Have you ever seen a fish wake up and say, "I don't know what to do today?" No, there are no confused fish. Every day, they wake up and they swim around. They act like fish because they know they are fish. A cheetah knows to run fast, and the impala knows to run faster than the cheetah or risk being lunch! The impala never gets confused, thinks it's a cheetah, and chases it. The impala knows it's not a predator. The lion knows to roar. The lion knows it's the king of the jungle. There is no confusion.

Once you know who you are, you can know how you should live, and you begin to allow God to restore you into that child of God he had in mind when God first created you.

Why I am Still a Pastor:

Like you, I could get paid to do almost anything, almost anywhere. Even my age, I have enough tread on my tires to do many different things.

I could sell cars.

I could sell insurance.

I could write books, including children's books.

I could travel the country and be part of the Speaker Lab or John Maxwell's Speaker Team.

I could be a Full-time Life Coach.

Did you know that 50 percent of all clergy resign from preaching and teaching within five years of ordination?

Why?

I am in year thirty of ministry.

But I have not quit.

One reason: **When has quitting ever helped develop more character?**

Why have I not committed to these other career paths?

It's not the money. It has to do with an email I got this week. It was the kind of email I printed out and put in my box of hope. It's not a chest, more of a shoebox.

It has notes, cards, emails, and reminders of why I am still a pastor. When I fire myself as I often have, I get my shoebox and start reading the notes. It reminds me of my calling.

The email I received is from a guest of Grace, someone I don't know. But she has been coming here for a few weeks and bringing along a family member who has experienced way too much pain and trauma that any soul should have to endure.

She was sexually abused and began to think of herself as "just damaged goods!"

But here's the good news. She told me that her family member had learned one thing in the past couple of weeks, and she's even begun claiming it. She's been going around the house saying a phrase that her family has never heard her say before she went to church, and here's the phrase:

"I am a child of God!"

Six life-changing words.

Do you know who you are?

You are not your job, your car, your bank account, your marriage (or lack of one), your gender, your sexual orientation, your khakis, or your IQ. You—yes, even you—are a child of the Almighty God.

He made in His image with love.

God thought of it before the beginning of time! (See Ephesians 1:4 for that)

God calls you his masterpiece, his Picasso, his Rembrandt!

God formed you and fashioned you in your mother's secret place! You are fearfully (with a sense of wonder) and wonderfully made. (See Psalms 139 for this)

It's such a simple message.

But so hard to believe.

Because what I hear from you are some different "I am" statements.

What are your most common "I am" statements?

You know, how you talk to yourself:

I am not enough.

I am weak.

I am scared.

I am afraid.

I am worried.

I am angry.

I am depressed.

I am concerned.

I am nervous.

I am weird.

I am small.

I am damaged.

I am messed up.

I am wounded.

I am hurt.

I am down.

I am fallen.

I wonder what your most common "I am" statement is?

What if this was one of yours?

Can you read these and say them out loud?

I am brave.

I am happy to be here.

I am always learning.

I am intelligent.

I am proud of who I am.

I am happy.

I am responsible.

I better hurry up. I only get to do this once!

I am strong.

I am going to get through this.

I am unique.

I am patient.

I am worthy.

I am loveable.

I am fun.

I am creative.

I am trustworthy.

I am a survivor.

I am loved.

I am "me."

Jesus had a few "I am statements" as well:

"I am the bread of life" (John 6:35, NIV).

"I am the light of the world" (John 8:12, NIV).

"I am the gate" (John 10:9, NIV).

"I am the good shepherd" (John 10:11, NIV).

"I am the resurrection and the life" (John 11:25, NIV).

"I am the way and the truth and the life" (John 14:6, NIV).

"I am the vine" (John 15:5, NIV).

If I could get you to believe and say only one "I am statement," it's this:

I am a child of God.

If you could base all your self-worth, let go of all the other "I am statements," and rest in this one, you are on your way to knowing God.

You are on your way to being healed of your past.

You are on your way to living an abundant life today, knowing you have a heavenly mother or father who empowers you.

You are on your way to knowing you have someone who will always love you, be with you, never leave you, and empower you to live an abundant life.

I am a child of God.

Can you say it?

Can you believe it?

Not just in your head, but in your heart?

It's so much better than:

I am damaged goods.

I am my wounded past.

I am what I am.

You are a child of God.

You are eternally loved.

You will have abundant life today, forgiveness for yesterday, and eternal hope for tomorrow.

Is there anything better than that?

If I can get strangers to our family of faith to believe this, to know this, to live into this identity, it's why I am a pastor.

I hope you get a shoebox explaining why you do what you do.

"See what great love the Father has lavished on us, that we should be called children of God! And that is what we are" (1 John 3:1, NIV).

If you want your life to be different, you must seek relief and restoration. What if you didn't let your trauma from the past negatively influence your future? What if you allow God's love and your hopes, not your hurts, to be your life's template?

Can you see it?

What if your only I am statement was: I am a child of God?

Pablo Casals, world-renowned cellist, once remarked, "Each second we live is a new and unique moment of the universe, a moment that will never be again. And what do we teach our children? We teach them that two and two make four and that Paris is the capital of France. When will we also teach them what they are?"

He continues, "We should say to each of them: 'Do you know what you are? You are a marvel! You are unique. In all the years, there has never been another child like you— your legs, arms, clever fingers, and how you move. You may become a Shakespeare, a Michelangelo, or a Beethoven. You have the capacity for anything. Yes, you are a marvel. And when you grow up, can you harm another who is, like you, a marvel?"[25]

What's he saying? **You're better than that.** Have you ever been told you're better than that?

You're better than that.

That's what my mom told me when I came home from college, ready to give up and work at Dairy Queen for the rest of my life. I worked at Dairy Queen throughout high school and during Christmas break in college. Richard Thayer, who owned eighteen Dairy Queens, offered me a regional manager job and to quit school and work for him at 55K a year and a company car. I owned five pairs of heavily used underwear and a 10-gallon fish tank with a slow leak. A company car was sounding good at nineteen. Having Dairy Queen money seemed better than no money. But it was not just about my major; it was my calling or career, grades, the right girl to date, what success is, and how to chase it. I was ready to lower the bar. I was prepared to quit dreaming God's dreams for my life and surrender to the current realities of my situation…and my mom said

---

25 Goodreads. (n.d.). *A quote by Pablo Casals*. Goodreads. https://www.goodreads.com/quotes/194563

these life-changing words: You're Better Than That. I didn't bring you into this world so you could put a curl on an ice cream cone! But at that point, that was my primary life skill. If you ever go to the Chinese buffet with me, trust me, you will want me to get your ice cream cone for you!

During her adventures in Wonderland, Alice comes across a caterpillar who asks, "Who are you?" Her response is interesting. Alice replied, rather shyly, "I hardly know, sir, just at present. At least I know who I was when I got up this morning, but I think I must have been changed several times since then." "What do you mean by that?" said the caterpillar sternly. "Explain yourself!" "I can't explain myself, I'm afraid, sir," said Alice: "Because I'm not myself, you see." "I don't see," said the caterpillar. "I'm afraid I can't put it more clearly," Alice replied very politely, "for I can't understand it myself to begin with, and being so many different sizes in a day is very confusing."[26] Alice didn't know who she was; she had identity confusion before it was cool! We find ourselves in a position like Alice's. This is who I am on Facebook. This is who I am at work. This is who I am on Friday night. This is who I am on Sunday morning. This is what sin does to us; circumstances can do to us—divide us and make us un-whole. So, if we are pressed, as Alice was, and someone asks us, "Who are you?" it is not surprising to see that we are confused. We are one person at home, another at work, and still another with friends. We have identities rooted in our careers, accomplishments, trauma, and failures. This is why David prayed in Psalm 86:11 (NIV): "Teach me your way, LORD, that I may rely on your faithfulness; give me an undivided heart...." Have you ever looked at your life, marriage, family, finances, service, and dedication to God, or maybe stood there right out of the shower buck naked and heard God say to you: You're better than that?

We have this jacket in our house. It's not a coat of many colors, but a cool leather jacket. My boys fought over who could wear it and who it belonged to. We solved the problem. We wrote Jacob's name on his jacket. Ever do that—write names on things you buy? This jacket belongs to Jacob. My kids fight all the time. That's mine. This is mine. Ever put your leftovers in your fridge and write your name on the box? This is mine. It has value. It has my name on it. God says of you, you're mine. That's why he put his name on you. God did it with the blood of Christ.

Our jobs, bodies, families, intellect, GPA, health, and usefulness define us. If anything makes us feel worthless, improving one of those qualities will make us more intrinsically valuable. If I can change something on the outside, it will make me better on the inside. Yet whether I'm amazing, or I'm worthless—either sentiment is pride. If feeling good about yourself is a mountain of pride, feeling worthless is just as much of a lie. It's an inverted mountain of pride. It's pride either way. C. S. Lewis said humility isn't thinking less of yourself but of yourself less. If I write a better book and buy that 21k

26 de Rooy, L. (2020, September 20). *Chapter V: Advice from a Caterpillar*. Alice-in-wonderland.net. https://www.alice-in-wonderland.net/resources/chapters-script/alices-adventures-in-wonderland/chapter-5/

Rolex watch, I'll be a better, more desirable, and more attractive person. It's a crisis of identity, a forgetting of who we are.

Remember the movie *Toy Story*? Woody thinks he's no longer worthy to be Andy's favorite toy, and Buzz thinks he's too good to be just another toy. Are you not good enough for others? Or are you too good to need others? Most of us fall on one side or another of that divide, sometimes switching sides in a day, depending on a well-placed compliment or an ill-timed criticism. Woody and Buzz's roles reverse in one of the movie's pivotal moments. The neighborhood boy, Sid, who likes to torture toys, has captured the two. While in captivity, Buzz sees a TV commercial advertising a new toy called Buzz Lightyear. And he realizes that Woody is right.

Buzz doesn't have any special powers. His laser is just a blinking light. His spaceship is made of cardboard. He's just a toy. And because of that, Buzz now thinks he's worthless. Buzz says, "I can't help anyone… I'm not a Space Ranger. I'm just a toy. A stupid, little, insignificant toy." Woody says, "Being a toy is much better than being a Space Ranger… Look, over in that house is a kid who thinks you're the greatest, and it's not because you're a Space Ranger, pal. It's because you're a toy. You are *his toy!*" Buzz looks at the bottom of his boot and sees that his owner, Andy, has written his name on it! Buzz realizes that his value, worth, and identity don't come from who he is. His value comes from the one to whom he belongs. The lesson they both learn is that it doesn't matter how important you are, that it only matters how important you are to someone.

In Romans 1:1 (NLT), Paul refers to himself as "a slave of Christ Jesus." If we live our lives as God intends for us to live them, we *belong* to God, there's a sense in which God now *owns* us. As Paul says in 1 Corinthians 6:20 (RSV), "You were bought with a price."

What *Toy Story* teaches is identity. Many people today are confused about who they are. They don't know how, what, or who defines them.

Everyone is looking for a nametag you can't take off. There's only one: You are a child of God.

Yes, you. Even you. Reread it. "See what great love the Father has lavished on us, that we should be called children of God! And that is what we are" (1 John 3:1 NIV).

Most of us answer the question of who they are with one of these three categories:

1. **We get our identity rooted in *stuff*** – what I have, money, cars, treasures, pedigree, education!

2. **Identity rooted in *action*** – what I do, and how productive I am, look what I bring to the table.

3. **Identity rooted in *existence*** – who I am, whether I am young or old, skinny or fat, working or retired, alert or asleep.

Some things are loved because they are valuable, but others are valuable because they are loved. We are valuable because we are all loved by God, regardless of category one or two!

The problem with you rooting your identity in stuff is this: All the things you have now will end up in a junkyard. You're just the middleman. The only difference between the merchandise in a junkyard and those at Nordstrom, Best Buy, or BMW is *time*. Treasure is junk waiting to happen. If you want the formula, junk equals treasure plus time. I saw an ad for an expensive watch not long ago that said, "You never actually own a Pat Philippe. You merely look after it for the next generation." This particular watch platinum version (no kidding) sells for $1,230,000. That's for a watch that will still end up in a junkyard.

Junk is just treasure plus time. That beautiful car is going to end up in somebody's junkyard.

The problem with rooting your identity in what you bring to the table is that eventually, someone else will do it better, be younger, hotter, sexier, and now what? I can remember a time when I was introduced as the "young" minister! No one introduces me that way anymore. I would say I am the pastor, and people would say, Youth Pastor? They don't say that anymore. Have you ever had your spouse look at you as you are in bed at 8 p.m. on a Friday with a heating pad and say you've changed? People look at you as if you are no longer young or full of potential. I'm sure you have plateaued out and quit growing there, older man. Not true. But our circumstances look that way, don't they? Our drawstrings start to frazzle, our joints begin to creak, and we're no longer the "young" minister, or we're no longer a parent of little kids, or we're no longer employed, or we're no longer healthy.

Like Woody, we know what it's like to have a life change and feel left behind. Life changes without consulting us first. Woody struggles because he no longer feels like he's important. Andy has a new favorite toy. Woody gets so jealous that he pushes Buzz out of a window to try and get rid of him. Remember, Buzz can't fly, but he does fall in style! Jealousy is a nasty animal. It's so easy to look around and see people who are wealthier, healthier, better looking, more successful, people who have it all together. What does that do to our self-worth? The less we think of ourselves, the less we think God thinks of us!

Again, we usually base our self-worth on stuff or what we can do while ignoring the greatest love of all just because of love! How does God love you just because? Not because you are productive or have cool stuff but because you are the mud He created. God loves you the same way he loves Jesus! God loves Jesus just because He is Jesus. Don't you believe me? When Jesus was baptized, The Bible says the clouds opened up, and God's voice from heaven said, "This is my Son, whom I love; with him I am well pleased" (Matthew 3:17, NIV). And guess what? Jesus had not done one miracle, one feeding, one Messiah-like thing. God didn't love him any more or any less because he had saved the world or not; he loved him just because! Jesus hadn't multiplied a Lunchable or healed a papercut yet! This was the beginning of Jesus's ministry, but God is saying I love him because of who he is...not because he's done anything. And God says the same about you.

Identity rooted in stuff or actions leads to mere functionality. I'm only valuable for the specific tasks I can do. And sooner or later, you get too old, or someone will come along and do it better; there will be a new toy, a new Buzz Lightyear.

Christian faith has a unique understanding of existence identity. Christians assert that I must first know "whose" I am to know "who" I am. We belong to God. We have been bought. Our trail and our past has been covered and forgiven. We don't live as if we are our own.

This is Woody's argument. And this is the core theme of the *Toy Story* trilogy.

Who I am is defined by who I belong to!

Did you know you have God's name written on you? It's not on the bottom of your shoe. It's in your heart. You are *that* important.

Books like this and the church are where we come together and remind each other of our true identities. Not so much out there in the world. Out there in the world, you've got to earn your place. You've got to do something to be special. I read this week about a chef in France named Benoit Violier, who took his life, leaving his wife and his young son without a provider, without a father, without a husband. And he did so because rumors started circulating that the Michelin company was entertaining the notion of taking away one of his Three Michelin Stars. They say retaining that star is the only thing harder than getting a third star. And the thought of what that would do to his identity as a successful chef was too much for him to bear. The person I heard talking about this, the head runner of the restaurant Eleven Madison Park, said he was so sorry to hear this happening because of his friend's pressure. And the worst part was that he said it was not true. They weren't going to take away that third star. But just the thought of having that blow to his identity taken away.[27] Isn't that just a tragic picture of life where you have to continue to be enough? I need to be pretty enough. I need to be successful enough.

I think the most challenging part of belief in God concerns identity. The hardest part of belief has never been believing in God but in believing in the God who says He is infinitely in love with me, all of me, just because! He's not ashamed of me, He believes in me, He showers me with honor, with kisses, with rings, with robes, with brisket, with a party, with dancing! It's the prodigal son coming home, and we all need to go home!

---

27 Bilefsky, D., & Severson, K. (2016, February 1). *Benoît Violier's death shines light on high-pressure restaurant world*. The New York Times. https://www.nytimes.com/2016/02/02/world/europe/benoit-violier-chef-dies.html

God promises to jiggle the wires, get out the wrench, and help us change our lives. God says to put away the can of paint. We must pray, "God, give me firm boundaries to love and give people what they need." You must ask God to give you the eyes of faith to see beyond what the human eye can see and to look with the eyes of your heart, not just at yourself but at others as well.

We are all children of God due to the love of the Father. We are all accepted because Jesus was condemned. The cross was the once for all event. Jesus's sacrifice is the one for all. All. There are no qualifiers here. All means all. It's a joy to the whole world. (See Hebrews 7:27, NIV.)

If we could know our identity, set boundaries accordingly, and live that out, our activity would be clear.

It will be nothing but *indiscriminate love.* Then you can say, "It doesn't have to be this way." It's a tall order, and none of us are there, but we can step toward that today.

When we allow God to restore us, he rewrites our story. It's a re-story-action of everything!

It's time to quit painting the piano and know who you are. Be courageous enough to play chess, not checkers, seeking restoration not relief.

CHAPTER SIX

WOULD YOU RATHER WIN THE LOTTERY OR GET CANCER?

Your happiness will not come to you. It can only come from you.

—Ralph Marston

YEARS AGO, WHEN WE LIVED in Missouri, I wanted to grow stronger. I wanted to grow in my physical well-being. There was an amazing guy at our church. His name was Doug. I will not tell you his last name because you could look him up online. He was the three-time Mr. Universe in the forty and over category. He did infomercials for home strength equipment. He looked like Popeye. Does anybody remember Popeye the Sailor Man? He looked like Popeye on steroids. I asked him, "Would you work out with me?" He did, and it was unbelievable. Doug was unbelievable. My wife asked me, "Could I come to watch you and Doug work out?" I said, "No, I can't make it today; it's just going to be Doug." She said, "That would be okay. Can I still come?" "No. No, you can't." I eventually told Doug, "What I want to do is look like you." Doug said, "Well, are you all in?" I said, "What do you mean?" He said, "Nobody just drifts into this. People get this goofy idea."

You don't just drift into this.

No one drifts into excellence. Are you all in? I began to hesitate as he described the steps he took to maintain the way he looked. He said, "I lift weights until I am so sore that my body is on fire. Sometimes I can barely tie my shoes after a strenuous workout the following day. Then I will go and do it again. I will monitor every calorie I bring into my body and not get any wrong ones. I sometimes set the alarm and wake up in the middle of the night to ingest protein when my body can absorb it. Mostly, I'm talking about pain, the ability to absorb searing, mind-numbing levels of pain. Are you willing to do that? Are you all in?"

I said, "Uhhh….ehhh…well, maybe."

Nobody changes their life with a wish to, want-to, maybe

That's why I look like this today.

Thank you for laughing.

No. See, I was an admirer, not a follower when it came to Doug.

Changing your life often involves knowing how to exit—an exit from the way you have been thinking, living, and trying. It might include exiting from clinging to previous identity statements and previous I am statements!

"Every exit is an entry somewhere else." (Tom Stoppard)

When it came to looking like Doug, I was not all in. I was in when it was convenient. I wouldn't mind looking like that, but I have to go to work sometime. (smile) I can't live at the gym. I am a trainer of the soul, not the body. I was not willing to pay the price to look like that. I liked how he looked, as did my wife, but I won't do what he did.

I have chosen chips and queso as my Friday night goal—a more reasonable goal, and they look good for your taste buds, all right! No judging!

That's not to say I don't have fitness goals, but I have two particular fitness goals: 1) I need to fit in my pants, and 2) I need to look good with a seat belt on. Have you ever been on a date and been conscious of your appearance with a seat belt on? I have. I don't want Dun-lap syndrome, where my belly has Dun-lapped over my waist. Okay, maybe one more goal: look good, not with a shirt off but with a shirt on! (Smile)

When Jesus was around, people admired him. "Well, that's good." You might be in that category. That's how any following starts with admiration first. He's looking for followers. Everyone online wants followers, so I must keep my image and brand up. Will you follow me, like me?

When you follow Jesus, your old selfish shadow self begins to look for an exit so you can drive down a new road in life called your greater self. This means a change in values, which always means a change in direction and living.

Mostly, what Jesus came to bring was life change on this side of heaven. Most Christians get so focused on the next life and getting to heaven that they forget heaven came to us, came to earth, to change us! Why do we first try and get people to trust Jesus for the next life before we trust Jesus in this life? Jesus told the disciples to trust him in this life first, to live the abundant life today, and then trust him for the next life, eternal life, later. We get it all backwards. Start following Jesus in this life before you try and trust Jesus in the next!

Jesus knew that not everyone who wanted life change was willing to move from admirer to follower. It is so easy to admire; you can do it from afar. But to follow, you have to do that up close and personally. Legend has it that one of the disciples' prayers was a follower's prayer: "May you follow Jesus so close that you will be covered in the dust of his sandals." That's not far off; read about him online admiration. That's taking the same steps he took, getting dusty!

My favorite healing story in the Bible is one where you have to ask yourself, what exactly did Jesus heal? What was the illness? What was ailing this man? He didn't wave a magic wand, spit, or put mud in the guy's eyes. He just told the guy how to think.

It starts with a conversation, like the one I had with Doug.

In chapter 5 of the book of John, Jesus found a man by a pool, where he and many others lay sick and diseased in various ways. The location was Bethesda, a supernatural site where legend said an angel would come down and stir up the waters, and the first person to get into the recently stirred waters was healed of whatever disease they had. Wow, instant healing, pop a pill, pour some hot water on it, instant transformation, that was the legend anyway. Jesus walked up to a man afflicted with a disease for thirty-eight years.

When Jesus saw him lying there and knew that he already had been in that condition a long time, he asked him a bizarre question. He said to him, **"Do you want to get well?"**

The first thing we can see here is that Jesus knew this man did not get sick a week ago. Thirty-eight years is a lifetime in Biblical times, and this disease had gripped this man for most of his life. When you read this account, it seems Jesus is being a little uncaring, at least by our modern-day standards. He doesn't ask for the man's story. He doesn't say how you lived this way for the last thirty-eight years.

He sees him living one way and asks: Do you want to get well?

He's saying: You don't have to live like this. Your life doesn't have to be this way.

Jesus knew that someone who has had a disease for a long time can end up wrapping their identity around their disease. What comes against us can become a part of our identity if we are not distinguishing.

You would think that after thirty-eight years, the man would figure out to slip his best friend a twenty and roll his lame body into the pool. But what if the main thing that was lame was his mind? What if this man needed to exit the pool of excuses in which he was taking shelter?

Can you hear Jesus ask you that question today?

Do you want to get well?

Do you want a healthy, loving, deep, intimate marriage?

Do you want deep, meaningful relationships with your kids?

Do you want to be sober?

Do you want to live generously financially?

It's a strange question asking someone if they want to stay wounded, stay sick, stay stuck, stay trapped in depression, or cycle of shame and a loop of anxiety.

Jesus would be canceled for questions like that today.

It's like asking a guy in a wheelchair: Would you like to do a cartwheel and a backflip? But Jesus knew something very important:

Not everyone who is down wants to get up.

Because if you get up, you can't continue to live like you are down.

Jesus is saying: It's not your fault that you're messed up, broken, and a train wreck. It is your fault if you stay messed up, broken, and a train wreck.

If the man says, "Yes, I want to be healed," he has now taken some responsibility to live in a new way. He has to leave the road of excuses he's pretty comfortable navigating.

If he says, "No," he looks foolish, and it's like a guy holding a sign will work for food, but in the end, all he wants is a handout, not a hand-up or a job.

I have counseled many down people who didn't want to get up. Some people have gotten so comfortable with disappointment that they've learned to manage their expectations, lest they dream big and get dashed again.

Well, I'll probably never get married.

Well, I'll probably never own a home.

I'll probably never actually get to have children.

I'll probably never get to start this business.

I don't think my dreams will ever come true.

I will work to pay my mortgage and take up the air!

So, we learn to live with what we can't rise above. We get comfortable on the ground.

Jesus comes not saying it's time to dream big. He says, do you want to stay there longer? Would you like to do some cartwheels, or do you want to remain paralyzed?

Do you want to dream of something better?

Do you want to let go of what the disappointment has done to you and learn to walk?

The most significant healing Jesus provides to this man is an alternative way for him to think about his future, which involves exiting the pool and getting back into the lane of life!

He doesn't touch the man and heal him. He tells him to get up, start living your life, and make sure you don't die before you live.

How did Jesus heal this man of physical or mental issues? What about both?

What was most paralyzing about this man, lying by a pool for thirty-eight years, was his thought life, his mindset that he needed to leave.

The man had been lying by the pool for thirty-eight years, and when he looked in the mirror, he saw a victim. Seeing yourself as a victim gives no room for the holy trinity of change to work: Love, hope, and faith. When we live as victims, we carry unbelief, which denies the possibility of our situation being changed. We lose hope and believe the lie that we have no more options. Often, part of our healing process involves exiting from the road of a victim mindset.

What kept him for thirty-eight years?

It was wrong thinking and the law of inertia. The law of inertia is often present in our lives: An object at rest tends to remain at rest until acted upon by an outside force.

Jesus was the outside force for this man, asking him to consider exiting his current coping strategies and trying another one.

When the man first answers Jesus, he doesn't say, of course, I want to be healed. Or duh. It would be like greeting you in the hospital and saying: "What should I pray for today? More time in the hospital, or do you want to be healed?"

(By the way, there is one good thing about hospital food: if you happen to be in the hospital and reading this, they bring you food. Take heart and have hope. They only bring a tray to folks they think will make it.)

The man says, "I am not quick enough to be the first in the pool when the water is stirred." Jesus says, "I am not asking if you are fast enough or too slow. I ask if you want to exit the pool of excuses and return to living an abundant life."

Sometimes we need an outside force to escape our inertia. God and others are often that outside force asking you to move, to quit resting. Do you want to get well?

When I was younger, my dad was an outside force! "Don't make me take this belt off."

Did you grow up hearing that? My dad was old school, and my crimes were always way worse than now. John goes to Time Out. Ha. My dad's idea of Time Out was how long it took him to get the belt out. Can anyone remember the sound of a belt coming out of six loops in less than 1.5 seconds? Renee and I were going to be "better in our parenting." We read all the books and attended parenting classes. We didn't spank like what we got growing up. We gave our kids Time Out. Jacob, our firstborn, would be on Time Out, and he enjoyed it. He would sit in the chair, read a book, smile, and laugh. We would have to say, "Okay, son, times-up. You can be miserable in your room now."

Our second son, Zach, not so much. We would put Zach in Time Out and he would excuse himself from it. One time, after he dodged the Time-Out chair, Renee broke down and was violating the no-spank clause, trying to spank his behind, and she was about a bag of Cheetos and a margarita short of one hundred pounds. So she's spanking, and Zach turns and looks at her and says, "You better get Dad. This doesn't even hurt. Ha!"

I remember I came in, physically picked Zach up, put him into the Time-Out chair, and said, "Now, ah, you sit here and think about what you did wrong for ten minutes." I left the room for maybe three minutes. I came back, and he had the chair facing the other way. He was leaning up against the window and kept saying something repeatedly. I got closer to hear what he was saying, and he was looking out the window and saying, "I got to get out of here!"

Have you said that?

He wanted to make an EXIT. I can't blame him.

Do you want to experience a resurrection in your life? Do you want to see yourself change? Are you willing to pay the price to achieve it? You have a role here; it's not all on God. I know, I know, we all want a shortcut. We all want instant healing pools of water to jump into and, poof, instant change.

Keep looking for that, and you will look for it for a long time.

James A. Garfield, before serving as president of the United States, was president of Hiram College in Ohio. One day, a father asked Garfield if there was a shortcut whereby his son could get through college in less than the usual four years. He wanted his son to get on with making money. Don't we all want the shortcut, the microwave fix in life? We think God is at the drive-through and always at the sit-down meal. God rolls with a slow cooker, and so does any lasting change in your life.

The college president replied, "Of course, there is a way; it all depends on what you want your boy to do. When God wants to grow an oak tree, he takes one hundred years. When he wants to make a squash, he only takes two months."

What do you want to be, a tree or a squash?

Real growth takes time! To grow is to realize we are products of our past, but we don't have to be prisoners of it!

Now, there are some important principles to follow when exiting pain, which are counterintuitive. Most of us want to exit our pain right away and make it quick, right? We all want to hurry up and get this over with. But again, nothing good comes in a hurry. Most wisdom is obtained from experience, and experience is a moment-by-moment teacher. What if I told you that you want to exit your pain only after you are done learning from your pain? Because after thirty-eight years laying there amid his pain, insight should have come, and wisdom should have been his. All pain can teach us something. We can all assign meaning to our pain, and it should come a little quicker than thirty-eight years if we take the right steps.

Have you ever tried to change a habit or workout program or decided to forgive your spouse and you thought, *Maybe it's not going to be as easy as I thought it was?*

Have you ever felt like you've been stuck for a long time?

When we lived in California, we didn't have a pool. Believe it or not, it got up to 90 degrees there on occasion. So, for fun, Renee and I would set up the sprinkler in the backyard, and Jacob loved to run through it. I did too, and then he swam in the kiddie pool. So, about the third time we did this, we were hanging out on the porch, drying off, and Renee had cut up some watermelon. It was like a scene out of Andy Griffith, right? Wholesome family time, and Renee was standing in the doorway of the sliding glass back door, and Jacob and I were standing there in our swim trunks, and a big bee landed right on Renee's naked foot. She jumped and flicked it impulsively, and the bee flew through the air and landed on Jacob's stomach.

I was wondering how that happened. She didn't even play soccer! And, of course, now the bee was all upset and stung Jacob, and he started bawling. He was four, crying and saying, "Mommy flicked the stinging bee on me." I was there on the couch, you know, with Benadryl because he's having an allergic reaction, and I am saying, "Yes, I am sorry, son. Your loving dad would never flick a bee on you." Of course, we took Jacob to the country club pool four years later and he was like, "Oh, no. I did the swimming pool thing once and got stung by a bee, Dad. If you look closely at my stomach, there's the scar." Now, there was no scar on the outside, but there was a scar on the inside, and it's the scars you can't see that are the hardest to heal! He had let trauma become his template when it came to swimming. I was like, "When was this?" and he was like, "Years ago, but I remember it." You could almost feel the bee sting so fresh in his system walking up to the pool. But he was so big. He took a deep breath and said, "It's time to conquer this fear. You know, let's go swimming." And as soon as he hit the water, the trauma was gone. He swam. He splashed around like a kid is supposed to. I was so proud of him.

When we finished, I asked Jacob, "Did you get stung?" He said, "I didn't get stung, and no bees landed on Mom's feet!"

And you laugh, but how does this show up in your life? Once stung, twice shy. And you can get this in your system where it's traumatic, right? The odds of ever getting stung by a bee again are that you would have to run through the sprinkler system for the next one hundred summers to see a bee land on Mom's feet. We can spend a lifetime trying to forget a few terrible childhood moments!

We know it's irrational, and we have these fears.

And yet, when are the traumatic things that we go through that get lodged into our memory response and our olfactory system and the smells and all of that ever rational?

But we can get to where we're walking up to swimming pools in life, afraid of the bee sting that will never come.

We can end up carrying in our system the trauma from the traumatic that we now feel is going to happen, however unfounded that might be. See, there is no time stamp on trauma.

We can get to a place where we will sabotage ourselves, hurting ourselves before someone else has the chance to do so, ruining our chances at a healthy relationship, and even potentially ending up in a dating relationship with someone we know is not good for us; they are toxic.

But we don't think we deserve any better; remaining in a job or a season of life that we've outgrown, fearing that something painful would be repeated, lashing out and hurting other people before they have a chance to hurt us, running the moment someone gets close, armoring up to protect ourselves because of something someone else did that's no longer even in our life anymore.

I was on Zoom this week with my counselor. I have a life coach. Every pastor needs a pastor friend, and I was on a group counseling Zoom call for grief. And the counselor in the little Zoom square says, "Pastor John, would you talk about how you moved through grief when your mom passed and went home to be with Jesus? What does grief feel like? What does grief smell like?" And I started to feel a little triggered. Do you want to talk about triggers? Every time I hear Christmas music, I have a bit of a trigger because I grew up listening to my mom play the organ and piano, and every time I heard these songs, it was Mom playing them. Then you hear those Christmas songs in the CVS, and every time I pray with my kids, I remember my mom praying with me every night until I was sixteen. At sixteen, I finally said, "I got this, Mom." Oh, and how about Christmas? It's the most wonderful time of the year. But it brings back to me all those memories. And you have examples of that everywhere. Renee had a very similar experience because she lost her mom five days after I did.

We lost the two women in our lives who gave us our faith. Our boys lost both their grandmas in one week. Then the pastor on Zoom said, "What did you do? How did you do that when it was so hard?" I told her we kept telling ourselves that we needed to lean into, not away from, our grief. We need to run toward the pain and the grief. The pain and grief make us feel afraid of Christmas, making us feel fearful of Christmas music and praying with our kids. It can make us feel afraid of whatever we associate this traumatizing experience with. But I will not run away from things that scare me. We're going to run toward the pain and the grief, and if it kills us, so be it. At least we don't have to live terrified anymore.

So, we will embrace it even if it's hard or scary. And we cried. Renee and I cried together right into our cereal the following day. I remember Raisin Bran, milk, and lots of tears. We didn't eat, but we cried. And Christmas, the first Christmas after my mom was in heaven, I cried every time Renee played a hymn. I cried all through "Silent Night" the first two years after my mom died. And decorating the tree and the house; my mom was there because my mom gave me an ornament for every year I have been alive. We could have thought that decorations, all of that, were too much. We put twice as many decorations, ornaments, and lights in our house and on the tree! And then the pastor said, "What was your conclusion?" I said, "I didn't want my trauma to become my template."

Friends, I wrote this book to tell you: **Don't let your trauma become your template.**

Because for me and my house, we will be people of hope, not hurts.

Healing, like happiness, is an inside job! Our trauma wasn't our template. God's love is our template.

Let's not get paralyzed and lay in our trauma for thirty-eight years. If God's love and truth are our template, then the bee sting doesn't get to keep us from the swimming pools of life. I refuse to wear a beekeeper costume every time I go for a swim out of fear of something that might never happen. And you don't need to either.

We can choose not to walk in dysfunction! We can walk, fearing disappointment that even if it does come, God will get us through if we keep walking with him. When the caterpillar thought the world was ending, he became a butterfly. What the caterpillar calls the end, the world calls a butterfly. Oh, come on.

Consider your ways. Take a moment and reorient yourself away from the trauma, the difficult, the pain, the loss, and the oh, I can't do that.

My anxiety would flare.

I can't go over here. That would trigger me. God wired us for life and love. Trauma rewires us, but we must return the wires to God and let him fix us.

Come on, let's trust God. Let's make His word, salvation, and healing the center of our lives. Trauma creates change you don't choose. Healing is about letting God's love change you!

Let your hopes, not your hurts, shape your future. Let your hopes, not your hurts, be your template!

You can see this in the life of people God calls. God calls Moses, right? Moses went through some trauma early on. Think about the family he was born into. He was born into a family where the safest thing your parents can do is to put you in a crocodile-infested river, where you get raised thinking your grandfather is the man who wanted to kill you, but your nanny is your mom. It sounds like a costly therapy bill to me. Moses. Moses. What does that mean? Moses means "drawn out." How did Moses have such a sense of strength? Because his name came from what he was rescued from, not what he was put into.

We've got to stop having our identity come from all the hard things we were put into and start taking our identity from what we were called out from. What trauma has the world put you in, and how has God called you out from that? It's funny that the word *church* means *ecclesia* or *called out ones*. We've been called out of the world. I don't cry or feel sad when I hear Christmas music because it's over. I smile because it happened. After all, God gave me a mom who taught me these Christmas songs, lived these Church songs, and believed these songs. I have her blood inside of me. I have her faith inside of me. What a gift.

Healing doesn't mean the pain never existed. It means the damage no longer controls our lives. Consider this: You didn't choose abandonment. It happened to you. You didn't choose trauma. It happened to you. You didn't decide to get stung by a bee. It happened to you. It can feel like everything has been taken away, but that's not true. You have the choice to let trauma be your template, or you have the option to allow God's love to be your template!

Let your hopes, not your hurts, shape your future. Let your hopes, not your hurts, be your template!

I was doing a counseling session this week with a young man who's been through some trauma, some pain, some hardship in his life. He told me of a painful childhood experience he endured. This guy, let's call him Gary, had a father who was a heavy drinker. Even as a child, his mother often turned to Gary to sympathize with her and help her in her struggles with his father. One night, Gary's father had been drinking and decided he wanted to go for a drive. Gary's mother refused to give him the keys. Instead, she took the car keys upstairs and handed them to Gary, the child, telling him to keep these keys away from his father. Gary clenched one little fist around those keys and thrust his fist under his pillow. Then he pulled the covers over his head. A minute later, his father came into the room, drunk and begging for his keys. Imagine the sadness of this scene: A father sitting on the edge of a bed begging his little son for his car keys. Tell me where the keys are, Gary.

Then, Mom came into the room and ridiculed her husband for being drunk, begging for keys. This sounds like a lot of therapy, and Dr. Phil to me! He's telling me this in my office, and it's just a flood of tears. You can spend a lifetime trying to overcome a few terrible moments in your childhood. He tells me that sometimes, when he sees car keys that look a certain way, or when he sees drunk people, or when he considers his drinking problems from the past, he gets triggered. Then he says something like this, and I will never forget it. He says, "Pastor, some memories are bullets, some whiz by you and spook you, and others tear you open and leave you in pieces."

We just sat silently for about ten minutes, tears, silence, pain. Then I told him—because trust me, this guy has been enrolled in the University of Pain and Hardship; they have been his distinguished professors. I tell him, "You have had a lot of pain in your life, and it wasn't all your fault, but you have been a good steward of your pain!" He's like, what? Steward of my pain? I don't want pain. I said, yes, I know that's why you drank for a long time. You drank to forget. I told him what I would say to you: Steward your pain. Don't release your pain until it has taught you what you need to know. Do you know you can manage, share, and develop your pain today so that it can help others tomorrow? Now, Gary's been attending AA meetings not just to keep himself sober but to share the wisdom he got from his pain. Trust me, those 12-step meetings are nothing more than people who are sharing the pain of their addictions, what that pain has taught them, and how God has redeemed that pain. The same is true with a good sermon! Don't throw away the lessons you can learn from your pain—steward your pain. Every effective priest, every effective pastor, every effective counselor, every effective Christian is nothing more than a wounded healer.

If we can let God heal and steward our pain, every one of us can become a healer!

What is an effective pastor?

These are the wounded healers of the world, and healers who have fully faced their wounds are the only ones who heal anyone else.

There are secret riches you only discover in dark places. David wrote most of the psalms in caves, on the run for his life. This proves that some of the richest treasures you will ever find are in the darkness of your life when you steward your pain.

Why do you think the best leaders of AA are people in recovery? Why is it that the best Christians are the ones who have had great brokenness?

No one leaves this earth without wounds, scars, or pain. Stay where the pain is. Wait, stay right there. Stay where the suffering is, where the struggle is. Stay there. That's where it's going to come—the insight, the knowing, the wisdom.

If you have chest pains, you should listen to them and get to the ER. If you have heart pains, you should listen to that, get with God, and ask God to help you make sense of what's going on here! Don't bury your pain; ignore your pain, drink away your pain, sex away your pain, and work away your pain. Embrace your pain because the pain is there and has something to teach us.

Studies show you grow the most in painful, not pleasureful times. But no one ever says, "God send me some pain." Strength is built, not born, and it's usually built through pain. We are healed of suffering only by experiencing it to the fullest! We find ourselves in an exceptional liminal space when we can hold our pain consciously and trustfully and not project it elsewhere.

I'm telling you, you are going through it. You look down at your wheelchair. You look down at your shaking limbs. You look down at your withered body. You look down at your depleted bank account. You look down at your empty home because you don't have a spouse, and you go, oh my gosh, it's so terrible. But I got out of bed this morning to say to you: God is going to remind you of the sadness and the sorrow, the loneliness and the fear, the crippling thoughts of sadness; these things are not yours forever. God is saying: What I'm going to do amid your pain, what I'm going to work amid your pain, that's yours forever: Wisdom, strength, grace, character, and integrity. You do get to keep these things forever. There are treasures in darkness, not just your fears!

I told Gary, and I will tell you, the value of what you have in your hands, pain, might not be visible, but don't let it go. Steward it. What if what you held that seemed worthless made you almost feel like you would walk out on trusting God? What if you look back upon it one day as if you were handed a rare treasure?

Pain (here's some good news) has a problem. Pain has a problem. Like the short shelf life of your body, hear me if you're in Christ, *pain is not forever.*

One of my favorite verses when I am dealing with pain is, "This too shall pass!"

When I preach this in church, I get a few raised eyebrows, but not many amens. I wish I had a church that said Amen, who was excited about the fact that pain is not forever.

Because as I read Revelation, you know that John of Patmos, after being boiled in a pot, wrote about eternity, our next life, and heaven.

I read this whole thing about Jesus wiping every tear from our eyes: there is no more darkness, no more pain or hardship, the sun never sets in heaven, and the gates of heaven are never shut. There is no death, no disease, no decay, no sin, no separation, no sorrow, no cancer, no statin drugs or antidepressants, no car accidents, no strokes, no dementia, no Alzheimer's, no asthma inhalers, no global warming, or forest fires.

There will be only righteousness, eternal life, abundant life, joy to the full, drinking from the rivers of pleasure. Come on.

We will be with Christ, like Christ, in a new body and world.

Don't let pain get into your identity.

I am just a wounded bird. I live hurt and cynical all the time because my past, my parents, or some dead people still affect how I live today. So, I project my hurt, pain, and cynicism on others. It's just who I am. Don't say, "This pain is who I am." Don't let trauma and pain become your template. Let your hopes, not your hurts, become your template for life!

Look what God did with Jesus's pain! We know very little about Jesus's resurrected body except that he still has the scars from the cross. There's a treasure in the scars of Jesus's hands! Every scar has a story. Jesus's scars are a story of love for you and me. Jesus's scars are reminders to anyone who ever doubted God's love for you! What was meant as signs of horror and pain, God teaches us, are signs of love. Come on, there are treasures in Jesus's pain, the treasures of his love for us. That's why he bears them in heaven today!

Do you want a Christmas example of pain and the transformation of pain into growth? Here it is:

God plans to find a willing soul, a young girl who's 13, a virgin, and she will have the son of God. If God wants to bring a baby into the world, of course, He's going to look for a virgin because otherwise it doesn't make sense. His ways are not our ways.

No one chooses pain.

Gabriel unpacks the plan. Mary's response: That doesn't add up. I am still a virgin, But I'm in.

That's what you need to get good at saying if you follow God and watch Him work in your life. Because a lot of us say, "That doesn't make sense. I'm out." But if we could pivot and say, "I don't understand it cerebrally, but tell you what, spiritually, I'm in. I'm down. I'm yours."

It's not great gifts that God is looking for. It's great that you're willing to be a part of Him working through you.

What Mary said to God more than anything, is *I am yours; let it be.* Let it be, as the Beatles sang. For the first time this week, I studied what it meant when the Bible says, "Mary treasured up all these things and pondered them in her heart" (Luke 2:19, NIV). What does that mean?

Let's think about Mary and her pain first. She's 13, has no money, is from a town with no name, and she's unmarried. Her community disgraces her for being an unmarried pregnant teenage virgin. She has to convince her future groom that she's pregnant by God above, not some other guy. She's traveling on foot at nine months pregnant for a first-ever nationwide census beyond her control. She's having to labor and give birth in a barn cave surrounded by barn animals. Finally, she has to host strange and unexpected visitors right after giving birth! Yeah, you're worried about having a terrible Christmas. Let's think about the first painful Christmas because that's what this was. She is also homeless, and she must travel to Egypt right after having the baby. Let's not forget a prophet told Mary, yes, you will have this baby, but a sword will pierce your heart because he's going to be born only to die a horrible death on the cross. Pain. Her response to all this pain was that Mary *treasured* all these things and pondered them in her heart (Luke 2:19, NIV).

I did some studying this week, brushing up on my Greek, and here's what I found. The word *treasured* in Luke 2:19 (NIV) means "to preserve knowledge or memories for later use." Have you ever used a memory of a loved one after they are gone?

You've got to frame your pain!

Did Joseph and Mary not have pain by saying yes to God's call on their life? We know Joseph faced shame and persecution and struggled to find work. Yet they stayed married. And how did Mary handle all this? She framed her pain.

Have you ever taken a picture of a holy moment?

The moment the shepherds left, Mary took a snapshot. Pain will change you, but you don't have to let it define you. Only *God* defines you! Frame your pain. Mary framed her heart with faith, awe, and a spirit of adventure and risk. And she chose to make the memories that spoke of God's goodness. She chose to ponder these things in her heart. The memory of this moment would give her faith as she stood looking up at the cross, seeing her son's arms spread wide.

Everyone loves that song, "Mary Did You Know?" Mary, did you know your baby boy would one day walk on water? Did you know your baby boy would save our sons and daughters? Did you know that your baby boy has come to make you new? This child that you delivered will soon deliver you! Can we quit singing this song?

Yes, she knew. The Bible says so in the first chapter of Luke! She pondered what the shepherds told her, what Gabriel told her, what God told her, and it was this knowledge, this framing, that gave her strength thirty-three years later when Jesus took our pain on the cross.

Frame your pain to transform your pain, or you will transmit your pain.

Invite God to help your wounds become sacred so you might become a wounded healer. If we do not transform our pain into something selfless, something that honors Jesus's sacrifice, then we will only transmit our pain. We will transmit it, usually, to those closest to us—our spouse, family, neighbors, church members, everyone!

Do you ever go to the gym? What's that pain? I wouldn't say I like Miss Elliptical. She's a wench. But my body takes that painful forty-five minutes and turns it into a healthy heart and fat loss. Assign meaning to your pain, framing it so you are letting God transform it into wisdom. Transform the pain of divorce into learned lessons that serve making better choices next time, or you will pass this pain on to the next spouse and have chosen no more wisely than the last time.

Transform the pain in your marriage to being a better spouse. Do the dishes. Quit being a jerk. Greet your spouse whenever you walk in the door like your dog does for you. Jump on her, kiss her, and let her know you missed her. We all know hurt people who don't transform their pain. They lash out. What do we say when we see someone going after someone in an unhinged way? They are hurt. They are just mad.

Most people are like electric wires, what comes in is what goes out. Someone calls us a name, and we call them a name back. Most people pass on the same energy that is given to them. Now compare an electric wire to those big, green transformers that you see. Dangerous current or voltage comes in, but something happens inside that green box, and what comes out is, in fact, now helpful and productive. That is precisely what Jesus did with pain: He did not return the negative energy directed at him. He held it inside and made it into something much better. That is how "he took away the sins of the world." He refused to pass it on!

Most of us can bear lots of pain if we frame our pain if it has meaning!

Pregnancy, childbirth, from what I saw with Renee, lots of pain. But it's transformed into a healthy child! Surgery has pain, but it's transformed into healing. Telling someone you drink too much and that you're a jerk all the time can be painful. But they can convert that into sobriety and personal growth.

You get to choose what goes in your frame.

I have a frame here with my mom in it, and it has times we did ministry together—weddings, times with my sons, and times when she was encouraging me in the faith! Is there pain sometimes when I look at this? Yes, she's gone on to heaven. But I have these pictures here because it's a memory of her telling me to preach the word. So today, as I preach, I remember what I ponder in my heart, that my mom is with Jesus!

As I think about 1,610 days since she died, I also think I am 1,610 days from being closer to her. I get to choose what goes in the frame. I'm not framing and holding up, just pain, difficulty, and darkness. I'm saying God was there. He was with me. And you can choose to do this. Don't let your pain get into your story of how you view the world. What is it with this bad thing that happens to you, and what do people say, "Oh, pastor, it's the story of my life?" It can't be—if your life is more than just your life on this earth.

Because it was my mom who taught me to sing: When we've been there ten thousand years, Bright shining as the sun, we've no fewer days to sing God's praise Than when we'd first begun. What about 10,000 years from now? How can something that measures only a blip on the Richter scale of our grand scheme of eternal life be that strong?

It's why it's so powerful that Paul said my citizenship is in heaven. You're not just a citizen here. Do you find your worth and value in this world? Paul said these trials are not even worth compared to the glory that shall be revealed in us. Paul said trials are just small potatoes when considering the joys, unbridled beauty, and bliss of paradise, being with Jesus. Paul said in Philippians it's far better to depart and be with Christ. The best description of heaven I can find in the scriptures are these two words: far better.

What is coming is better than what is gone.

Paul got to go there one time. He got to go there just for the day. His life was weird. A snake in Malta bit him, and he got to go to heaven once. Many people think it was when he was stoned…with rocks. I've got to clarify. It's 2023. You're like, "Wow, Paul did that?" He was high on the most high only. And he got to go to heaven. And then God was like, "Sorry, you've got to go back to earth." And he was all bummed about it, emotional. He was like, "I would rather be in heaven because it's far better having seen it. And yet, I'm willing to come back to this world, be here on purpose, and be on a mission. But my life's not here. My heart, my citizenship, my thoughts are in heaven. Only my feet are presently here. While my feet are here, I will do as much for the Kingdom of God as I possibly can. But I'm not going to be defined by this world. I'm going to enjoy its blessings. I will be as happy as the next person with a good meal, a great trip, and a scenic view out of a hot air balloon. But that's not going to fill any emptiness in me. Only Jesus can do that. And I get to be his son and his daughter."

Most of what we think will make our life better, won't.

Would you rather win the lottery tomorrow or get cancer?

Someone just in my life, literally two weeks ago, told me I would start playing the lottery because my life would get so much better if I just won a big payout. So, I'm going to set aside a little. And because it's natural for us all to think winning the lottery would be a jackpot, cha-ching. Everything's better. And if you do, remember, my church friends, 10 percent, please!

Most of us, all of us, would say that cancer would be the worst thing I could get.

Yet I was reading an article by Arthur Brooks, who pointed out that psychologists have repeatedly, conclusively determined that winning the lottery brings no lasting satisfaction and almost always brings unbridled misery to the recipient. He found researchers have consistently pointed out that survivors of illness and loss experience what they describe afterward as *post-traumatic growth.*

We are a culture obsessed with post-traumatic stress. How about post-traumatic growth? It was hard, but I grew. It was hard, but then I trusted. It was hard, but then I grew.

He said explicitly that those who had to deal with cancer and survived on the back-end report higher levels of happiness than demographically matched people who never had to have cancer. So, what we think will bring us joy brings us misery. What we believe will be the worst thing causes us to walk away grateful!

Why?

When people survive cancer, live through an accident and pain, or focus on the brevity of their lives, this causes them to appreciate what they have previously taken for granted.

This perspective prompts us to appreciate every sunset, every smile, and every aspect of life we may have previously overlooked. It is a truth that individuals experience the most profound growth during challenging periods in the face of trauma, grief, and whatever other adversities life presents. However, it is rare for someone to seek out difficult times or actively pray for trials. We do not choose hard times; instead, they choose us. Despite this lack of choice when facing adversity, we have the agency to determine growth during challenging circumstances. Rather than merely complaining about our pain, we can undertake meaningful actions that contributing to our personal development.

Steward your pain. Stay where your pain is. Pain is not forever. Don't transmit your pain. Frame your pain, give your pain to God, and let him transform your pain and you!

CHAPTER SEVEN

YOU ARE ONE FRIEND AWAY FROM CHANGING YOUR DESTINY

True friends stab you in the front.

—Oscar Wilde

I CONTEMPLATED THE FUTURE AT TWENTY-ONE, on the brink of graduating with a psychology degree. My father humorously remarked, "You can always say, 'Tell me about your mother,' as you hand them their fries,"—a playful jab at the prospect of me working at Burger King. While I chuckled at his wit, I realized that pursuing a master's degree was essential for meaningful career prospects in psychology.

Faced with this decision, I narrowed my options down to two paths: the first involved obtaining a PhD in Psychology, which would allow me to charge $300 per hour to listen to people's problems. The second path involved obtaining an 86-hour Master of Divinity degree, allowing me to delve into pastoral care. In this realm, I could listen to people's problems for free, relying on the generosity of church members. The latter meant potentially making less money, but it was uniquely appealing.

Choosing the less conventional route, I embarked on the journey. It almost didn't happen, but as a pastor, I can't help but share that I prayed about it. It's a cliché, but what else does a pastor write? But it was more of a deal-maker prayer when I prayed about it. Have you ever prayed that kind of prayer: "Oh God, if you will just get me out of this mess, I promise you I will become a monk or at least go to church once a month!" My prayer went like this, "God, whatever door you open the widest, I will go through, so if it's PhD and Psychology or Ministry, you have to open the door."

I applied to two schools and got partial scholarships to both, with the leading candidate being a PhD program at St. Mary's University in San Antonio. When it looked like Freud would win, my friend, Rev. Bill Henderson, who was also my pastor when I attended his college ministry in San Marcos, told me, "Let's take a trip to SMU," where he was an alumnus. This guy worked full time and had a busy schedule but took two days off to drive me in his vehicle, on his dime, from San Marcos, Texas, hours up the road to Dallas, Texas, paying for all the hotel, meals, and gas. We toured the campus, and I met with Rev. Dr. Harry Wright, Director of Admissions for SMU, Perkins School of Theology. I walked alone into Dr. Wright's office, and we had a nice chit-chat about how good my grades were in undergraduate and how they would love to have me attend SMU. Honestly, I was their idea of diversity.

See, SMU was nothing but rich white kids, and they were not ready for compelling diversity, but a poor white kid, well, there you go! They were so willing in their quest for qualified poor white guys that they offered a partial $6,000 scholarship. How nice. Problem: SMU runs about $55,000 a year.

I walked out into that lobby where my friend Rev. Bill Henderson had waited for me, and he said, "Well, are you going to Seminary? Are you going to be a preacher?"

I said, "I don't think so, Bill. SMU is expensive, and I can't graduate with $250,000 in debt. It looks like I am heading to get my PhD. That's the direction God is leading me."

He told me to sit in the lobby and went into Rev. Harry Wright's office for twenty minutes. I could have sworn I heard some swearing, but who knows when two preachers are in the same room! Then he came out of the office and told me to return to Rev. Wright's office to meet with him again. He said, "Let's pretend the first meeting didn't happen."

Huh? I walked back into Rev. Wright's office, shut the door, and he stood up and said these eternally life-changing words: "Congratulations, John, you are the next *Presidential Scholar.* You will be given a full academic ride if you maintain an eighty-five average. We will get you a job as hall director, which comes with an apartment and meal plan, and you will graduate with no debt from Southern Methodist University!"

Now, how did I go from partial, in debt the rest of my life, to red carpet rolling out Presidential Scholar with full academic ride, job, and a meal plan? I had a friend who changed my destiny, which means you are only one friend away from changing yours! The door had swung so far open that the hinges came off.

I walked out of the office with a stunned look and asked Bill, "What did you say to Rev. Wright?" No response, just congratulations! Thirty-four years later, I still don't know the content of that conversation between Bill and Rev. Wright, *but I know that a friend changed my life.* A friend who cared enough to take two days of his life to go and "testify" on my behalf that I would be worth the investment. It's probably the biggest compliment I have ever received from a friend. When people invest their time, talents, and love to make you a better person, to give you a better future, that's a friend. Not only that, but SMU also gave me a $1,500 scholarship in the form of a check to buy my first year's theology books. Let me tell you a secret. I never bought any books. I went down to Jared's and purchased an engagement ring with the best cut, color, and clarity a man could buy for $1,500 in 1993 and borrowed my first year's set of books from some rich white kid! On my wife's hand, that ring is much more valuable than any book from thirty-four years ago! Let's see, education and a wife are all due to a good friend.

A friend recognizes that the greatest enemy of your future success is your current success.

When you're perpetually afraid to risk what is for the sake of what might be, you might as well cue the funeral music now.

My friend convinced me to risk everything I was to become what I could be, but it took an investment on his part. Without that friend, I would not be writing this book today. You can see how one friend changes another's destiny in people in Scripture. In Acts 9:26 (NKJV), we learn that the whole trajectory of the Apostle Paul's life was changed by one friendship. It says, "And when Saul had come to Jerusalem, he tried to join the disciples, but they were all afraid of him, and did not believe that he was a disciple." You see, before Paul was the Apostle Paul, he was Saul, known as the chief persecutor of Christians. He not only persecuted Christians but he killed them. So now he's a Christian and he's like, "Hey, I want to preach," and all the Christians are like, "I don't trust you. Last week you were killing us. I don't want you to come to my small group!"

Then Acts 9:27 (NIV) says, "But Barnabas took him and brought him to the apostles." Barnabas, his friend, brought him to the apostles! Barnabas put his credibility on the line to vouch for Saul. Barnabas had a conversation with the director of admissions, and suddenly, Paul is the Presidential Scholar for preaching! Barnabas told them how Saul had seen the Lord and that the Lord had spoken to him and how, in Damascus, he had preached fearlessly in the name of Jesus. The Bible says Saul stayed with them and moved about freely in Jerusalem. What happened?

Don't miss it. God used one person, Barnabas, to change the course of Paul's destiny. Now, Paul wrote over half of our New Testament and impacted millions and millions and millions of people. The course of history was changed because God used one friend to change the course of one man's destiny.

And the same thing could happen for every single one of you! A friend is someone in your life who says, "I will do what I can to bring out the best in you!" You cannot discover yourself alone—you need others to help you!

True story. In Paraguay's impoverished South American country, there is a slum called Cateura outside the capital of Asuncion. This poorest shanty town is built on a landfill where the city's 1,500 tons of garbage and waste is dumped each day. Despite the filth and stench and the contamination it breeds, about 2,500 families live in Cateura, making their only hand-to-mouth living by sifting through the trash and selling anything recyclable. Twenty-four hours a day, people are going through the most feeble of waste of others, cashing in on ten cents for a pound of plastic and five cents for a pound of cardboard. The children are all barefoot and don't go to school, can't read or write, have no medical care, and are forced to sift through the trash from a young age just like their mothers and fathers. There is no hope for escape to a better life in the landfill community. Joining a gang, becoming a criminal, or becoming a drug addict are usually the only other options. They don't have time to read books called *It Doesn't Have to Be This Way* because their lives certainly feel like it *has* to be this way. The inhabitants don't usually have electricity or plumbing, and their drinking water is dangerously polluted. That was the only life they knew in Cateura…until one person said, "Wait, who is my Lazarus?"

Remember when Lazarus came out of the grave after four days and was all mummified and bound up? What did Jesus tell his friends? You unbind him, you unwind him, you unwrap him. Lazarus had to smell, you know, like people living in a trash dump.

Do you know what it's like to live among the tombs? Some people don't want to come out. They like the tombs. It's safe and secure. There are no surprises in this lifestyle. We all have attachments to tombs. There are two steps to sanctification. Once Jesus tells Lazarus to come out, he turns to his disciples and says, "Unwrap him."

There is a division of labor in sanctification. God's power alone can bring the dead to life and save sinners, but it is up to us to untie those bound by sin, to free those chained to addictions, and to heal the ravages of absence and death. God frees us from the grave. But we have *got* to take the grave clothes off of each other! This is what real friends do. They help unbind us. They open up doors for us. They talk to the director of admissions. They help us to a better future! This is where the church comes in. This is where the twelve-step programs come in. This is where real friendships come in. God releases us from being wrapped up. Perhaps one of the most sacred roles of a true friend is that we get to take the wraps off of others, the character defects. We get to be honest, true friends and stab someone in the front, as Oscar Wilde says, not stab them in the back. A true friend tells you when your fly is down and also when your character sucks, but they do it in an un-binding manner. A true friend helps people get unwound and unbound. God gives us breath. We provide each other with mobility. "I'll lose him from death," Jesus said. "You loosen him for living!"

So, how tightly wound are you? What are you too wrapped up in? What's binding and confining you? What's hamstringing your hands for ministry? What are you so wrapped up in that you can't come out and be all God calls you to be? Maybe you need a friend?

When environmental technician Favio Chavez visited the landfill community years back, God told him *it doesn't have to be this way*. He had an idea for a music school to help lift the children out of their wretched conditions. He quickly realized that buying new instruments or using used ones was not an option. "A violin is worth more than a house here," said Chavez. So, instead of generating instruments for the music school, he turned to a resource they did have in abundance, which was trash. Why not make the instruments out of all the recycled materials and garbage? So, he turned to another friend, local trash worker and carpenter Don Colá Gomez, for help, asking him to make a violin. Though Gomez had never seen one, they started going to the dump together three days a week as friends to scour for things they could use to construct their patchwork instruments: oven trays, oil cans, recycled string, drainpipes, bottle caps, forks, metal scraps, and salvaged pieces of wood. They brought everything back to a cramped workshop at the dump's edge, where they went to work. Soon, Gomez produced three violins weekly and taught himself to make cellos and guitars, trumpets and saxophones, and drums and basses.

The instruments were given to the children during free music classes; thus, the Recycled Orchestra was born. The availability of instruments and the new presence of music in their lives inspired the children and reinvigorated the community like no one could have imagined. Finally, someone saw the invisible people and the divine mud that they were! Most parents in the landfill community had never heard their children play, so they set up a concert at the local church, with banners in the street and regional radio stations advertising it. The concert was packed with humble parents, swelling with pride and hopes for a better life, rising with each musical note. The children kept playing and became quite adept. Favio Chavez began music school and said, "Having nothing is not an excuse for doing nothing." Sounds like the words of an amazing friend. The amazing story of a children's orchestra from the poorest places, playing with instruments repurposed from trash, spread like wildfire and soon they were invited to play in the main city, then to other countries in South America, and now all over the world. "People realize that we shouldn't throw away trash carelessly," said a young man nicknamed Bebi as he plays the Prelude to Bach's Cello Suite No. 1 on an oil can cello. "Well, we shouldn't throw away people either." There's a movie called *The Landfill Harmonic: An Orchestra Built from Trash!* and a children's book, *Building an Orchestra of Hope.*[28]

Today's friendships determine tomorrow's destiny. What you do today for a friend or a friend does for you can echo into eternity!

Just think about the most amazing and blessed moments in your life. What did they always involve? Did they affect other people or friends? When I think about the most amazing moments in my life, I always include others—friends, my spouse, my kids, and my parents—my best days, graduating from college with my friends, getting married and having my groomsmen there, the day my boys were born and my best friends celebrating those moments, picking a destiny changing career moment and having Bill there, celebrating my parents' fifty-fifth wedding anniversary on a cruise. I can see the faces of my friends, smiling, laughing, and encouraging me all along the way. Even in the most challenging moments, I can see my friends being there saying, "Me Too!"

---

28 Tsioulcas, A. (2016, September 14). *From trash to triumph: The recycled orchestra.* NPR. https://www.npr.org/sections/deceptivecadence/2016/09/14/493794763/from-trash-to-triumph-the-recycled-orchestra

"You are going to get through this!" "I am here for you!" "I have your back!" "I will do what I can do!" "How can I help you?" These moments with my friends and others have been my life's best moments!

As I think back and scan through the inventory of the pits of my life, the moments that were the most anxious, the moments that were the most fearful, the moments where I felt like the despair was going to swallow me alive, I realized I was always alone in those times; alone because I had chosen to self-isolate, or alone because I had the wrong people surrounding me in my life at that time. I was alone because I didn't share what was on my heart and how I struggled in that season. You can be surrounded by people and still be very alone. How would you define loneliness? The best definition I have ever read was this: *manmade misery*. God made us for community and wired us for relationships. Often, trauma rewires us for isolation and protecting our hearts and ourselves. God made us to be in relationships. The first time God says in the Bible that it's not good is when he sees Adam alone.

God immediately gives Adam and Eve a helper, friend, and companion with whom to walk through life. Loneliness is manmade misery. When I talk to my Roman Catholic Priests, who are friends, they often tell me about the crushing loneliness they live under because they can't have a lifelong companion to give their hearts to. It's also more challenging to make real friends as you get older. Why? We are so busy paying for life that we fail to make time for those who bring us life. Have we all turned into Kevin McCallister from *Home Alone*? We have Alexa and Siri to keep us company, and we've shut the garage door before we're out of the car!

We are now backyard people, not front-yard people, as our cultures used to be.

We order our food via DoorDash, talk to others through the safety of the apps on our digital leashes, and shop alone on Amazon! We text instead of talk, email, Zoom, or face-to-face meetings. We are reticent to leave the great indoors! As of this writing, it's been raining for five days in Corpus Christi. That's very unusual. I hate getting out in the rain—I might bump into a friend. But then I get hungry. I'm going to DoorDash. I'm not going to a restaurant. I will only proceed from my *lair* when I see on my ring camera that they are gone. I might wave at them as they drive off, but that is as much social contact as I'm getting today, people. How crazy that that kind of life is possible? We can work from home with Zoom. My son currently works at home without putting on a pair of pants. He's "zoomed" for work, meaning you are professionally dressed from the waist up. We are all swimming around with our VR goggles on, giving us the idea that this is real. This is real life.

We have begun to see friendships as optional, not essential to our souls and physical well-being. Then we wonder, *Why am I so lonely?* In September 2023, the US Surgeon General reported that misery now affects more than half of American adults. Fifty-eight percent of American adults are now considered lonely. And younger Americans are almost twice as likely to be lonely as those over sixty-five. Seventy-nine percent of people between the ages of eighteen and twenty-four are lonely, disconnected, and suffering in silence! Almost 80 percent of young adults have their whole lives in front of them, and their future is so bright that they should need sunglasses, as Corey Hart once sang. They are connected digitally to more people than anyone has ever been linked to in the history of humankind, but they are lonely because those connections are hollow. Why does life feel so hollow if this is how life should go?

Men have it worse than women. Studies bear witness that men have seen a much sharper decline than women in their close friendships over the past thirty years. A higher percentage of men say they have no close friends at all. Fifteen percent of men say they have no close friends, compared to only 10 percent of women. This is why magazines like the *New Yorker* publish articles titled "Can Pickleball Save America from Loneliness?" Men receive less emotional support from friends than women. They are also less likely to admit loneliness, making it challenging to gauge. And they are much less likely to address their suffering. They would rather soldier on through it alone, the tough, independent Marlboro Man!

"Loneliness crushes the soul but does much more than damage your spirit. Loneliness has been correlated with strokes, heart disease, dementia, inflammation, and suicide. It breaks the heart and the body equally powerfully." Of course, you've heard the anecdotal comparison that helps us understand how big of a crisis this is. The Surgeon General now says that loneliness is about the same as smoking fifteen cigarettes per day or drinking six alcoholic drinks every single day, right?[29] So you have the devastating effects. We all know obesity is a problem. They say that being lonely is worse for your longevity than obesity is. The Alameda County study, headed by Harvard social scientists after studying seven thousand people, concluded that eating Twinkies with friends is better than eating broccoli alone![30]

Toward the end of 2023, the Surgeon General, in collaboration with popular figure Matthew McConaughey, addressed the pressing issue of friendship during an event at the University of Texas. The Surgeon General asserted that we are currently facing a friendship crisis and a friendship recession, highlighting the severity of the situation. This concern stems from the fact that loneliness has reached epidemic proportions in the United States, with more than half of the population grappling with this emotional isolation.

What makes this matter even more critical is that loneliness has unexpectedly become the foremost mental health crisis in America, as stated by the Surgeon General when he

---

29 Murthy, V. H., Our epidemic of loneliness and isolation: The U.S. Surgeon General's advisory on the healing effects of Social Connection and Community (2023). Rockville, Md; U.S. Public Health Service.

30 Housman, J., & Dorman, S. (2005, September). *The Alameda County Study: A systematic, chronological ...* Education Resources Information Center. https://files.eric.ed.gov/fulltext/EJ792845.pdf

assumed the role. The levels of loneliness, anxiety, and depression in the nation have surged to unprecedented highs, and a significant contributing factor is the inclination toward navigating life in isolation. Creating friendships and deeper, more meaningful social connections is crucial in addressing this epidemic! The US Surgeon General said he did not anticipate loneliness to be the number one mental health concern that he would be wrestling with first. Yet, loneliness, anxiety, and depression are at all-time highs, and the primary reason for this is that we are trying to get through life alone. True friendship—the kind that drives to Dallas and spends two days of unhurried time, money, and gas to bless someone else who can never and will never repay that—is in peril, in serious trouble. A true friendship where you help people give up lives of digging through the trash to play around the world in a children-led orchestra is rare air!

How many friends do you have right now? I am not talking about your five thousand digital "so-called Facebook, Instagram, or TikTok friends," but the ones you can call at two a.m. and they will answer and say, "I will do what I can!" There's lots of digital connectedness in our day. Still, perhaps there are fewer personal connections than ever before because there's an illusion of friendship, like a mirage in the desert. There's water, palm trees, and an oasis, but that's untrue. I grew up on fourteen different Air Force Bases, so I learned how to size someone up and determine whether a person was worth the investment of my brief time in each state. But today, it's all about the phone and online. We have become a swipe-right culture.

We're connected digitally to everybody with LinkedIn, Instagram, and TikTokers! Because now I'm connected to you on some level, we must surely be friends. Proverbs 17:17 (FBV) says, "A friend is someone you may or may not know well who accepts your friend request on Facebook. This person is born to like and comment on your posts to make you feel good about yourself." That's a bad joke, by the way. Three thousand, five hundred years ago, it was actually written as, "Keep company with the wise and you will become wise. If you make friends with stupid people, you will be ruined" (Proverbs 13:20, GNT). Today, secular humanists echo God's Word with people like Dan Pena concluding things like, "Show me your friends and I will show you your future." The implications are: "Your friends are your future you." Your mom was right all along—you become like those you hang out with. If you have five friends who smoke, you will be the sixth. If you have five friends who are in shape, you will be the sixth. If you have five friends who drink, you will be the sixth. Did you know that a person's chance of becoming obese increases by 57 percent if a close friend is obese!

Friendship is so weird. It's the family you choose. You pick a human you've met, and you're like, *Yep, I like this one*, and so you do stuff with them.

Ralph Waldo Emerson said, "It is one of the blessings of old friends that you can afford to be stupid with them."[31] I have a good friend, Brek Blair, and I wanted to be stupid

31 *Ralph Waldo Emerson - it is one of the blessings of old...* BrainyQuote. (n.d.-a). https://www.brainyquote.com/quotes/ralph_waldo_emerson_105261

with him and tell him how much I loved him, so I texted him, "I'd walk through fire for you, my best friend. Well, not fire. That would be dangerous. But a super humid room… but not too humid because, you know, my hair…" He called me up, laughed, connected, and we had lunch together.

What can you expect from a real friend? You can expect them to encourage you when you are down. You can expect a warning about going in the wrong direction. True friends help you navigate life. They tell you things like you can do better than this and live better than in a trash dump! True friends mean you should expect wise counsel when you're making decisions. They will connect you with people they know to help you have a better God-given future. With real friends, you can expect support in difficult times. You should expect a common purpose with the people you're doing life with! You should sometimes expect to see God living in them and through them! You should expect someone who knows all about you and loves you anyway! The Bible says in Ecclesiastes 4:10 (NIV), "…But pity anyone who falls and has no one to help him up!" Basically asking: Who's there to catch you when you fall?

Ecclesiastes 4:9–12 in *The Message* puts it best:

"It's better to have a partner than to go it alone. Share the work, share the wealth. And if one falls down, the other helps. But if there's no one to help, tough!

Two in bed warm each other. Alone, you shiver all night.

By yourself you're unprotected. With a friend you can face the worst. Can you round up a third? A three-stranded rope isn't easily snapped."

It turns out friendships are more than just the spice of life. It's not just this luxury thing. It's necessary for your mental health; it's like food for the soul.

What can you expect from a good friend? The use of their mouth!

I remember going on a fishing trip with two close friends and one guy who taught me about friendships. It looked like rain and thunderstorms as we were getting into the boat. I was spooked and ready to head to Lake HEB for my fish. As I got into the boat, I said, "I'm afraid we're not going to catch anything today." One of the old fishermen, not a friend, started cussing me and saying, "Don't put a bad mouth on this fishing trip." I'd never heard that term used that way…bad-mouth on a trip? Bad-mouthing? *Bad-mouth* means to talk badly about someone or something, to criticize or run down by abusive language. Have I ever been bad-mouthed by someone? I remember when someone was talking to me about another person in their life who didn't like them. They said, "Pastor, my name is not safe in their mouth." With a true friend, your name is always safe in their mouth, right? Have I ever bad-mouthed more than a fishing trip?

Between 1605 and 1615, the Spanish author Miguel de Cervantes wrote a book about an aged idealist named Don Quixote and his comrade Sancho Panza. Don Quixote set out on a campaign to restore the age of chivalry, battle evil, and right all wrongs. He was a hope dealer to the hundredth degree. When Don Quixote arrived at a roadside inn, he met a barmaid and prostitute named Aldonza. He never called her by that name. Instead, he *good-mouthed* her.

If you can bad-mouth someone, you can also good-mouth someone!

He envisioned her and named her Dulcinea, his ideal of a lady. She was bewildered by the older man's behavior. She shouted at Don Quixote in anger and disillusionment, "Oh, don't call me a lady. I'm only a kitchen slut reeking of sweat, a strumpet men use and forget. I'm only Aldonza. I am nothing at all!" She found it hard to love because no one loved her back. However, this changed after she met Don Quixote. Using his charm, using the hope he dealt into her life, she turned in the card of whore for one of a child of God. What a way to change her hand and her perspective. Love changed her perspective on herself and others!

Her rough exterior masked Aldonza's gentle heart, but his love for her allowed her to see herself through his eyes. Don Quixote good-mouthed her into being. Don Quixote is the Christ figure of the story. He loves an immoral woman with an indiscriminate love! The years of her mistreatment are washed away by Don Quixote's captive heart. The good name that Don Quixote put on Aldonza is the opposite of the act of bad-mouthing another person. He good-mouthed her, regarded her, and treated her as good and upright. He named her a person of wholesomeness and integrity.

Every church, every 12-step group, from Alcoholics Anonymous to group therapy that I know frees people from hang-ups, is an attempt to good-mouth a person, to enable them to accept themselves by being accepted. It's an attempt to tell you what your true identity is, that you are mud but Holy mud, God breathed into the dust of the earth, a child of *the King.* A true friend always good-mouths you! A true friend tells you when you have broccoli in your teeth, rather than let you embarrass yourself! They tell you your fly is down. They tell you when you are being egocentric, prideful, and selfish! They remind you that you can, in fact, do better than this! They do it by good-mouthing you and encouraging you to improve.

The New Testament word for this good-mouthing is *logidzomai,* meaning to regard and treat as good. That word appears in Paul's Letter to the Christians in Rome as the word *reckon.* "Likewise also reckon yourselves to be truly dead unto sin…" (Romans 6:11, JUB). To reckon ourselves in this way and to give ourselves a good name is to consider ourselves a specific value. We become able to good-mouth ourselves in this way because God has reckoned us to be good and acceptable in company with Jesus Christ: "to the praise of the glory of His grace, by which He made us accepted in the Beloved" (Ephesians 1:6, NKJV).

Doesn't Christ on the cross take our bad-mouthing and give us in return his excellent mouth? Doesn't Christ on the cross take our poor hand life has dealt us and give us a new set of cards? Come on, who here needs some hope and a friend? Christ is the classic example of one who used the power of a good name. Our records about Christ show him using good names to build a person's sense of worth. For example, among his twelve apostles was a weak, vacillating, undependable man named Simon. What did Jesus do for this man? He gave him a good name, a nickname. Christ renamed this shifting, redneck, impulsive, and fickle fisherman by calling him "The Rock—the stone upon which Christ builds the church!" Christ had no silver or gold, but he gave Simon what he had. He gave him the undeserved gift of an unexpected lift through a new name. This is what Isaiah of Babylon meant when he wrote, "You will be called by a new name, a name given by the Lord himself" (Isaiah 62:2, GNT).

What a lift that must have been for Simon because "a good name is more to be desired than great riches; esteem is better than silver or gold!" Christ did the same thing over and over again for people whom he met. Remember the woman who was caught in the act of adultery and dragged before Christ by scribes and Pharisees who wanted to use this abused woman as a way to trap Jesus? When Christ saw the bystanders weighing the stones in their hands, the stones with which to kill this lawbreaker, he "said to them, 'He who is without sin among you, let him throw a stone at her first'" (John 8:7, NKJV). The crowd of accusers dissolved as one by one, beginning with the oldest, the men dropped their stones and left the scene. He took the bad mothers and sent them away. Then, for the first time in the encounter, Christ addressed her. Please think of the names he could have used. Instead of using the bad, hurtful names people have created, he chose to dignify her by the power of a good name. "'Woman, where are those accusers of yours? Has no one condemned you?' She said, 'No one, Lord.' And Jesus said to her, 'Neither do I condemn you; go and sin no more'" (John 8:10–11, NKJV). Woman here means daughter or beautiful lady, the same term he calls his mother from the cross. It's a term of respect, of endearment. Jesus good-mouthed her as Don Quixote did.

Jesus traveled through the city of Jericho. In that place was a man named Zacchaeus, the superintendent of taxes. Such Jewish tax collectors, willing helpers of the hated Roman occupation force, were despised by their fellow Jews, who would not accept their testimony in court nor their money in the synagogues. When Christ spotted Zacchaeus, who had gone on a limb to see this popular figure, our Lord invited himself to dinner at the tax collector's home. When the townspeople saw Christ befriend this man, they put Zacchaeus down by placing on him the bad name of "sinner." In contrast to the crowd's judgment, Jesus chose to elevate Zacchaeus by bestowing him a good name and demonstrating compassion. While society sought to put him down, Christ's gracious gesture uplifted Zacchaeus, illustrating the transformative power of acceptance and kindness.

Jesus said of him: "Today, salvation has come to this household because he too is a son of Abraham." (Luke 19:9, CEB).

"Man lives by affirmation even more than by bread," said Victor Hugo.[32] Yet, how important is the basis of that affirmation? One time, I read a true story in a magazine that reported an older man named Candelario had found a $700 gold nugget in the gulches of Sandia Peak near Albuquerque. "As soon as my luck was known," he said, "I became Don Candelario; within a week, I was Don Juan Candelario, then Don Juan de Candelario, Caballero. My name grew for three weeks till my gold was gone. Then I became simply Old Candelario again." He enjoyed a good name for almost a month, but it didn't last. How human it was for him to want that good name! "A good name is more desirable than great riches; to be esteemed is better than silver or gold" (Proverbs 22:1, NIV). Yet, how undependable was the basis of that old fellow's good name? The affirmation he received from other people was based on his monetary worth. In contrast, it is the glory of the gospel that in a world where many factors today conspire to put us down, Christ lifts us by putting on us a good name and raising our sense of self-esteem.

"You are salt…light for all the world." (Matthew 5:13, 14, NEB) And best of all for our good name is this: "You are now my friends" (John 15:15, TLB). God wants you to experience the fullness of it! Yet even within Christianity, we have this mistaken notion that it's just all about me and my walk with God. I don't know about all the church because there's drama, and I've been hurt. And there's messed up people, and they smell bad, and there's a bunch of hypocrites. So I don't go to church! Or if I do go, I stay in my pajamas and watch online from home. Really? I am glad we stream our worship services, but watching a service online is like watching a fireplace on your TV. You can see the fellowship, but you can't feel the warmth of the fellowship. You can see the fire, but you can't feel the fire. The same is true with your digital friends. To me, it's like watching a fire on the TV screen. You just can't broadcast fellowship or friendship. But, no, no. Your relationship with God is intended to be experienced communally. Didn't Jesus say, "For where two or three are gathered in my name, I am there in the midst of them" (Matthew 18:20, LEB)? There are aspects to your relationship with God that you will never be able to experience alone. So many things have become more accessible and more manageable, but friendship has gotten more challenging!

Why is friendship so hard? First, we are more "mobile" than ever! Who puts down roots anywhere anymore? Throughout most of human history, you ended up dying not far from where you were born. You didn't walk around back in the day asking people: Where are you from? I'm from right over there; that's where I was born! It's John Mellencamp's Song, Small Town, right? You know me. We've lived next to each other all of our lives. But we're so transferable and mobile and lacking roots today. It is more affordable than it's ever been to go live wherever you want to go. Hundreds of years ago, it was costly if you wanted to go to Europe and live abroad. You had to get on a ship, and it would take months. During the potato famine, people fled Ireland because there was no food.

---

32 *Victor Hugo quote: "man lives more by affirmation than by Bread."* Quotefancy. (n.d.-b).
https://quotefancy.com/quote/926480/Victor-Hugo-Man-lives-more-by-affirmation-than-by-bread

They had to get on these pricey coffin ships to try and seek a better life. Of course, they called them coffin ships because of how many died on these boats. Just the hope of life in a new world, the costs, and the time it took, it was months of this dangerous ocean crossing. Today, if you want to, you can go live somewhere else. You can get a Southwest Airlines ticket and ding—"You are now free to move about the country!" Or, you can take your life into your own hands and go on Spirit Airlines. Has anyone here flown Spirit? It's cheap for a reason. Their slogan should be: Fly Spirit, We May or May Not Get You There! This nomadic lifestyle would have been foreign for most of human history. That works against friendships. When you live in a camper van or RV and work remotely, it turns out that you don't put down great roots, shockingly. I live here this season, but I live here during the winter. Some of my congregation, Winter Texans, are only here half the year. I follow the sunshine, or I follow the waves, or I need a Wi-Fi connection in a coffee shop where I can do my work. We have personalized former community activities like going to the movies now just downloading or streaming them on Hulu, HBO Max, or Netflix. Unlike in the past, I will binge-watch my shows when you might be hanging out on the front porch talking to someone and not texting them. *We have entertainment options that can keep us sort of in this medicated coma inside of our homes.*

What's another foe of friendship?

We only try to connect with friends through our strengths instead of our shared vulnerabilities. If you want to make friends, get off the four-hours-a-day addiction to social media. If you give a phone to a fifteen-year-old—like if you are a phone Nazi who believes "No Phone for you until you are fifteen, as too much of today's society looks at it"—at an average life span of seventy-five years, that person (at four hours a day on the phone) will spend ten years of their life scrolling and staring at a screen. Can you imagine standing before God, and God says to you, "Well, what did you do with that extra ten years of health, vitality, talents, and strength I gave you?" Will you respond, "Well, I spent it all on my phone, mindlessly scrolling and watching Tik-Tok videos! It was so rewarding, God!"

Is it the life we want, to be so addicted to our digital pacifiers? Do we really want to waste four hours a day, ten years of our lives?

God said it's not good for us to be alone, and we are more digitally connected than ever and lonelier than ever. It would be best if you had an anti-social media mindset. Social media is built around this idea: We show the best and hide the rest. For every photo you see on Instagram, think of the other thirty pictures on their camera roll that will get deleted because they were not deemed good enough. Oh, no. That's not true. I have my vulnerable posts. We know that because you wrote "vulnerable post colon." And then now comes a carefully calculated algorithm-smashing vulnerability that's all been sanitized. So now, we can't even trust our vulnerable post moments. We want to show people our filtered selves while our real lives are full of blooper moments. If you want a real friend, they see your bloopers and love you anyway. Blooper reel moments, I said the wrong thing. Blooper reel moments, I put my foot in my mouth. We got red-faced and embarrassed in those moments, and it didn't go well. We tend to run away from that. But don't resist that. We impress people with our strengths, but we connect with people through our weaknesses! This is vulnerability. This is a real friendship. We live in interconnected networks of terminally casual relationships. We live with the delusion that we know one another, but we don't because we never get vulnerable and say this is where I need help; this is my struggle. We call our easygoing, self-protective, and often theologically trite conversations 'fellowship,' but they never reach the threshold of true fellowship. We know cold demographic details about one another, like married or single, type of job, number of kids, general housing location, etc. Still, we know little about the struggles our friends are going through every day behind well-maintained personal boundaries or filtered posts on social media. This is where we want to get to, where those friendships can be vulnerable. Come on, enough with the church talk. I get so sick of church talk. How are you doing? So good. Great. Yeah, you're doing great. Great. Everything's great. Yeah, because everything's perfect because you have a halo. Yes, because God's good all the time, and all the time, God's good. Enough with all that. Where's the place where we can tell people that we love and are connected to? Here's what's going on? And I won't be afraid that my mess and weakness will repulse you! We need to be comfortable feeling uncomfortable, exposed in that way, and vulnerable in real friendships! People need to see us living in the trash so they can lift us to a life out of the garbage!

Another hurdle to friendship: We've been burned in the past! A friend has burned us, so that means I will probably get burned again!

Friendships are challenging and often not sought after when we get a little mileage on us because they have gone or can go wrong. You thought you knew a guy. You thought you had made the right choice for that business partner and lifelong friend. Then they ended up stabbing you in the back. They ended up betraying you. They ended up gossiping about you, and you found out later. This happens to everybody, but never let what happened to you with one friend stop you from making another!

Ulysses S. Grant was asked at the end of his life: In all that you went through and experienced, what was the most painful part of your life? Think about Grant's life. There's much pain, considering he was the commanding general during the Civil War. How many people under his command died? That's painful. While he was president of the United States, his daughter married a British guy, and there's the pain of her moving to England. He couldn't FaceTime with his daughter! Grant didn't want it to happen and didn't like the idea, but she fell in love. He had a few red flags with this guy, and of course, what he feared was justified! The British guy ended up being a bad guy, betrayed his daughter, and was a philanderer all around the world, and the marriage did not go well. He failed to have what every man must develop: sexual discipline. Quit acting like you are a young lion once you are married! History has well documented that Grant had an alcohol problem. Turns out, he had a tough time with a drink. And Abraham Lincoln was asked about it. "Why can you trust this guy to run our nation through the war? He has alcoholism." Lincoln said, "I'll tell you, if I find any other generals that do as well as he does, I will send barrels of alcohol to them too." Lincoln was like, the positives outweigh the negatives. But it was hard because even when there were seasons of his life when his addiction was under control, there were always rumors about the alcohol. His political opponents would just say, oh, the drunk, the drunk, you can't trust the drunk. That's painful. How about the fact that he was friends with Lincoln, who was assassinated? Grant experienced some pain, so I was surprised when the question was asked, "What was the most painful thing you experienced in your eventful life?" And Grant responded, and I quote, "To be deceived by a friend!" His secretary in the White House turned out to be a rat. There's this enormous scandal, ironically, called the Whiskey Ring Scandal. I know we can't imagine presidential scandals in the puritanical times that we live in, right? It turns out that Lincoln paid for the Civil War by imposing a massive tax on whiskey. But then, after the war, the tax had not been removed yet, but it was susceptible to corruption because people could, for favors, say that the tax due had been paid when it hadn't but siphon much money off for doing that favor. And they suspected someone close to Washington DC was involved at a very high level. When rumors began circulating that it was President Grant's secretary, the president said, "No, there's no way! This guy is true blue; he's the real deal, and we are close friends." Grant's friend was taken to trial, and Grant volunteered to give testimony on his behalf, and everyone said he couldn't do that. Presidents can't go on trial. I mean, can you imagine that in our day, presidents are on trial (smile)? Grant said, "No, I'm doing it for this guy because he's my friend; he's my ride-or-die friend. I will die for this guy. He's my real deal friend." The bad guy got off, and right after the fact, Grant found out the guy was a snake in the grass, lying and double-dealing under his nose. He counted that betrayal of a friend, of someone who served him, as the most challenging thing he had endured.

King David went through some difficult things, some hard days. And yet David, in Psalm 55:12–14 (NIV) said, "If an enemy were insulting me, I could endure it; if a foe were rising against me, I could hide. But it is you, a man like myself, my companion, my close friend, with whom I once enjoyed sweet fellowship at the house of God…" He's talking about that pain we all know if we've been betrayed. He had this friend named Ahithophel. He said I can handle enemies. I've been having enemies come at me since Goliath. But to have someone who I thought was one way end up being another way hurts. It's the "Et tu, Brute" that rings out throughout history, and Jesus himself experienced this through the betrayal of Judas and the kiss of deceit.

The question in relationships is, will I get hurt or not? Inevitably, you will. It's always about what you do with the hurt. Do you let it define you? Do you nurse it? Do you let it consume you? **The question is not "how many times will I get hurt?" but "how soon can I get over the hurt?"** Do you say, "Well, since I can't be friends with them, I probably can't be friends with others?" I would tell you that you must continue to let people get close, even when you've been hurt, even when it's been hard, even when you've been stung by that kind of pain! The only other choices are bitterness and resentment. Every time you have a conflict with a friend, it is an opportunity to leave the relationship because that's hard and start over new with someone less drama. Or you can go deeper and persist through the difficulty and get your relationship to another level. *Welcome to marriage and genuine friendship.* Now, there has to be some discernment here, and you can have people in your heart but not in your life anymore. Don't just let your friends fall away because things have got tough.

With all of my heart, I still say they're worth it. Why? A Harvard study was begun in 1938, at the height of the Great Depression and the Dust Bowl, which is this dark, challenging chapter in our history. Some scientists and sociologists at Harvard University said we should study what makes people happy. The best way to do this would be to track people through their entire lives, a longitudinal study. Then, look at what was different about their lives and if there was any commonality in the happiest, healthiest group. Sounds good. The only problem was whether the researchers would die or retire before the subjects of the study and who then would continue their work. However, they launched this project, the Harvard Study of Adult Development, and got this group of 724 men, half of whom were going to come from Harvard University, and that grouping included John F. Kennedy. The other half would be based on sampling the poorest neighborhoods in the inner-city district of Boston. In the Great Depression, you had people living in slums without running water, and they found half of the group from that sampling. These two groupings of people were as different as any could be. One group consisted of wealth, privilege, opportunity, and Ivy League, while the other group had bleak possibilities for better lives.

One group was trying to decide to be a psychologist, and another was trying to figure out how to live in the middle of a trash dump!

This is a long, old study; the original researchers either died or retired. The baton has successfully changed hands to the current one, who just released a book called *The Good Life!* The author is the fourth director of the program. Every two years, they call each of these men and interview them about their health and every detail of their life, and they compile it all. It's literally in human history that the most extended study on human thriving has ever been done. At this time, 59 of these men are still alive and in their nineties. They now have an accurate picture and an understanding of what leads to happiness. What's shocking is how it has almost nothing to do with the number one, number two, and number three things that most people, millennials and Gen Z alike, say that there are goals in their life, which usually are somewhere in this order: Money, great job, ability to travel, being famous. These are the TikTok goals of our current culture! They found that those who lived the longest were the healthiest and the happiest, but they didn't have any of these things like money, great jobs, traveling, or fame. Having a fat 401K and having a mansion on the beach is not what the happy ones all have in common. Not even having a six-figure income made them happy! How about good cholesterol? Shockingly, in your 40s and 50s, good cholesterol does not predict whether you will be thriving, happy, healthy, and living a very long life! Access to a country club was not on the list. College education is not even on the list at all. Those who are happy and healthy and thriving all have one thing in common:

They have deep, meaningful friendships and relationships! Rich or poor, employed or unemployed, the one key to happiness you can have is deep friendships![33]

It's not about more money.

It's not about having a prestigious job.

It boils down to friendships.

Friendships, they say, seem to delay mental health and physical decline of aging and are better predictors of long and happy lives than any other single thing. Friendships not only change your career from psychologist to pastor, but they also change every day and every year of your life. Friendship is one of the keys to pursuing happiness. Secular scientists conclude what the Bible says all along: It's not good for man to be alone. Remember: You may only be one good friend away from changing your life—it's not easy, but it's possible!

For me, friendship is a little like falling asleep. You cannot enter it by sheer willpower, but I can take the initiative, be vulnerable, be a plug and help, and choose not to let the pain of previous failed friendships stop me from reaching out for new friends today.

I was thinking this week about the miracles of Jesus: Walking on water, water into wine, feeding 5,000, amazing miracles. However, one of the least appreciated miracles was when he had twelve close friends in his 30s. That's a miracle. He's a man with twelve close friends in his early 30s. But how did he get there? He got to the end where, at dinner, everyone was swearing; they were his ride or die. And you know what? Every single one of the apostles who made it through to the day of Pentecost did give their lives for Jesus, except for the apostle John. How did he end up with such close friends? Well, it was unhurried time. *It was three years of spending every day together*. We are culturally obsessed with speed and hurry.

33 Liz, M. (2017, April 11). *Over nearly 80 years, Harvard study has been showing how to live a healthy and happy life*. Harvard Gazette.
https://news.harvard.edu/gazette/story/2017/04/
over-nearly-80-years-harvard-study-has-been-showing-how-to-live-a-healthy-and-happy-life/

You can't hurry and love at the same time. *You can't rush relational intimacy. That doesn't happen in a day. Building a friendship is like building a fire—good fires take time. It's just this tiny little thing, some kindling; you add twigs and a little kindling. You can't get to the big logs right away. It'll put the fire out. That little flame is not enough to take on that big log, so you need friendship kindling, which takes time.* So friendships are built like bonfires, one moment, one spark at a time!

The question then becomes, **how do I be a good friend?**

How do I be a good friend? First of all, you have to **take the initiative.** Take the initiative. Proverbs 18:24 (NKJV) says, "A man who has friends must himself be friendly." How does it start? Well, hey, you have got to be friendly. Ralph Waldo Emerson said, "The only way to have a friend is to be one."[34] *We don't make friends; we MAKE THEM!* I love this because it brings it back down to you having agency or control.

Are you lonely? Well, *it doesn't have to be this way*! It starts with you being a friend to another.

It's easy to walk into a church and go away and say no one was friendly there. No one was nice to me there. I left that church. Why? It wasn't a friendly church. Were you friendly? Have you been friendly at your church today, your workplace today, your home today, your neighborhood today? A church is just people; we're as strong as our weakest link. So if you want to have friends, it's back on you, Buster. It would help if you chose to be friendly. Someone has to take the initiative.

In 2000, Gabrielle Reece did for women's beach volleyball what Shaun White did for men's snowboarding, what Tiger Woods did for golf, and Lance Armstrong did for professional cycling. She brought it to the edge of popularity. I read an interview recently with Gabrielle. She was asked, "What's something that's helped you in life that maybe other people would need to hear?" She said, "I've just decided to be the one to go first. I'll say hello first if I'm checking out at the store. I'll smile first if I come across somebody and make eye contact. I've been experimenting with that, just a little bit at a time. Not all times but most times, it ends up in your favor." She then said, "I was at the park the other day. My kids were playing. These two women were a little older than me, standing there, and on the surface, we had nothing in common. I walked by them, turned around, looked at them, and smiled." And she said that immediately, a smile of relief came over their faces.

The realization is people are ready, but everyone's just waiting for someone to go first because we're being trained in this world to opt out. Nobody's going first anymore. That's what scripture is saying. Do you want to have friends? Be friendly. Go first. Come on. Let's take that initiative. Let's not wait for someone else to notice us.

---

34 *Ralph Waldo Emerson - the only way to have a friend is to...* BrainyQuote. (n.d.-b). https://www.brainyquote.com/quotes/ralph_waldo_emerson_100740

Look for ways to add value. Look for ways you can be a "plug" for someone. My son Jacob taught me that term. A plug is someone who says, "How can I help you get what you need?" My good friend Bill was for me. That's what people who cared about children living in a trash dump were! You'll have to look for and take good notes in your mind. As you meet and talk to people, think as they say things. Who do I know who could help you with the problem that you've just admitted to having? How can I be a connector? Hey, I noticed you mentioned you are not handy with tools, but I have a friend who is, who might be able to help you. Let me connect you two! That's how friendships are formed because the gifts you have, that you're strong in. aren't necessarily going to be for me and vice versa. So, as we have a budding relationship, we need to look for ways to add value.

Proverbs 18:16 (NKJV) says, "A man's gift makes room for him and brings him before great men." And this is an opportunity you have in the friendship phase to ask: What can I do to help you somehow? And that's intuitive because we get it. It makes sense to me. Someone I've done something for will look favorably on me. And that's true. Proverbs 19:6 (NKJV) says, "…every man is a friend to one who gives gifts." Maybe the harder part then is the reverse of this. How do we build a friendship when the other person is helping us? That's the harder one.

We're all looking, oh, I've got to introduce you to so-and-so. Let me open that door for you. Is there something I could do for you? Hey, you mentioned you're having difficulty with your miniature schnauzer. I know of a great invisible fence. And hey, I'd come over, and we could dig that thing. Do you see what I'm saying? And they say that to you. And you're like, oh, no, no. All of our pride kicks in, and then I think: If I invite them over, they will see my house, and I won't have time to clean it up. And I may not have the right music on, and I may not have my stuff in order, and now I feel vulnerable. You must be willing to be on the receiving end of someone helping you, even if it shows your vulnerability.

Read the room. Do you want to have friends? Social smarts cannot be overstated.

John Rockefeller, the richest guy in the world at one point, would take guys golfing. And he just wanted to have friendships. But he had a rule that he didn't tell anybody. It was an unspoken rule. If you brought up work or asked for a job or a favor for so-and-so, or you asked for a loan or subtly hinted at a bit of funding for your dream thing, you would never get invited back again. You were just crossed off the golf list. He was looking for people who could golf with him and be in the moment and read it, and those were the people that he began to confide in and trust and who knew the moment that he wasn't there to have a meeting. He wasn't there to do any Shark Tank investments. He was there because he liked golfing.

During my tenure as a pastor at First Congregational Church in Escondido, California, the men's ministry presented an interesting proposition: every Monday, they insisted that the pastor join them for a game of golf. They generously covered the country club membership fees, creating an initial impression of a delightful arrangement where I could be paid to play golf. However, what unfolded on those golf outings was quite different.

The men's ministry meetings on the golf course discussed church matters. For the entire round of golf, spanning five-plus hours and nineteen holes, the conversation revolved around church-related discussions, strategies, and suggestions for how I should lead the congregation. While I initially saw it as an opportunity to enjoy golf and engage in fellowship, it evolved into a platform for them to share their perspectives on the church's direction. There were Mondays when all I craved was the camaraderie of a friend, someone to share personal moments rather than someone constantly advising on church matters. This experience underscored the importance of recognizing and respecting individual needs and understanding the context of the moment. It emphasized the need to "read the room" and be attuned to what people genuinely seek: professional guidance or friendship.

"He who blesses his friend with a loud voice, rising early in the morning, it will be counted a curse to him" (Proverbs 27:14, NKJV).

Some would say the Bible isn't practical. Is this person an early bird or a night owl? Are they caffeinated enough yet? You know what I'm saying? Like me, please don't talk to me until I have had at least one cup of coffee under my belt! *Ah, this person seems to back away slowly whenever I walk toward them. Maybe I'm doing something annoying.* Reading the room means not overdoing it or coming on too strong. Proverbs 25:17 (NKJV) says, "Seldom set foot in your neighbor's house, lest he become weary of you and hate you." What does this passage say about reading the room? Maybe not being so needy always, and your friends get compassion fatigue! We don't want to have that impact on people. We want our friends to have Wi-Fi rights in our homes and their phones so that they do not need our passwords. Yes, but we don't want to overstay our welcome. We want to sort of leave them wanting more. You get invited to someone's house, the art of knowing when the night's over when the host stands up and says, well, thank you for coming. That's your cue to go. It's like, it's a Monday. They have to work tomorrow. Just mellow, right? This is just so important. I remember taking Zach camping, and we were splitting and kindling off logs for firewood. And he asked: "Why do we need to do this? We have so many logs." I tell him—you can't shove these big logs into a little fire. It'll smother it. It'll suffocate it. So it takes a little kindling and is a little bit bigger. Eventually, the flame will be so powerful that it can handle that big log. But I think some of us are trying to leap forward two decades out of our camper van friendship that we just formed into this beautiful thing that will stabilize us in life's hardest trials. But that friendship is weak. You can't handle that kind of flame. And it won't work if you repot the tree and move it to a new nursery every two years. It will not work if you keep on with this nomadic life, where you're on to the next friend whenever any difficult thing ever appears because there's too much drama!

Do you want happiness? You don't want to be lonely anymore? You don't want to face life alone anymore? It does not have to be this way. You are only one friend away from someone who will pull you out of the muck and the mud of life, set your feet upon the rock, and help you to become all God intended for you to become!

CHAPTER EIGHT

10 WAYS TO MAKE LOVE, BETTER!

Love is when the other person's happiness is more important than your own!

—H. Jackson Brown, Jr.

AHH, LOVE...REMEMBER THE FIRST TIME you felt it?

The sky seemed a bit bluer, the sun seemed brighter, and birds landed on your shoulder, singing sweet love songs in your ears. Is that the feeling of love?

Love calling? I got a call this week that still makes me laugh. It was on Tuesday, the day after Christmas. It was a woman on the line; we'll call her Barbie. Barbie called me and asked if I could conduct a spur-of-the-moment wedding for her this Friday at Grace Church. I told her, for the most part, I do weddings, *but not spur-of-the-moment weddings*. I asked if she and the groom would come in, and we met and set a date. You know, I like to counsel couples who want to get married in a church because getting married in a church implies that you are inviting a third party into the marriage, you know, God. When you ask God into your relationship, it changes you and the relationship! Barbie was irritated at my response. After a pause, she continued, *"Well, I'll find someone else to perform the ceremony, but I want you to know something: I believe you are wrong about spur-of-the-moment weddings. Some of my BEST marriages have been spur-of-the-moment."* I laughed out loud and said, "Well, how many times have you been married?" She says, without skipping a beat, "Five times!" Wow. Maybe you need to slow your giddy-up on the way to the altar.

Look, I do a lot of weddings, and it helps pay some of my son's college expenses. If you need to be married, man, I am your huckleberry. I will do what the couple wants to make their day, including letting them write personal vows. Usually, vows are what? "In sickness or health, until death do us part, we will make it work." But this bride last week sent me her vows that she got out of *Cosmo*, and this was just one line, but do you think this marriage is going to last or if I should have felt good about them saying, "We don't need any preachy pre-marriage class from a pastor." Here's a snippet from their vows. "We'll stay together as long as we have feelings for each other. When the feelings go away, we're not obligated to stay." Do you have an attorney on speed dial? Love is always more than a feeling; it includes feelings, but it's not held hostage by feelings. Today's view on dating and relationships is all about the microwave—instant gratification, just getting what you want!

Proverbs 23:7 (NLV) says: "For as he thinks in his heart, so is he."

In other words, *the kind of thoughts you think will determine the kind of person you become.*

You've heard it said you are what you eat, and that's true. But to a greater degree—because you are not just body but are also spirit, mind, and emotion—*you are what you think!*

I am not saying hate the world or never hear what the world says. The moment we start "the world's got cooties," we can't reach the world. Yet we must learn to think right, or we'll never be able to live or love right.

An unfaithful heart cannot create a faithful life.

An undisciplined mind cannot create a disciplined life.

I will repeat it, not only because repetition is one of the marks of good teaching but because it is that important. We will never be able to live or love right if we don't think right about love!

I saw that you were perfect, and so I loved you. Then I saw that you were not perfect, and I loved you even more.

Don't we all want that sort of love, or at least be the recipients of it? Our number one need in life is to love and be loved. Some things are loved because they are valuable, right, expensive car or house, but some things are valuable because they are truly loved. That's the love we all long for, the "just because love." I always thought they should teach Relationships 101 like Algebra or History. Can anything give us more joy or pain than our relationships?

Love, we all long for it. Whether single, divorced, married, or remarried, we chase it. We all long for love; what I learned about love as a kid was from fairy tales that start with "Once upon a time…" and end with "They got married and lived happily ever after." In between, they meet, fall in love, and get into trouble; she eats the fruit she wasn't supposed to eat, the carriage turns back into a pumpkin, and she pricks her finger against the spinning wheel and sleeps for a hundred years. Then things work out, and Snow White eventually marries Prince Charming, Cinderella marries Prince Charming, and Sleeping Beauty marries Prince Charming. There were no laws against bigamy back in the old days. I always wondered, "How come it's always Prince Charming? Why did

Prince Charming's wife end up happily ever after when he married all these women?" How about Prince Charming falling in love with and kissing Snow White while she sleeps? It seems a little bit aggressive these days. Is it in this "MeToo" world? It's like, wait, he fell in love with her after she eats a poisoned apple, and while she's comatose, cupid strikes? People say to follow your heart, and you will find love, but what if your heart is more confused than what's in your head?

Where does one turn in this world for the most important matters of life, the issues of the heart? Maybe social media can help.

I came across an article about some of the top tweets about marriage.

Marriage is two people taking turns mashing down the garbage, hoping the other person will fold it first and then empty the bin.

As a thirty-year veteran of marriage, this is true. One man said all the premarital courses I took, counseling we endured, and books we read failed to mention that husbands would be expected to know the difference between regular and good tweezers, right? I've had my hand slapped more times for using good scissors. Then I'm like, all scissors are scissors.

This one, though, is my personal favorite.

One man's wife had to unexpectedly stay overnight in the hospital because her mom had been hospitalized. She was going to stay and sleep in the room with her. And so she sent her husband home with a list of things to get for her. And on the list, he was shocked. It said comfortable underwear. *Comfortable underwear?* And he didn't want to get this wrong. And so he texted her, how will I know when I find your comfortable underwear? She said, "Simple. Just pick them up, imagine me wearing them, and if you smile, you got the wrong one, so put them back and get the other ones."

Marriage is confusing. Relationships are confusing.

How about history? Maybe it can help us with relationships.

Sir Walter Raleigh is one of my favorite explorers from the Elizabethan age. He was an explorer, going back and forth to South America, looking for mines and gold. But he despised Sir Walter Raleigh under King James I, the same King James whose name is in the Bible (the King James Bible printed in 1611). He had him locked up in the Tower of England. Eventually, he sentenced him to die by beheading. At the critical moment of Sir Walter Raleigh's death, the executioner, who didn't feel like Walter deserved this, gave him a tip. He said, when you kneel at the block, and your head is on this thing, orient your head in this way because it will cause it to be over quicker, and you'll feel less pain. And some of his last words before he died were this: It matters not the condition of my head as I die. All that matters is my heart is right! There is some truth in that for all of us. And that message in the last moments of Sir Raleigh's life came right to us in God's Word 3,000 years ago when Solomon wrote these powerful words. In Proverbs

4:23 (NIV), Solomon writes: **"Above all else, guard your heart, for everything you do flows from it."**

Has anyone here ever had relationship problems? If you are not saying Amen, we know who the liar in the relationship is. Here's the good news about relationship problems: Relationship problems can be a catalyst for profound personal and spiritual growth!

The First Way to Make Love Better: Get Your Heart Right!

Guard your heart! The rest of your life will follow if your heart is in the correct position. If your heart is full of love, you are relationship-ready. If your heart is loving, your feet will follow love.

Why guard your heart?

Because it's the well that you pour into others' lives.

The greatest part of a person is unseen, and it's your heart, your love, your true essence, so you better guard it and make sure you are good with what lies within it.

It's what you give to others—your heart, your love!

What comes out of your heart?

Everything. All the issues of life.

So, if you want to change your relationships, it starts by examining your heart—your capacity to forgive, try over, get over the past, make amends, and love again like it was the first time you loved. We all know how difficult it is to change ourselves, let alone someone else, so if you want to change your relationships, *focus on the one you can change, you and your heart.*

My wife taught me this. She always says to me, **"When I change me, I change we!"**

Love is more than a feeling. Love, as I know it, is a decision, at times even independent of feelings.

It is an attitude from which we operate. It is a way of behaving toward others. It's a state of being loving, like being healthy or sick.

We may not always feel love, but we can do the loving thing.

Can you think of someone at work, a spouse, a friend, or one of your relatives you don't feel loving toward? I'm sure we all can. Your feelings toward that person are perhaps negative or suspicious. That person may have hurt you. Their words may have cut you down. They don't deserve your love. If you allow God to claim over your heart, God has given you a command to love that person. *That doesn't mean you have to feel a certain way, but to do the loving thing, to respond from a stance of love.* That might mean forgiving, giving that person another chance, and sacrificing pride. It might mean deciding not to pay that person back or putting them down to prove you are right. You may choose not to criticize or talk about that person behind their back.

You can practice the discipline of not having the last word.

We don't have to wait for a feeling of love before we love.

We can decide to love without feeling love.

Love doesn't always change the other person but it will always change you.

But to do this, you have to guard your heart and not allow painful experiences in the past to make you lock your heart away or let it become cynical, jaded, or full of resentment. This is where you must guard it, protect it, and evaluate it.

Guard it.

Why is it important? One simple reason:

Your love life is going to impact all of your life!

I just conducted a wedding for an eighty-four-year-old woman; her prince charming is eighty-six! I conducted it at the Viera Nursing Home. It was a beautiful ceremony. The whole community was there, along with Channel 6 News. But they didn't meet at the nursing home. They met, fell in love, married, and moved in. They met on a dating app called *Silver Singles*. They didn't understand how to fill out the questions on the app, but their grandkids did. Why does someone who is 84 or 86 get married? Because your love life will impact your whole life!

It would be tempting to think I can honor and love God, but I also have "this" here. I can do this over here; it won't impact anything. But our lives cannot be segmented like that, bifurcated like that. You can't compartmentalize your life; you can't compartmentalize your heart. Your love life will impact your whole life because it flows from your heart.

God's word says to keep your heart diligently for life issues out of spring.

What you do when it comes to your heart is going to impact every part of your body. What goes into your heart gets to your toes. What goes into your heart gets to your head. What goes into your heart goes everywhere. You must keep your heart with all diligence. We can't just take what our heart tells us to do and say to ourselves; the heart wants what the heart wants. No. You have a job. And it is to steward your heart, to shepherd your heart.

When your heart speaks, take good notes.

Proverbs 23:19 (NLT) says, "My child, listen and be wise: Keep your heart on the right course."

Did you notice who is supposed to keep your heart on the right course? Not someone else, not your spouse, not your lover, but you!

Your heart is your responsibility!

It must not be followed blindly. It must not be given into. It must be forced to submit to God. We must continually keep steering our hearts back to God through repentance, wise counsel, and listening to the Holy Spirit. Jeremiah 17:9 (KJV) says, "The heart is deceitful above all things, and desperately wicked: who can know it?" What is this text in Jeremiah telling us: *Your heart can get you into a whole mess of trouble.* Does anybody want to say Amen? God's word says that there are many things to watch out for when it comes to the heart, like the double heart, as opposed to the double chin. There's the double heart, the hard heart, the proud heart, the unbelieving heart, the cold heart, and the unclean heart. If you want to audit what's happening in your heart, you don't have to get a blood test. All you have to do is audit the words coming out of your mouth. Jesus said in Matthew 12:34 (NKJV): "For out of the abundance of the heart the mouth speaks." You can say, "No, you don't know my heart. I do. I know exactly what's in your heart because I follow you on Instagram and Facebook and get your texts!"

As the mouth speaks, so the heart does! As you talk, you and I listen to each other's hearts!

So, we have to constantly be doing what David did in Psalm 139:23 (KJV), praying to God: "Search me, O God, and know my heart: try me, and know my thoughts." In AA and NA, they teach a step called taking a daily inventory. It's asking yourself: Where did my heart go wrong today? Where was I rude? Where was I off balance when it came to letting something go instead of insisting on the last word? How could I change this tomorrow? You can even have a heart journal to record your thoughts and actions, examine them, and move toward growing in love. So, the first way to make love better is to focus on becoming the right person and having the right kind of heart for that person. This means, ladies, it's not your job to be a rehabilitation center for bad men. It's not your job to fix him, change him, parent him, or raise him. You want a partner, not a project!

Marriage does not create problems. It reveals them.

The more you can deal with emotional problems before you get married, the happier, more God-honoring, and more fulfilling your marriage will be. I am saying start with yourself and focus on your heart. *If you are not in a relationship, you should become the person you want to date.*

Look, let's be honest: marriage is a mixed bag. Some days it's sunshine and some days it's cloudy. Ultimately, you want a love that ends up in the oak barrels, not stuck in the honeymoon stage of the "feels!" Because if you run out every time the "feels" run out, you will repeat that quite a bit! Happiness is an inside job. It's a choice: You either choose to be happy or not. You must own your own happiness. Some of my favorite definitions of marriage are:

A good marriage is two independent pillars holding up the same bridge.

A good marriage is the union of two good forgivers!

A good marriage requires falling and growing in love often, always with the same person!

A good marriage is two people with short memories!

Or how about this one Khalil Gibran from his famous book *The Prophet:*

> "Love one another but make not a bond of love:
> Let it rather be a moving sea between the shores of your souls.
> Fill each other's cups, but do not drink from one cup.
> Give one another your bread, but eat not from the same loaf.
> Sing and dance together and be joyous, but let each one of you be alone,
> Even as the strings of a lute are alone, though they quiver with the same music."[35]

Read that again and ask yourself, is this how my marriage looks?

Or how about this gem from the Bible, from 1 Corinthians 13:7 (MSG):

> Love never gives up.
> Love cares more for others than for self.
> Love doesn't want what it doesn't have.
> Love doesn't strut,
> Doesn't have a swelled head,
> Doesn't force itself on others,
> Isn't always "me first,"
> Doesn't fly off the handle,
> Doesn't keep score of the sins of others,
> Doesn't revel when others grovel,
> Takes pleasure in the flowering of truth,
> Puts up with anything,
> Trusts God always,
> Always looks for the best,
> Never looks back,
> But keeps going to the end.

---

35 Gibran, K. (2019, January 1). *The prophet.* The Project Gutenberg eBook of The Prophet, by Kahlil Gibran. https://www.gutenberg.org/files

Is this describing your marriage? What if you took your name and substituted it every time you see the word "love" here? Would that be true of you? Most of us would say we have got some work to do! There is one name that works here for the word love: Jesus. Jesus never gives up. Jesus cares more for others than for self. Jesus doesn't want what he doesn't have. Jesus doesn't strut… go on down the list. We need to have the same mind of God and the same heart of Christ.

Get your heart relationship ready. The ideal time to learn about love, relationships, marriage, or commitment is like learning to fly a helicopter. Don't you want to learn to fly before you are up in the air? The best time to prepare for marriage is before you're in one, but the second-best time is when you are in one. But it starts with examining your heart. What areas of your heart most need to improve? What are the tendencies of your heart that have shown up consistently? When's the best time to plant a tree—spring, fall, winter, or summer? No, ten years ago! What's the second-best time to plant a tree? Today, the same is true with love.

Get your heart ready. Maybe some things in your heart don't fit anymore, like resentments, grudges, and previous relationships. Grow. Don't date unless your emotional hurts are healed or in the healing process. God can't heal what you hide, so don't hide your heart defects. Name them, claim them, let God heal them as you get honest about them. Do you struggle with bitterness or anger problems? Work through those before you start dating. Please get rid of your emotional baggage, and then, when you begin dating someone, size that person up quickly, particularly concerning their emotional health. Don't be afraid to ask questions like, "Do you have uncontrolled anger?" "Can we talk about me?" or "Will you pick up the tab?" If you see warning signs of unresolved emotional difficulties, ask yourself what you see happening here, whether it is a change or more of the same. Maybe you're already in a dating relationship and now see the signs of emotional unhealthiness in your partner. If so, talk with your partner about it. Every couple needs counseling, but not all couples get it. "But I won't have anybody to go out with on Friday night," you say. Here's the truth: A bad marriage is a million times worse than not going out on Friday night! And the longer you stay in a dead-end relationship, the more difficult it is to get out of it. Proverbs 28:23 (NLT) says, "In the end, people appreciate honest criticism far more than flattery."

No matter how much it hurts, be honest with yourself and your partner today. In the end, you both will benefit from it.

Back to our caller Barbie, wanting to do a spur-of-the-moment wedding, you might say her picker is slightly off! Her selector is a bit off. But why? Validation. She's looking for validation from these marriages—someone to tell her she's pretty enough, tall enough to ride the ride, qualified enough, but these guys are empty wells because they can't fill the hole in her heart; only God can. She needs to work on herself instead of hoping the marriage altar will alter her heart.

The Second Way to Make Love Better: Quit Putting the Keys to Your Heart in Someone Else's Pocket!

People believe marriage will be easy if you find the right person. What do you think? True or false? False. This notion is: "Someplace out there is my soul mate. When I see them, I'll know. I'll know, and then it will all be so easy!"

We all want someone to say to us: You complete me, but then around year seven, we hear these words: You deplete me!

Happiness in our relationships does not come by finding the right partner; it requires you to become the right partner. Happiness is not about finding the right person; it's about becoming the right person. This requires massive personal spiritual growth. Your relationship allows you to learn how to control your anger, reactions, and defensiveness. Why would you put the keys to your heart and happiness in someone else's hands and give them that much power over you? If they don't love, accept, and validate me, I won't be happy! Silly. That kind of commitment is reserved for God. Remember, ladies, don't believe the lie that you tell yourself: "If I give him my body, maybe he will give me his heart!"

Here's what I love to teach married couples in counseling, and they hate it. Still, it's necessary: You can either work on "your stuff" in the relationship you're in, or you can work on it with someone else, but you will have to work on it if you want a healthy, long-term relationship.

Everyone thinks I want to leave. I want someone else at some point.

It's very interesting in the Bible. The Bible has a lot of characters. Many of them are married, so it describes a lot of marriages. If you asked, "Who in the Bible has the best marriage? Who has the happiest marriage in the Bible?" it turned out to be a tricky question. There are not a lot of them. Some say, "Jacob and Rachel," because he greatly loved Rachel. Now, if you know anything about the Bible, you know Jacob was married to Rachel and loved her. He was also married to her sister, Leah, and to both of their maidservants. They had a contest to see which of the four women could bear Jacob the most children. That is not a happy marriage! The Bible never has a story that ends, "They got married and lived happily ever after." In the Bible, marriage never delivers happily ever after. Only Jesus delivers happily ever after. Can I get an Amen from anybody on this? It's an interesting thing.

Marriage does not exist to make you happy. According to the Bible, marriage exists to make you like Jesus. It exists to sand off the difficult edges, be used by God, and make you more and more the kind of person God designed you to be!

Now, God can also use singleness for that, but that's part of what marriage is about. It's a great tool of God for spiritual formation. We all need this because I'll tell you a little secret. If you are married, when you get married, the most important thing for you to know about that person you married is that you got married to a sinner. Then the other thing you need to know is that, if you're married, the person you married, married a sinner.

Paul wrote this to the church in Colossae: "When Christ … shows up again…" Jesus is coming back again. "…you'll show up, too—the real you, the glorious you." Colossians 3:4 (MSG). Now, this is a fabulous idea.

What Paul is saying here is that there are two "yous."

There is the current you. There's sinful you, flawed you, messed-up you, junked-up you, immature you, but then there's glorious you.

The glorious you is "you" as God intended you to be!

The glorious you is the "you" with all the sin and junk purged away.

Now, when you fall in love, part of what happens is you get a little glimpse of the glorious you, the person you've fallen in love with. That's why falling in love is kind of a gift of grace. We can't control it, but part of what's going on is we get this glimpse of the glorious person God created that other person to be. You fall in love with them, and you get married to them. Who are you married to when you marry them—the glorious or the current sinful them? Well, you married the current sinful them, and you see them so close up that you cannot help but see the junk and the flaws and the "messed-upness." Every person is imperfect, and every single person will cause you to want to push them away, dump them, or leave them.

Every relationship demands an effort to keep it on the right track; there is constant tension between the forces that hold you together and those that tear you apart.

The trick to making love last is to discover—and to continue to discover—reasons for staying together—and it starts with you being a child of God, and your purpose is to glorify God. If you want to fight, fight for the marriage, not each other.

Again, the Bible is clear about this. The Bible often warns people, basically saying be careful when choosing who you're going to marry. This is one such verse, and there are a lot of them. It is rich: "A nagging spouse is like the drip, drip, drip of a leaky faucet; you can't turn it off, and you can't get away from it" (Proverbs 27:15–16, MSG).

Welcome to marriage!

That's in the Bible.

I go to the dermatologist every three months because I have bad skin, and it got damaged a lot from getting sunburned. Every time I go there, the dermatologist has this magnifying glass and this compelling light. He goes over every pore. Every time he sees another flaw, I hear, "Hmm. Hmm. Hmm. Hmm." It gets depressing. I can't count them after a while. Being married is like going to the dermatologist. By the very nature of the closeness of marriage, we get naked (emotionally, spiritually, physically) and we become vulnerable. Our spouse sees us without the makeup and clothes of the day. They see the warts and moles we like to hide. We don't like to get close to people because they see stuff in us that we don't want them to see, that we spend most of our lives trying to hide from other people. This is the human condition. There's an old noir detective writer, Raymond Chandler, who has a line in one of his books that I love. This hard-boiled detective sees a blonde, and he says, *"From thirty feet away, she looked like a lot of class. From ten feet away, she looked like something made up to be seen from thirty feet away."*[36]

I love that because that's all of us. We're all made up to be seen from thirty feet away.

Marriage is the great flaw detector.

See, marriage doesn't create flaws; it exposes flaws. It reveals flaws.

The task of marriage is not primarily "Make me happy." So please don't put the keys to your happiness in their pocket. It's to help as God is turning the current sinful me into a glorious me.

It's glorious, but it isn't easy.

Almost everyone will one day wake up next to their partner and think, "What was I thinking marrying this person?" But if you have the right kind of love, agape love, which is a stubborn love, you can make it work. Why? You begin to realize over time with your marriage partner that you *will have many relationships within your one relationship.* You will fall in and out of love with your partner over time (and perhaps many times). The shift and balance of power and roles in the relationship may change as you two navigate different life stages, and, almost certainly, you will feel ebbs and wanes of attraction to them. Who you fell in love with in the early days of your relationship may change, and likely so will you, as well as how your partner feels toward you. That's okay as long as you two are willing to grow and get to know the new versions of your partner over time. We have to ask ourselves the question: What would a person who's bringing glory to Jesus Christ and thankful to God the Father through him, what would that person do? Ok, I'm going to choose to live that way. Why? Because knowing who you are determines everything about your relationships!

I am going to be all about letting my identity determine my activity!

Listen, this is critical to your relationships:

Knowing whose you are and who you are!

I am a child of God. I am here to give God glory. What gives God glory? An amazing marriage between Renee and me that is full of forgiveness. That gives God glory. I want the kind of marriage that when people see Renee and I together, they say, "God is a good

36 *Quotes from Raymond Chandler's Writing.* Chandlerisms - Quotes. (n.d.). https://www.shamustown.com/quotes.html

God to bring these two hearts together! I want them to see the forgiveness, grace, and love of Jesus between our hearts."

Let us remind ourselves who we are, children of God, who *He says* we are, not how *we feel we* are. We will let that lead to our daily lives; *our identity determines our activity.*

So this means, as a Christian in a marriage, God's word says, "[Love] keeps no record of wrongs" (1 Corinthians 13:5, NIV).

If I am going to be a Christian husband, it means I need to have a short memory of my wife's wrongs and vice versa. Proverbs 17:9 (TLB) says, "Love forgets mistakes; nagging about them parts the best of friends." So when our spouse does something stupid, we will not (for the next twenty years) remind them that what they did was stupid on April 8th, 1999. Right? We don't say, here it is, honey, your mistake from twenty years ago. I brushed off the dust from the file. I played part-time archaeologist, and I rediscovered this and dug it back up right now so we don't have to address our current issues!

In a good marriage, there are no part-time archaeologists; the past stays buried!

Because my identity as a Christian means I am a forgiver. I am going to let that determine my activity—i.e., forgiving.

See, regarding my marriage, I am more concerned about having a future with Renee than declaring a winner in our past! While her forgiving me for something I did twenty years ago won't change the past, it sure enlarges and makes possible our future.

Does anyone remember God's calling on Jeremiah? Jeremiah was stressing that he didn't have the goods to do what God called. Do you remember what God told Jeremiah? He said, I can't preach; I'm too young. I can't do this; I'm not a good enough speaker. God said, Jeremiah, "Before I formed you in the womb, I knew you" (Jeremiah 1:5, NIV). We're dealing with something outside of our ability here. "I knew you before you were in the womb, before you were even born. This is a big word; I sanctified you." The word sanctified is the Greek word *Hagiaz*—not Haagen-Dazs, that's a delicious frozen treat. It's *Hagiaz*, which means *set apart*. I mean, that's special. It's the China that you only bust out on Thanksgiving. If something's been set apart, it's reserved for a particular use, reserved for royal use. God told Jeremiah and spoke to you, for you are a chosen generation. You are a royal priesthood. You are God's special people called out of darkness into marvelous light that you may proclaim his praises. You are Holy. You have been called Holy by the blood of Jesus shed for you. God sees you as Holy. So now I'm not trying to do something to be something. I remember I am something; therefore, I get to do something from the response.

A Christian's life aims to bring your conduct up to the level of your calling, not vice versa. Religion says to "do" and you can "be." God says you already are; now live out of that truth. Live out of that every single day. Remember, God has a purpose and plans for your life, including when you say, "I do!"

God only gives good gifts. Every perfect gift comes down from the father of lights in whom there is no variation or shadow of turning. So, marriage is good. Marriage is a gift from a good God. Proverbs 18, and, again, take anything Solomon says with a grain of salt. He was the wisest man ever, yet he had over 1000 wives. His life was a total hot mess. What am I to do with that? You're to do this. God can draw a straight line with a crooked stick. God used Solomon to give us great truth even though he needed to read a bit more of what he wrote after writing it. "He who finds a wife (notice it's singular Solomon) finds a good thing." "He who finds a wife finds a good thing, and obtains" what? "Favor from the Lord" (Proverbs 18:22, NKJV).

I can believe one day at a time, one step at a time, as I ask myself: How do I give glory and honor to God in what I'm about to do? How will God participate in and work it all out? When it happens, it's his Favor, his goodness in my love life. Again, if you are single and trying to find someone, maybe God is saying trust me more. Trust me more, and work on yourself to become the right person so you are ready when God gives you a person. I'll go along for the ride. I still have a part to play, but I trust he's working it out.

The Third Way to Make Love Better: Remember No One is Completely Compatible!

If you love God with all your heart and then do as you please, you can find love.

This means I love God and trust that God will help me prepare my heart. I will work to keep my heart ready for love throughout the relationship. There's all this pressure in our society to find someone and not be single. You can be single and be happy—Jesus was!

If we remove the pressure we're trusting, we can rest in God. And in due time and season, he'll bring it to pass if that's God's will for us and if we work for it. It also takes away the rushing that I often see in Christian engagement. I feel like there are a lot of times when people say to me, I've never had a love like this pastor. You don't understand, we have to get married now! And I'm thinking: "Hey, slow your roll. Have you thought about premarital counseling?" No. You're trying to keep us from each other. You don't understand. But have you talked about it? Have you thought about it? Have you worked it out? No, that doesn't matter. It won't be an issue for us. No. None of the marriage or family of origin issues will be a problem. No talks about finances could be good, and comparing notes on strategy for childbearing? No. What will sustain you? Love. Just love, pastor. Oh, God. You grimace on the inside like you're watching a car accident happen in slow motion. Just this rushing, this pressure, you need to get married. Hold on—pause. Should you make it to eighty and get married at thirty—that's fifty years. Maybe three or four pre-marriage sessions about money, sex, and kids might be good! Oh, Pastor, we want to be married. We want to unpack the stuff from Williams-Sonoma. We want to cuddle together. We rush, but we can take that pressure off because we need to give enough time to find out if what they advertise online or who they are is just excellent creative writing and fiction. Do they know they have a God-given purpose? Anybody can suck it in for a minute, but we need to give enough time and not be in a rush to the altar. What do you do under pressure? Is there a temper there? So we're taking the pressure off of rushing to the altar, giving time to see who they are, but we're also stretching that period out almost infinitely. The other side of the spectrum is that sort of dating and engagement that's everlasting, and this engagement goes on and on because you want to make sure, based on what you saw with your parents' divorce, that they are the one. So, we're almost too nit-picky about that. I wouldn't say I like the way they eat their soup. We just might not be compatible. I like it. Are you guys still engaged? Yep. See you at the same time next year. All right. Are you still engaged? Yep. Right? It's almost like a mini marriage with no end and no sense. Couples are dating forever today, like they are afraid of commitment. I do weddings today, where they have been together ten years, have three kids, two cars, and a house, and now we can get married. Huh? I just officiated a wedding of a couple engaged for fifteen years.

"No two people are compatible."

Newsflash.

Some people are the wrong person to marry. Everyone else is still naturally incompatible!

You know who gets along with me, me.

You know who I never irritate, me.

My wife and I are incompatible. She's a turtle. I am a gorilla. I had to learn to speak turtle, crawl into her shell, and find out what makes her tick. She had to learn to beat her chest and fight like a reformed gorilla. What animal are you in the marriage?

Compatibility. Ha!

We do not agree at all on the volume of anything being played.

I want it loud.

She wants it soft.

We don't always agree on how we should pressure our kids when they don't want to do something they should do. And I'm of the kick the baby bird out of the nest, and they'll learn to fly on the way to the ground kind of variety. And she's more of the, "Oh, how are you doing? Can I give you a hug?" variety. "And hey, honey, I paid the kids' Discover bill again, okay?"

We have different thoughts on how the house feels and what we should do. And we're incompatible in a million different ways. And you know what? Thirty years into being incompatible in many ways, we are still both running toward the same God and fulfilling the purpose he put in our lives. And our sex is better than ever, our friendships better than ever, we work together, and that's better than ever. We're watching God do incredible things, but we are completely incompatible in many different ways. Renee's idea of a good time is on the couch alone, reading a book. My idea of a good time is having thirty friends at my house tonight to laugh and eat together. That's the problem with an Amazon order approach. This is precisely the kind of girl I'm interested in. But we both know we have a purpose, and it's not about us; it's about giving God the glory. How would dating and married life look different if it was all about giving God glory?

The Fourth Way to Make Love Better: Be A Curious Scholar of the One You Love!

You've got to be a scholar to try and understand what makes this person tick. What are we to study about our spouses and our significant others? Listen to me—everything.

Become an expert in your husband. Keep a note about your wife on your phone. What's her love language? What's her spiritual gift? What's her fighting style? What makes her smile? What makes her frown? What makes his day? When do you see the light in their eyes? Be a full-fledged PhD in your spouse. Study them. Love like a scholar would. What if someone was launching an investigation into your spouse? Pretend you are a private investigator, but don't stalk them, be curious. You have this person. And you know what? We can become blind to things we see every day. We can take them for granted. What did your spouse wear yesterday? We just become blind and get stuck in a routine and a rut when it comes to home. Do a staycation. Investigation. Do you know what their favorite kind of coffee is? Do you know what kind of toaster strudel your spouse likes every morning? I do—strawberry with extra glaze.

It's an old story: A man went to the sheriff's department to report that his wife was missing. "My wife is missing," he reported to the desk sergeant. "She went shopping yesterday and has not come home." The sergeant asked: "What is her height?" The man said, "Gee, I'm not sure. A little over five feet tall, I suppose." The sergeant asked, "What about her weight?" The man looked helpless. "Don't know," he said. "Not slim, not fat." The sergeant asked, "What's the color of her eyes?" The man answered, "Never noticed." "The color of her hair?" the sergeant asked. "It changes a couple of times a year," said the man. "Maybe dark brown." "What was she wearing?" the sergeant asked. "Could have been a skirt or shorts," said the man. "I don't remember exactly." The sergeant asked, "What kind of car did she go in?" The man said, "She went in my truck." "What kind of truck is it?" the sergeant asked. The man glowed and said, "It's a brand-new 2017 Ford F150 King Ranch 4x4. It has custom leather seats and Bubba floor mats. It has a heavy-duty towing package with gold hitch, a DVD with navigation, a 21-channel CB radio, six cup holders, and four power outlets." Then he paused for a moment. "My wife put a small scratch on the driver's door," he said. At this point, the husband started choking up. "Don't worry," the sergeant reassured him sympathetically. "We'll find your truck."

You are in trouble if you know more about your truck than your wife and men. Come on. Be a student of the person God has placed in your life. Psychologists and physiologists call the phenomenon HABITUATION. We must avoid it in our marriages, taking each other for granted.

Imagine you are in your backyard when you hear a loud banging noise from your neighbor's yard. The unusual sound immediately draws your attention, and you wonder what is happening or what might be making the noise. Over the next few days, the banging noise continues regularly and constantly. Eventually, you tune out the noise. This is an example of habituation in perception. It's not only sound that prompts us to become habituated. Habituation can also affect other senses, such as eyesight or smell. Another example would be spritzing on some cologne before you leave for work in the morning. You know what I wear as a pastor. The only cologne a pastor should wear is Eternity! After a short period, you no longer notice the scent of your perfume, but others around you may notice the smell even after you've become unaware of it. We are "used" to it. Habituated. Habituation is growing so accustomed to something that we no longer even realize they are with us. You are just scrolling on your phone, not paying attention to them at the restaurant!

In the same way, we can get habituated to needy people or the homeless people we see on our drive to work every day, and we can get habituated when it comes to the loves of our lives. We lose compassion for people experiencing homelessness because we can't solve it all, and we lose compassion for our spouses because we can't seem to make it work. We get compassion fatigue from habituation and from giving up. We take them for granted. We don't even know what kind of coffee they like. Their work wife knows more about them than you do. This is why you must study, ask, learn, and care. You can't take care of something if you don't know what makes it tick. Part of what happens is people allow their hearts to get compassion fatigue; once our hearts are tired, our relationships suffer.

I started 2024 with a phone call. Here's how it went: "Pastor, I feel like I am being pulled in 1,000 directions. You ever feel like that?" I'm just being pulled in 1,000 directions. There's a great line in Tolkien's Lord of the Rings where a fatigued Bilbo Baggins talks to Gandalf at the end of this old time on Earth. He's just trying to explain how exhausted and depleted he is, and the line is: "*I feel thin. I feel like stretched like butter scraped over too much bread.*"[37] Does anybody feel like that? Do you have more bread left at the end of your butter when it comes to your time? Just so much to do. When it comes to your finances, there are just so many things, so many things, so many things. There's a fatigue we feel when it comes to our attention, compassion fatigue, which is *that I am out of "cares" today*! But when it comes to my heart, when it comes to enthusiasm, so many things we should care about, it just feels like, my gosh, I'm just depleted.

Ensure you have enough butter for the bread of your marriage and relationships!

---

37 Rubin, G. (2015, July 29). *Butter Scraped Over Too Much Bread.* Psychology Today. https://www.psychologytoday.com/us/blog/the-happiness-project/201507/butter-scraped-over-too-much-bread

Do you want a better marriage? A better relationship? Have a curious heart.

Curiosity is a superpower of love! This is why Einstein once said, "Imagination is more important than knowledge. Knowledge is limited. Imagination encircles the world."[38] Renee and I have been through some things and seen some things. We've been with each other for over 30 years. I'll give you a little confession, and I'm not proud of this, but I've been ridiculously frustrated with myself lately. And maybe some of you can relate, but I'm just not happy with how I've responded to so much happening in the world. I am not satisfied with what is going on with this horrible war in Ukraine. With all the world events that are taking place, I am a Christian and a pastor. I should be full of faith, but I have been unsettled, which is a spiritual way of saying I've been worried. I'm baptizing the word a little bit. I have been anxious and trying to trust God, but I haven't been feeling comfortable with what I've been seeing.

To add insult to injury, I've been way too self-centered in my leadership and caring for people. I want to be a servant, and I want to be others-focused, but I've just been too busy with myself. On top of that, I've been inconsistent, meaning I have a lot of goals to improve, become better, and be more like Christ. And then I can crush it for a little while, and then I fall back, and I try not to work too much, and I don't, and then I do. And I try to be loving at work, and I am, and then I come home, and I'm impatient. And I'm just not proud of my inconsistencies. And then, on top of all of that, some of you wouldn't understand this, but I'm just really aware of my mortality. I look like I'm 28, but I am aging so fast. (smile) My eyesight is just like going. On the iPad I preach with, I might have the font so big that I may have three words on the page before long. I've got prescriptions. I don't even know how to pronounce what they are. I'm not even sure what they're for. And I drink a lot of water, like all the time. I have to go to the bathroom so much, and it's embarrassing. Renee is starting to treat me like a grandkid, saying, *"Hey, you need to go potty before we leave?"* I'm like, "Lay off me, and maybe I do! It's none of your business." If any of you can relate, say Amen!

But Renee, like a good turtle, taught me the power of curiosity. She is always curious about what ails me, and she knows about me! Curiosity spells love. You are curious about what you care about.

You want some great marriage advice. Be curious.

Curiosity, curiosity, like, what's that? Do you know how kids are curious? What's that? Why's the sky blue? Why can't I eat Twinkies all day? All two-year-olds say, What's that? No one has to teach them it. They're just curious because they don't know anything. I always tell parents to relax. Your kid knows nothing, and neither do you. You'll figure it out together. So, curiosity, curiosity like a child! Jesus said, if you want to be great in God's kingdom, be like a child. If you want to be great in your marriage, be

38 Nilsson, J. (2018, August 24). *Albert Einstein: "imagination is More Important Than knowledge."* The Saturday Evening Post.
https://www.saturdayeveningpost.com/2010/03/imagination-important-knowledge/

curious. If your spouse goes freaking out, be curious about it. *Instead of responding to the energy they meet you with, be curious. What's going on here? That seems like a two-alarm fire, yet it's like an eight-alarm response. Why do we have a SWAT team in our driveway?* We were burning the waffles. You know what I'm saying? Like, hold on a second. But instead of meeting it at the eight-alarm fire, ask yourself: I wonder what's the thing under the thing? Because anger is a secondary emotion, there's probably some hurt behind the hurt! It would help if you shifted from responding with *fire to fire to with curiosity to fire.* Are they tired? Are they worn out from a long week? Do I need to have some curiosity-based compassion here? A gorilla responds to fire with fire, but a turtle sticks their head out of its shell and asks: How can I help? What's going on here? Renee taught me to shift into curious mode. I'm putting on my curiosity hat. If it keeps you from divorce court, I say you do it, ok? Say something like, "So, I am curious, what's going on here?" Try to figure out what's provoking them. Ask yourself, *What could I have done? How might I have played a role in this?*

Be curious about your responsibility and how your heart, perspective, and happiness belong to you. Again, don't place the keys to your happiness in your spouse's pocket.

How could I be complicit in this? Curiosity, be curious about yourself. Be interested in your spouse. It's a superpower. Have you ever been to Napa Valley and sipped some wine, friends? Come on, I am not Baptist! Renee and I did when we lived in California. I learned that the vine owners were always curious when I was there. Curiosity leads to better wine in your marriage. Did you know that Napa Valley hires NASA companies and NASA subcontractors? Wineries will hire NASA-based companies that typically study the surface of Mars and the moon using thermal and other technologies. They send planes up into the air to study the ground. They're looking for water. They're looking for this on the planets. And so they send these planes up to 10,000 feet, and they take these incredible pictures of Napa Valley. *Why? They are curious. They want to understand the soil, what's under the ground, and how topography and sun exposure change* grape-growing dynamics. And they say every time they send the plane up, they learn something new about different sections and blocks of their vines. Some areas need more dirt, some need more water, and some require more fertilizer. *Their curiosity leads to better wine! You can't have a "one size fits all" approach to improving your marriage. And you can't also look at what's working for another couple as to what's working for you. You have to hear the spirit of God speaking to you. Be curious; it leads to better wine!* You have to know what your marriage needs. And it starts, I think, like sending that plane up to see what's happening underneath. How do you figure out what's going on underneath your marriage?

So, when was the last time you sent the plane up? When was the last time you checked in with your spouse? How can I be a better husband? What's going on in your heart? How's the soil of our marriage?

As part of curiosity, **every couple should do a weekly check-in and a weekly date night.**

Read that again. Like any good thing, **good marriages require regular maintenance, such as changing the oil, checking the engine light, being curious, looking under the hood once a week, and asking: How can I do better? How can I be better? What do you need from current me?**

Don't mix up the two—the weekly date night and weekly check-in.

The weekly check-in that's like going to the dermatologist.

The weekly date night that's chips and queso, wine, and a hotel room!

Have you ever seen someone super triggered and all excited in an airport, miss their flight, and they are yelling at the agents? You think—what a jerk. But if you're curious, you think—*I wonder if their wife is in the hospital?* Curiosity helps you to be excellent. I wonder if they just lost their job because if they're belligerent and yelling at the hostess at Chili's, chances are things aren't going great in their life. You know what I'm saying? *If you start being curious, it puts you in a greater place of empathy.*

The Fifth Way to Make Love Better: Accept Each Other as an Unconditional Gift from God!

When did you last argue about a sunset, sunrise, or rainbow? I wouldn't say I like all that purple or orange here. When did you last argue with a sunny or rainy day? You accept each day as a gift. Likewise, you have to take each person God has placed in your life as a gift and then look for the gifts in them.

Don't marry or commit to someone and then say now that we are married; I will try to change them.

This is the person you chose. Can all people grow and change? They can grow and become your soulmate. They can grow and become a more loving spouse, but global personality shifts, like taking a turtle and asking them to be a gorilla, nah. You are not making an introvert turn into an extrovert. They were good enough to marry, so don't expect them to change now.

Don't give up who you are for the person you're with.

It will only backfire and make you both miserable.

Have the courage to be who you are, and most importantly, let your partner be who they are.

Those two people fell in love with each other in the first place. I am saying to have realistic expectations about your relationship and romance. You will not be gaga over each other every single day for the rest of your lives, and all this 'happily ever after' Disney fairy-tale is just setting people up for failure. They go into relationships with these unrealistic expectations. Then, when they realize they aren't 'gaga' anymore, they think the relationship is broken and over and need to get out. No! There will be days, weeks, or maybe even longer when you aren't all mushy-gushy in love. You're even going to wake up some morning and think, "Ugh, you're still here…." That's normal! And more importantly, sticking it out is worth it because in a day, or a week, or maybe even longer, you'll look at that person, and a giant wave of love will inundate you, and you'll love them so much you think your heart can't possibly hold it all and is going to burst. Because a love that's alive is also constantly evolving and growing!

It expands and contracts and mellows and deepens. It won't be how it used to be, and it shouldn't be. It's going to be better as you work to make it better! If more couples understood that, they'd be less inclined to panic and rush to break up or divorce. Did you know that in ancient times, people considered love a sickness? Parents warned their children against it, and adults quickly arranged marriages before their children were old enough to do something dumb on the back of their out-of-control emotions. That's because love—though able to make us feel giddy and high, as though we had snorted a shoebox full of cocaine—can also make us highly irrational. We all know that guy who dropped out of school, sold their car, and spent the money to elope on the beaches of Tahiti. We all also know how that same guy ended up creeping back a few years later, feeling like a moron, not to mention broke. Unbridled love like that is nature's way of tricking us into doing insane and irrational things to remember to procreate. If we stopped long enough to think about the repercussions of having kids—not to mention being with the same person forever and ever—few would ever do it. It's been rumored that the late and great Robin Williams once said, because it's true: "God gave man a brain and a penis and only enough blood to operate one at a time."

Blind romantic love is a trap designed to get two people to overlook each other's faults long enough to do some baby-making. It generally only lasts for a few years at most. That dizzying high you get staring into your lover's eyes as if they are the stars that make up the heavens—yeah, that mostly goes away. Once it's gone, you must know you've buckled down with a human you genuinely respect and enjoy being with. Otherwise, things will get rocky. True love is deep, the kind of abiding love that is impervious to emotional whims of feelings.

True love is a constant commitment to a person regardless of present circumstances. It's a continuous commitment to someone you understand isn't always going to make you happy, nor should they be! That form of love is much harder because it often feels bad. It's unglamorous. It's lots of early morning doctor's visits. It's cleaning up bodily fluids you'd rather not be cleaning up. It's dealing with another person's insecurities and fears even when you don't want to. During COVID, my wife cleaned up my vomit with Clorox Clean Up, and I told her that's enough bleach; I can still smell, and she discovered she had COVID because she could not smell it. (Smile)

But this form of love is also far more satisfying and meaningful. And it brings true happiness, not just another series of highs. True love knows: "Happily ever after doesn't just happen!" Every day you wake up and *decide* to love your partner and your life—the good, the bad, and the ugly. Some days, it's a struggle, and some days, you feel like the luckiest person in the world. Most people never reach this deep, unconditional love. They get addicted to the ups and downs of romantic love. They are in it for the "feels," so to speak. And when the feels run out, so do they. Some people get into a relationship to compensate for something they lack or hate within themselves. This is a one-way ticket to a toxic relationship because it makes your love conditional. You will only love your partner if they help you feel better about yourself. You will give to them *only as long* as they give to you. You will make them happy *only as long* as they make you happy. This conditionality prevents any true, deep-level intimacy from emerging and chains the relationship to each person's internal dramas.

The Sixth Way to Make Love Better: Take Responsibility!

Take responsibility for your heart and your relationships! Have you taken responsibility for your marriage? Or is it just all out of your control? **I have a red flag I throw up when I hear people talking about their marriage as though it's like an inanimate object they're not connected to. Oh, my marriage is not going well. You're half of that, right? Oh, you know, my marriage is in shambles. I don't know how it's going to go. Like, so you have no control?** Ah, I just fell out of love with her. If you fall out of your truck, don't you stand up and get back in it? You don't just abandon it by the side of the road. You've invested time and money in that truck. Your relationships are you. Marriage is you. How are you? What are you doing? What are you going to do?

Oh, the coins all fell out. Pick 'em up. Right? Take some responsibility. No one can love your husband for you. No one can take your wife to bed or lose her forever but you. And if you don't take her to bed, someone will. If you don't date your mate, the devil will find someone who will. It would help if you took responsibility for your life. It would help if you took responsibility for your future. It would help if you took responsibility. Unless the Lord builds the house, the builders build in vain. But you still have to build! You still need to watch. You still need to build. You still need to work. You still need to fight. You still need to forgive. You still need to care. It would help if you still showed up. Are you showing up in your marriage? Take some responsibility. Are you willing to fight for your marriage as hard as you fight with your spouse? Say about your marriage—this won't fail because of me. It might fail, but it will not because of what I did or didn't do. Do your best. Keep fighting. But they might not reciprocate. Do it anyway. But they always… It doesn't matter. Still do it. Be able to say one day, hey, the marriage fell apart, didn't work, but I fought until it was over. And then I fought some more!

The Seventh Way to Make Love Better: Get Good at Fighting!

Your relationship is a living, breathing thing. Much like the body and muscles, it cannot get stronger without stress and challenge. You have to fight. You have to hash things out. Obstacles make the marriage. John Gottman is the best psychologist in the world on relationships and a researcher who has spent over 30 years analyzing married couples, looking for keys to why they stick together (and why they break up). When it comes to why people stick together, he dominates the field. Gottman puts married couples in a room, puts some cameras on them, and then asks them to fight! Notice: he doesn't ask them to discuss how great the other person is. He doesn't ask them what they like best about their relationship. He asks them to fight. They're told to pick something they're having problems with and talk about it for the camera. Gottman then analyzes the couple's discussion (or shouting match) and can predict with startling accuracy whether or not a couple will divorce. But what's most interesting about Gottman's research is that the things that lead to divorce are not necessarily what you might imagine. He found that successful couples, like unsuccessful couples, fight consistently. And some of them fight furiously. Gottman has narrowed down four characteristics of a couple that tend to lead to divorces (or breakups). He has gone on and called these "the four horsemen" of the relationship apocalypse—Criticizing your partner's character ("you're so stupid" vs "that thing you did was stupid"); Defensiveness (or blame-shifting, "I wouldn't have done that if you weren't late all the time"); Contempt (putting down your partner and making them feel inferior) and Stonewalling (withdrawing from an argument and ignoring your partner) So what's the takeaway? Don't avoid conflict; lean into your conflict but get good at fighting and have ground rules for conflict!

Never insult or name-call your partner. Gottman's research found that contempt—belittling and demeaning a partner—is the number one predictor of divorce.[39] Now that you hear that, how many of you have some shutting up to do? Do not bring previous fights/arguments into current ones. Tear up the scorecard! This solves nothing and makes the fight twice as bad as before. Yeah, you forgot to pick up groceries on the way home, but what does his being rude to your mother last Thanksgiving have to do with that or anything? If things get too heated, take a breather. Be able to call a Time Out!

Remove yourself from the situation and return once your emotions have cooled off. This is a big one for me. Sometimes, when things get intense with my wife, I get overwhelmed and leave. I usually walk around the block 2-3 times and let myself seethe for a bit. Then I come back, and we're both a bit calmer. We can resume the discussion with a more conciliatory tone. Remember that being "right" is not as important as both people feeling respected and heard. *You may be correct, but if you are right in such a way that makes your partner feel unloved, there's no real winner.* When people talk about the necessity for "good communication" all the time, this is what they should mean: Be willing to have uncomfortable talks, have fights, and get it all out in the open,

---

39 Lisitsa, E. (2024, June 25). *The Four Horsemen: Contempt.* The Gottman Institute. https://www.gottman.com/blog/the-four-horsemen-contempt

but do it lovingly. This is why the Bible says: "Speak the truth in love" (Ephesians 4:15, NLT). It's not avoiding the truth out of love!

The Eighth Way to Make Love Better: If You Are Going to Be First at Anything in Your Marriage, Be First to Forgive!

You can always come in first if you are the first to seek forgiveness.

When you end up being right about something, then shut up. You can be right and be quiet at the same time. Your partner will already know you're right and feel loved knowing you didn't wield it like the sword of shame!

In marriage, there's no such thing as winning an argument because there is no I or you, just we!

Perhaps the most interesting nugget from Gottman's research is that most successful couples don't resolve all their problems. His findings were completely backward from what most people expect. People in lasting and happy relationships have problems that never completely go away, while couples who feel they need to agree and compromise on everything end up feeling miserable and falling apart. This comes back to the respect thing. If two different individuals share a life, they will inevitably have different values and perspectives on some things and clash over them. The key here is not to change the other person—as the desire to change your partner is inherently disrespectful (to both them and yourself)—but rather it's to abide by the difference, love them despite it, *and when things get a little rough around the edges, to forgive them for it.*

Everyone says compromise is vital, but that's not how my baby doll and I see it. It's more about seeking understanding. Compromise is usually nonsense, leaving both sides unsatisfied, losing little pieces of themselves to get along. On the other hand, refusing to compromise is just as much of a disaster because you turn your partner into a competitor ("I win, you lose"). These are the wrong goals because they're outcome-based rather than process-based. When your goal is to find out where your partner is coming from—to truly understand on a deep level—you can't help but be altered by the process. Conflict becomes much easier to navigate because you see the context. It needs to be clarified, or I've preached before that the key to happiness is not achieving your lofty dreams or experiencing some dizzying high but finding the struggles and challenges you enjoy enduring. It's an inside job. It's your responsibility, just like having a forgiving heart. Relationships are the same: your perfect partner is not someone with no problems. Instead, your ideal partner has issues you feel good about dealing with.

But how do you get good at forgiveness? How do we become the first to seek forgiveness?

What does that mean?

When an argument is over, it's over.

Baby Doll and I have gone as far as to make this the golden rule in our relationship. When you're done fighting, it doesn't matter who was right and wrong; it doesn't matter if someone was mean and nice; it's over. And you both have to agree to leave it there and not bring it up every month for the next hundred years.

There's no scoreboard.

No one is trying to "win." There's no—"You owe me this because you screwed up the laundry last week." There's no—"I'm always right about financial stuff, so you should listen to me." There's no—"I bought her three gifts, and she only did me one favor."

Everything in the relationship should be given and done unconditionally, *without expecting reward or manipulating feelings*.

When your partner screws up, you separate the intentions from the behavior. You recognize what you love and admire in your partner and understand that they were doing the best they could yet mess up out of ignorance. This happened *not* because they're a bad person, *not* because they secretly hate you and want to divorce you, *not* because there's somebody else in the background pulling them away from you. They are a good person—that's why you are with them. If you ever lose faith in their goodness, you will begin to erode your belief in yourself.

The Ninth Way to Make Love Better: Remember, the Little Things Always Add Up to the Big Things!

Pick your battles *wisely*.

You and your partner only have so many cares to give.

Make sure you both are saving them for the real cares that matter. I talked to one gentleman this past week who's been happily married for forty-plus years. I asked him, "What's the best advice you can give a preacher preaching forgiveness?"

He said, "Choose your battles. Some things matter and are worth getting upset about. Most do not. Argue over the little things, and you'll find yourself arguing endlessly; little things pop up all day, taking a toll over time. Like Chinese water torture: minor in the short term, corrosive over time. Consider: is this a little thing or a big thing? Is it worth the cost of arguing?"

The Bible says the little things add up to the big things when it says, "Catch the foxes for us, the little foxes that spoil *and* ruin the vineyards [of love]" (Song of Solomon 2:15, AMP)

Speaking of little foxes that can destroy our love, the biggest "little thing" that can kill love today is a cell phone!

If you touch, respond to, interact with, scroll, and troll with this phone more than you feel, interact with, and respond to your partner, you are doing it wrong!

It's just a little phone, scrolling and distracting. It's four hours a day, the average screen time a person spends. Most people are more committed to their phones than their spouses. Try spending four hours daily with your spouse rather than screen time. *If you don't take the time to meet for lunch, go for a walk, or go out to dinner and a movie with some regularity, then you end up with a roommate.* Staying connected through life's ups and downs is critical. *Eventually, your kids grow up, your obnoxious brother-in-law will join a monastery, and your parents will die. When that happens, guess who's left? You got it—Mr./Mrs. Right!*

You don't want to wake up twenty years later and stare at a stranger because life broke the bonds you formed before the storms started. Don't ever stop doing the little things. They add up. *Put the phone down at dinner time, look at each other, talk to each other. Look into each other's eyes. Say I love you every day. I took my wife out to eat on our date night and read her a list of ten things I love about her! Do you know how much that did to bond us, unite us, smooth over the week we had?* Holding hands during a movie, doing the dishes, putting the toilet seat down, making the bed, mowing the lawn, and kissing: All these little things matter and add up over the long run. *Pay attention to how you greet each other when you walk in the door; it sets the tone for the evening.*

This becomes particularly important once kids enter the picture. The big message here is to put marriage first. Children are worshipped in our culture, and parents are expected to sacrifice everything for them. However, the best way to raise healthy and happy kids is to maintain a healthy and happy marriage. Good kids don't make a good marriage; a good marriage makes good kids. So, keep your marriage the top priority.

The Tenth Way to Make Love Better: Make Sure Your Partner Never Feels Invisible!

I had a conversation with a lovely person in our church. She's been going through a tough time, a difficult time of divorce and all that it entails. Whose friends are his friends, and which friends are your friends? How will the kids and grandchildren respond to me when I get divorced? A lot of collateral damage and collateral hurts come alongside a divorce. It got to a point where she said something compelling to me. She says: "Pastor, sometimes I just want to scream, 'Here I am!' Because I feel so invisible these days."

Have you ever felt invisible?

Does it matter if I get out of bed today? Will anyone miss me? I imagine the widow or widower might feel that way sometimes. Sometimes I have felt that way. I was reminded of a song by Joshua Kadison called "The Invisible Man." He sings about how he woke up and, instead of feeling alive, he felt like he was "disappearing so [he] ran to the mirror to check it out." And he looks at himself and asks, "Why do I feel like the invisible man?" Later in the song, he says, "Sometimes I think we all need to say, 'Here I am, here I am, here I am.'" Why? Because "life makes us feel like the invisible man." There's so much in life that can make you feel like a number instead of a child of God.

I still remember the phone call. It was the day after we buried my mom. Renee's dad told me that Renee's mom had passed. I kept saying on the phone, "Oh no, don't say that...don't say that..." If the words were taken back, it would change reality. I was already lost in grief, and now Renee was as well. Renee lost two moms that week. She said to me one night the week we buried her mom:

"I feel invisible. I feel like I am trying to be everything to everyone, but nobody is trying to be anything to me." "I feel depressed," I confessed in return. "When my mom died, it's like a part of me died too." We ping-ponged confessions back and forth that night through tears until I was struck with a startling realization. I couldn't rescue my wife. And she couldn't rescue me. We each desperately wanted to be healed, loved, noticed, and understood in that season, but our eyes were turned sideways instead of upward. We were both looking for a Savior, something we would never find in each other. There is no substitute for Jesus. When we look to a spouse, a friend, a child, or an Internet audience for the love, healing, and recognition only a Savior can offer, we'll always come up short!

Are you feeling invisible today?

Unnoticed and unseen, desperate for someone to meet you exactly where you are?

> You are not invisible.
> You are valuable.
> You are a helper.
> You are a hope dealer.
> You are a lover of their soul.
> God wants you and a relationship with you.

One of God's names in the Bible is El Roi; it translates to the God who sees you even when you feel invisible. Roi in the original Hebrew can be translated as shepherd or seeing, looking, or gazing. In other words, when we think that we are most invisible and forgotten by everyone else, we can remember that God does see us. He sees you and hears your cry. If you think that you are too naked, ashamed, and afraid to come to him, he looks at you and sees Jesus.

I remember reading this verse and feeling God wrap his arms around me: "Look up toward the sky. Who created everything you see? The Lord causes the stars to come out at night one by one. He calls out each one of them by name. His power and strength are great. So none of the stars is missing" (Isaiah 40:26, NIRV).

Whether you're crying in the bathroom at seven a.m., folding the ninth load of laundry at 7 p.m., rocking your baby at three a.m., or walking out onto your back porch, you are ready to scream, "Here I am, Here I am." Please rest in this: God sees you, God notices you, God loves you. Every single minute of every single day, you are fully known and loved by Him. After all, if God calls out every star in the sky by name, how much more must He know and love you?

The cure for feeling invisible?

Receive God's unconditional love and give God's love unconditionally.

It's hard to talk about unconditional love because everyone thinks it has limits! No.

Love is stronger than cancer, death, or anything we know of. Even 1 Corinthians 13:13 (NIV) in the book of faith says, "And now these three remain: faith, hope and love. But the greatest of these is love."

The book of faith says love is greater than faith!

If you look at your life, perhaps the answer is yes: love has limits. But if you look at Jesus's life, the answer is *no*. Jesus loved and touched and healed those with leprosy. Jesus loved indiscriminately. I am good at loving with discrimination. I am good at loving those who I know can do something for me. Jesus loved someone when they could not do anything for him or love him back. That's love. Jesus loved everyone because he saw everyone as a child of God.

Only the eyes of faith will allow us to see everyone that way.

Love's greatest challenge is loving people who are hard to love. Sometimes the ones closest to us are the hardest to love, so we ignore them. We make sure we come home when they are asleep, and they become invisible.

False love is conditional love; it expects something in return. Unconditional love, or true love, loves people regardless. Yet, *there's no section in CVS of the Hallmark cards for loving your enemies, right?*

Everyone becomes visible when you love unconditionally and with agape, especially the one you chose.

What is agape love? This love has been described as unconditional love: love without condition, love that is not earned, love that we did not see coming and did not have coming. It is unexpected. It is unannounced. It is unmerited. It just comes to you.

When you think about it, most love in the human realm is conditional. It's an if/then. If you love me back, do nothing to forfeit my love, or if you're beautiful, if you're something, then I will love or continue to love.

Human love tends to operate because of a feeling of attraction, thankfulness, or some emotion, and the fruit of that emotion is a decision: "Because I feel this way, I will love you." The decision can transcend the emotion, but it's never very far from that emotion. It's the "if" thing: "I feel attraction; therefore, I choose to love you. If I stop feeling attraction, my love will maybe shrink in proportion to that."

You must move on from the "feels" of love to get to the oak barrels of maturity. Nothing good comes fast or easy in life—not food, music, sermons, good scotch, or love.

Agape is not emotionless; it's just that the emotion follows the decision. In other words, the emotion is a fruit of the decision. There's a choice that's been made: I choose to love. Based on that choice, emotion rises. But the choice is fundamental. The choice is a thing that's in place regardless of the emotion. The emotion rides on the decision.

Here's where agape gets very interesting: It's far more stubborn than simply that I choose to love and feel loving.

It pursues the object of its love. People who are chased by love don't feel invisible.

This is why the father is always running in the Prodigal Son story. Running to meet the lost son, his first son, and running to meet the older son when he refused to come to the party (see Luke 15:11–31, NIV).

It is loving even in the face of resistance, even in the face of behavior where another emotion might be more expected.

Agape will love in the face of rebellion, in the face of rejection, in the face of rank badness, in the face of being invisible. This amazing form of love has made a decision, and the decision is final. It's set. Based on that decision, whether it's met with loving, good behavior or not, it continues to pursue love.

Agape is unprovoked love.

Usually, when we hear of something unprovoked, we think of anger, attack, aggression, or violence. When we hear about that unprovoked aggression, we say there was nothing in the victim that in any way had this coming to them. We have to ascribe the act of unprovoked violence to the perpetrator. There's something twisted and wrong in them. There's something broken and skewed in them; they're working out this deep anger, and you just happened to be in the wrong place at the wrong time. It's in them. That's how we account for unprovoked violence.

I want to call agape unprovoked love, which works on the same principle—just in the opposite direction.

What if we spread love like violence?

As with unprovoked violence, when we seek to understand unprovoked love, we look for the explanation not in the object of love but in the one who is loving. We say there must be something going on in them, something deep down that accounts for this act. (Curiosity, anyone?)

God is an agape lover. The Father is a lover who loves what he loves not based on the loveliness of the object but on some quality within himself.

In a sense, he can't help himself, though he does choose it. He loves, 1 John 4:16 (NIV) says, because "God is love."

God is love.

God does not try to love, but God is love. Present tense, continually.

(See 1 John 4:7–16, NIV.)

That's what the Good Book says.

When you truly love someone, you chase them, tell them, run after them, build your life around them, and make sure they are not invisible.

When you run after someone with unprovoked love, they know you care and don't feel invisible or like a roommate!

What if?

What if, beginning today, you treat everyone you love as if they were going to be dead by midnight?

I bet they would not feel invisible if you did.

Can you imagine how that would change how you dealt with others?

Imagine that invisible expiration date on everyone's forehead: tonight at midnight!

What if?

What if you gave them all the care, kindness, and understanding you can, knowing they will be gone soon?

If you did this today, your life will never be the same again!

Just try it for a day and see how it goes.

I guarantee your relationships will improve.

If you do these ten things, you will make love better.

CHAPTER NINE

EVERYONE GETS A BURNING BUSH!

Earth's crammed with heaven, And every common bush afire with God: But only he who sees takes off his shoes.

—Elizabeth Barrett Browning

A PROFESSOR AT THE UNIVERSITY OF Tennessee wanted to see if his syllabus was being read. His name is *Kenyon Wilson*. He felt like none of his students were reading the *syllabus*. Can you imagine a student not paying attention? He tucked an Easter egg into the middle of it: all this stuff about what books to read, and how stuff's going to be graded, and the curve, and blah blah, blah, blah, blah. But then he put some directions in the middle of the syllabus: Go to this common area, and there's a set of lockers. If you go to this locker number, you'll open it. The combination is this, this, this, and there's a little surprise for you. If any of you find it, it's my gift to you. And he was thinking to himself, indeed, they're going to skip through the syllabus. He even told them, so that you know, there's something *special in the syllabus.* It's not just a normal one. You should check this out. Seventy-one of his students nodded their heads, Amen, professor! We'll check it out. We'll read that syllabus.

Final exams came and went, and the whole semester is now over. He went to the locker and spun the combination everyone had had in their hands all semester. And when he opened the door, he still found waiting precisely as it was when he put it in there, the fifty-dollar bill with a note saying basically this: "This goes to any one of you who finds it first along with an A in the course."

All his students had access to the code. All his students knew where the locker was. But none of them bothered to go and open the door.

How often does God try to say to us: Hey, read the syllabus. Is there something special here? Pay attention. God places an "Easter Egg" or a burning bush in everyone's life, but not everyone listens, looks, or pays attention. God is always present; what is lacking is our awareness. God is always calling; what is lacking is our listening. God is always working; what is lacking is our participation with him.

I hope and pray that you will recognize that God has placed something special in the syllabus of life, Jesus.

Jesus said in Revelation 3:20 (NIV) that *"I stand at the door and knock."*

I pray that all of us would open that door and that there would be none of us who think we're okay just because we have the instructions in our hands. It's not enough to know.

You have to act on it. Love, life, living—all three are verbs, not nouns! Could you prove me wrong? How long will you drink from the well of comfort, knowing you are constantly thirsty afterward?

Have you ever thought you would wow someone, and then they go, "Eh?" *(Not impressed)* I remember being sixteen, getting ready for a blind date, combing my hair in the mirror, arrogantly smiling back at my reflection, thinking, *Okay, mystery woman, this is your one big shot to date a true stud. She is going to be impressed. This girl, whoever she is, look out, she will be wowed!* (My parents were overachievers when it came to building my self-esteem.) I went on one blind date, thinking she was going to love me. Look at me—what is not to love? Eh. Let's not date again. I think it became a pattern in my life. Thoughts were going one way, but reality was going another way. I graduated from school, got a master's degree, and had enormous money on the way. Look at my accounts! Eh. Please wake up and fill out my to-do list. I am ready to finish so much, and the day says, "Eh." Show up at work, "Hey, staff, I am here. Let's have a great, productive, amazing day!" Eh. Show up at the gym and play some basketball. "Hey, guys, I am here. Can I get in the next game?" Eh. Got married, come home from work. "Honey, I am home. I know you missed me, give me a kiss!" Eh. Kids, your rockstar dad is home! Eh.

Church here's another sermon that could change your life. Eh. Write a book—it will be more popular than *Fifty Shades of Grey* or *Fifty-One Shades of Do Me Now*. Eh. I woke up one day, fifty years old, looked in the mirror, and said, "Eh."

Can you relate? **Most people don't want to spend their lives fidgeting until they die.** When they reach fifty, most people realize there are fewer Christmas Eves in front of them than behind them, and they don't want to die the second death, the death of being forgotten. We all want to be remembered. That's why we put tombstones up and our names on them. We are all like that twelve-year-old kid carving his name into the desk, carving our names into this world, "I was here!" And we want the world to go, "Wow!" Not, "Eh." But when heading to college, you think differently than when you are fifty. Maybe that's the problem. I was born on a Saturday and in church on Sunday because my mom was the church organist, and my dad was a betting man. He always bet there was a 60 percent chance God existed, so get to church, put some money in the plate, and tell your mom she played well. So, I grew up going to church my whole life, but much of it was empty because I went to earn God's love. It was done out of a kind of religious duty. As I grew up, I got pulled into all sorts of sinful things, especially during college. It's like when my dad was going to college, his mom said to him, warning him: "Son, there are bad girls at college!" My dad said, "Where? What are their names?" I think I said the same thing. I don't want to list my sins or those less-than-holy things but use your imagination. Remember, when I went to school, Southwest Texas (now Texas State University) was ranked the number one party school by the leading authority on parties: Playboy Magazine. I remember reading that one day in between classes. I only looked at the articles, right? Ha! Incidentally, Playboy Magazine was also the first to get Jesus right. You know the Laughing Jesus, the Joyful Jesus! Google it—that great painting of Laughing, Joy filled, and Playboy Magazine first published Joyful Jesus. How did the church mess that one up? Why didn't the church publish that? Didn't they hear Jesus was, first and foremost, a joyful, loving savior? That love and laughter were common in his life? Why does the church prefer to paint this picture of sour-grapes Jesus? I joined the most popular fraternity and had all these "friends" and social life, school grades were straight As, and I remember lying in bed feeling miserable, empty, dead! I was at a crossroads, and the crossroads I was at was where I believe many folks who call themselves Christians end up living, at this address:

I knew too much about God to be happy in the world, but I had too much of the world to be happy with God.

Can you see that in your own life? It's like sitting in two chairs. Eventually, you fall between the two chairs! At some point, you have to pick one chair to sit in, one direction, and one shepherd for your life, and everyone has a shepherd. Everyone has something that points them North or South. For David, he said The Lord is My Shepherd, but for most people, it's money or seeking that WOW factor, validation instead of "eh!" I was trying to figure out that amazing question: What in the world am I doing here? Like beyond, what the hell is my major? My son Zach is going through a similar thing right now. He's in his second year at the prestigious University of Texas. He called me up last week, ready to quit. I told him, "Son, there are no refunds for the money I have spent on your tuition, but more importantly, today comes with no refunds. Today is not your practice life. This is your only shot on this side of heaven. Yesterday went with no refunds. Dreams come with no refunds. There is no money-back or satisfaction guarantee for what you hope to do with your brief 27,373 days this side of heaven. You might get life, liberty, and the pursuit of some happiness right!"

Jefferson, so smart, knew it was merely the pursuit of happiness. It was the chase, not the capture, that is guaranteed. The chase is often more fun than the capture; I mean, what's next right? My son Zach is struggling in college. Not with grades; he's a straight-A student. It's the major—that is the problem. What's the major going to be? What should I do with my life? It's a defining question for most people. "What do you do with your life, or maybe how do you pay the bills?"

I asked someone the other day, "What do you do for a living?" They said, "As little as possible!" Well played. When you are young, you can't wait to grow up. Then, when you are grown up, what do you want to be? *Younger.* Ha! So I told Zach to quit worrying about your major and focus on you and who you are. The focus should not be on what door you go through *but who exactly is walking through the door.* Who are you when all the veneer is peeled away, and you stand there naked? Who are you? When you walk through your chosen door, guess what you find on the other side? You. You take you everywhere; for some, that's the problem. You are not happy with you. Like Popeye used to say, when you see your shortcomings, you say: "I yam what I yam!" He always said it to say, "Hey, don't get your hopes up when it comes to me! It's just me, and I come with *spots,* and I don't think I can grow any *stripes."* Yet God says to you today, as you read these words: *I know who you are. But that's not all you will be! Who you are today is not who you will always be; you can be more. Let's face it:* You can get paid anywhere doing anything, but who you become is always with you. *Who you become is what we will talk about at your funeral.*

Focus on a funeral resume, not a career resume. Who you become is what you take to eternity. You aren't taking your car, your job, or your money. The richness of being is so much better than the richness of having. Who are you becoming? **We are never done becoming, are we? We are never really all grown up. At least, I hope not.** A true story from what was going to be an epic concert in Philadelphia, Pennsylvania, illustrates this. One of the pieces played by the orchestra featured a flute solo. This solo was to be played offstage to sound like it was coming from a great distance. The conductor had instructed the flutist to count the measures precisely to arrive at the exact time. After all, with the flutist offstage, there could be no visual contact between them.

On the night of the performance, when the time came for the flute solo, the flutist counted perfectly and came in precisely at the right time. The light, lilting notes floated out beautifully across the theater. Suddenly, however, there was a terrible shrieking noise, and the soloist went silent. The conductor was outraged. At the end of the piece, he rushed off stage to find the poor flutist. The flutist was ready for him. "Maestro," he said, "before you say anything, let me tell you precisely what happened. You're not going to believe it."

"As you know, I arrived on time, and everything was going beautifully. Then suddenly, this enormous stagehand ran up and grabbed away my flute. Then he pushed me back and snapped at me, 'Shut up, you idiot!' He said, 'Don't you know there's a concert out there?'" The poor flutist. He was only doing what he had been told by playing offstage. Can you relate?

There have been times when I thought I was doing all the right things, and then suddenly, life has taken a sharp turn, and I have been as startled as that flutist. What just happened? Ever been tempted to ask, "What in the world am I doing here?" What does it all mean? What is expected of me? Often, it bleeds over into my role as a pastor. "Things aren't going the way I expected," I think. *"How much does God demand out of me?"* "I thought everyone was going to like me!" I had the confidence to spare when I started ministry. Where did it go? Is it finite? "What do you mean love and pray for my enemies?" "What does it mean to be a Christian in this situation?" Being a Christian means you have to do the right thing regardless of personal feelings. Because it's always kingdom over personality, but sometimes I want to put John ahead of God! It took years to come to these conclusions, and I wasn't there yet in college. See, the real class that was happening was going on in my soul, my heart, and my head. You know that emptiness you feel at two a.m. in the morning? That nagging sense that not all is as it should be? What is the answer to that ache within? To that loneliness, I felt even in the middle of a crowded room. The nagging sense of meaning and purpose you feel as you lie in bed, awake, wondering at night. Why do we all long for glory? Why do we all long to WOW the world when it goes, "Eh." Why do we all love stories about people who sacrifice themselves for the good of others? It all hints and echoes the great story of a Savior who saved what was lost at his own expense.

After seven years of ministry, I quit. I had left the ministry. It's 2001, and I am in sales, and I am making a ton of money; I mean, for me, 16k a month in sales. My first check, take home, was 17k. I was like, there's been a mistake but let me head to the bank right away. I made 200k a year. I don't make that money now. After two years of one hundred-plus hour weeks, never seeing Baby Doll or my kids, I was lying awake at three in the morning, stressed, miserable, overworked, and fat because I never went to the gym; I mean fatter than I am now, and sad, because I knew God did not call me to sell. He called me to be a hope dealer. I remember thinking about my life plans and dreams and how they had not gone as planned. What did Mike Tyson, the infamous boxer, say? Everyone has a plan until they get punched in the face. Life has a way of punching us in the face more than once.

So I laid in bed, not the walking dead but spiritually dead, recalling all that had gone wrong in my life, how unhappy I was. I was in the middle of a poor me pity party, immobilized with emotional despair and brimming with anxiety. I hit bottom as I shouted, "God, this is a joke! My life is a joke!" Then, clear as my voice is coming to you right now, God said to me, and I can still hear it, *"It doesn't have to be this way!* There are three categories of people that exist in the world and all start with a W: The wanters, the wishers, and the way-makers. Which one do you want to be, John, because you can't be all three?"

It doesn't have to be this way! What you are facing right now: You were born for this, made for this, strengthened for this. You can change. Your life can change. It can be better.

Has God ever spoken that over your heart? It doesn't have to be this way. It was my burning bush moment. It was the syllabus that I had read and could never forget. God was calling me back to being a hope dealer.

I'm not telling you it will be easy; I'm telling you it will be worth it. What's that? *Leaving your comfort zone* at least enough to read and act upon the Easter egg inside the syllabus. Leaving the wells you've been drinking from, called your safe spaces. I had to leave the comfort of being in sales, at least the money side of that comfort, and go back to making much less. Should I give up more money to fulfill my purpose?

Comfort is like an octopus in our lives. It has a lot of reach and a lot of arms.

Comfort.

If you want to change your life, understand that change does not happen sitting in your lazy-boy, America's number one bestselling piece of furniture. It's not called the Risky-boy or Restoration-Chair. It's called the Relief Chair!

We must sometimes be called out of comfort for God's will.

Moses read the syllabus. At first, he didn't like what it said, but he was willing to act on it. Moses argued with the syllabus. Moses disagreed with the syllabus. But that's true for most of us *because the syllabus is always about others, not ourselves.* We get our life scripts from God and cry out, what about me? Why am I not the star here? Why do I get this small part? What about my dreams and my hopes? You don't think Moses had hopes and dreams? Do you think he was living his best life at 80, working for a family tending sheep that were not his? No one grew up in Moses's time and had career aspirations for shepherding sheep that didn't belong to you! Moses's dreams were eclipsed by the burning bush God placed in his syllabus.

The Bible says Moses slowed down enough out of the busyness of his life to *turn aside.* He *turned aside* from his everyday life to see the extraordinary life God called him to live. We all get this call! It's not based upon talent, just willingness to listen and say yes. Not everyone is willing. Yet you've read the syllabus, you've listened to the burning bush. This is why we lay in bed at two in the morning and wonder, *What does it all mean? Why am I here?* This is why we all yearn for greatness, for something in our lives to outlive the 3,910 weeks that the average person gets this side of heaven. We all have this divine spark inside of us. Some of us let God build it into a fire!

Moses felt that burning desire in his life from God to do something with his life finally. He was eighty years old now, working for his father-in-law, tending his sheep, living paycheck to paycheck, amuck in sheep crap.

Is this your life amuck in crap? Look around.

God told Moses that your life doesn't have to be this way. But remember, God doesn't call us into personal comfort. He calls us into living beyond ourselves for something greater.

Is there not, has there not, at least been those holy nudges to be more, seek more, and live for more than paying your bills? I know everyone today has TikTok goals of retiring early, being rich (FIRE), and being famous. But we can't all be TikTok famous. Not every video goes viral for the right reasons. Usually, they go viral for the wrong ones. So, Rev. Martin Luther King, Jr. once said, before TikTok, "Not everybody can be famous, but everybody can be great because greatness is determined by service."[40]

Moses was not seeking fame, but God called him out of comfort into service.

He didn't have much of a life, but he was comfortable. He had food, shelter, and a job. Comfort is the enemy. Your bed, the older you get, is the devil. You sleep your life away with a little more sleep and slumber. You don't sleep in; you sleep it away! It is ironic to me that when someone passes during hospice care, the main thing the doctors say, if they feel like they were successful, is: They were comfortable, they were not in pain, and they were resting when they died.

Yes, physically, that's a great goal in death, comfort. But it's a terrible goal in life!

The comfort zone is the graveyard of your God-given dreams. Your body can sleep forever, but your soul was made to live not in comfort but in a soaring, daring adventure called life! Moses, at 80, hiding there with his family, hiding from his fugitive past and his life on the run as a murderer, turns aside and has a conversation with a bush. Call the white coats, right? But you hear the voices too, don't you?

I believe we get to a point in life, sometimes before 80 years old, where we see our burning bush and finally read the syllabus. We see God's calling in our lives, but that doesn't mean we all act on it. Not all of us spin the numbers on the locker and get the prize. Let's hope we turn to the side, take off our shoes, put down our phones, and go and hear what God calls us to.

Let's think about this as if you were Moses. If you had a desert to live in for forty years and wandered around with 1.2 million people complaining about your leadership or a palace to live comfortably in for the rest of your life, which would you choose? Steaks and fajitas, life in the royal family, or manna with whiners? Does anybody want to guess which would be more comfortable? Any doubts as to why Moses was a bit reticent?

So many of our decisions are based on comfort and preference.

Moses took the exit on comfort, and he chose to suffer with the people of God over enjoying the passing pleasure of sin. At one point, he could have chosen to live with the

40 King, M. L. (n.d.). *A Quote by Martin Luther King Jr.* Goodreads.
https://www.goodreads.com/quotes/147771-not-everybody-can-be-famous-but-everybody-can-be-great

elite of the Egyptians. He was raised in their courts. He knew a life of privilege. Now, on paper, it was a crazy decision. *Moses could have lived like a king, but instead, he chose to live like a runaway leader of the enslaved people.* Why?

Purpose!

If your why is big enough, you will endure any "how"! If the why is engaging, your how will be revealed. The burning bush gave his life meaning and purpose. It was the Easter egg in the syllabus. Once purpose or meaning gets a hold of your soul, it will always outweigh the comfort trappings. Burning bushes become burning fires within us. Once you read the syllabus, you can't act like you've never read it.

Don't forget to factor in forever. Moses was also factoring in forever. Moses was factoring in the long game. I'm thinking about that moment when I stand before God, and He says, well done, good and faithful servant. You ran your race. You fought your fight. You did things that, in the moment, pulled you away from comfort, but it was what I had for you. David said he'd rather be in God's courts for a day than a thousand elsewhere. He would rather be a doorkeeper in the house of his God, which wouldn't be comfortable, than dwell in the tents of wickedness (Psalm 84:10, NIV). Paul, again in Romans 8:18 (NKJV), says, "For I consider that the sufferings of this present time are not worthy to be compared with the glory which shall be revealed in us." Moses chose God's will over comfort. Comfort is one of the "gods" Americans worship!

God, I confess I am quick to forget You.

I am so quick to forget the slavery you brought me out of and to even wish things were as they used to be. I quickly forget that you made me more loving and less hateful. I promptly forgot that you encouraged me to forgive when I wanted to hold onto a grudge. I quickly forget that you encouraged me to stay in my marriage during difficult seasons. I quickly forget that you gave me my parents, who loved and encouraged me even when it was difficult to love and nurture.

I'm just the Israelites who wished they were back in Egypt, where they ate good food, forgetting that's where they were enslaved! I look at the manna you have given me, God—food to eat, a house to live in, a loving wife and amazing church to serve in, two amazing boys. God, I confess I am quick to forget you, and I find myself wanting more—better food, a bigger home, more alone time, more money, and the ability to travel!

I turn to other gods in worship. I want my comfort, my control, my security. I think I can live under my roof and my rules, which will make me happy. I confess, God, that you have given me my daily bread, even when I ask for a year's worth at a time. I see the sunrise, and instead of being reminded of how great you are, I think about all I must do today. Yet you made the sunrise, not me. You made the seasons come, not me. Your mercies are new every morning. How quickly I forget, If your highest value is comfort, it will always keep you back from your calling.

Comfort zones don't keep your life safe; they keep your life small.

Moses could have chosen the comfort of living as an Egyptian, but he decided the discomfort of leading his people against the most powerful man in the world! When God first called Moses to the burning bush, Moses was unwilling to go. Moses said, "Who am I?" Such a good question to ask yourself. Who am I? It's possible to get so busy with life that you fail to ask the most important questions: Who am I? Whose am I? Does anyone besides me have a claim on my life? Often, the burning bush, the syllabus from God, tells us who we are and what we are to do with who we are.

Moses didn't have a hearing problem or seeing problem. He saw the burning bush. He heard God's call, but *he had an identity crisis!*

God told him Moses, here's your syllabus. Here's what I want you to give your life to. Moses's response was ahh—I don't think so.

He had all the wrong I am statements:

I am a murderer.

I am a fugitive on the run.

I am a slow thinker.

I am a stut-stut-stutterer.

I am old (and he was 80).

I am not able.

God said back to him, "I AM the Great I AM, and you are my Child. I made you, and I can remake you! Now quit seeking comfort, and this lame-ass job tending sheep that are not your own, and get out there and live the life I am calling you to live."

Please remember ass is a Biblical word.

So, it is with us, the walls of our comfort zone are lovingly decorated with our lifelong collection of favorite excuses.

To follow God meant giving up all that Egyptian wealth and money and living in the court of the Pharoh. Had Moses kept all the riches, he would have had to drop the purpose.

God intends for us to hold money in our hands and to hold purpose in our hearts. When we get those two mixed up, we lose in life.

Let's keep a light touch on this world's dust collectors, trinkets, and shiny objects as we keep a firm grip on purpose, the syllabus, and the burning bush. Let's hold the shiny objects in our hands, not in our hearts. The Egyptians did try that. They tried to keep the shiny objects in their hearts. They buried their kings with all kinds of loot. A thousand years passed, and the British archaeologists busted in; King Tut hadn't been playing with any of his shiny toys.

We don't get to keep what we put into our hands, what we accumulate.

But what we put into God's hands is ours forever. We get to keep that for all eternity. In Luke 12:15 (NKJV), Jesus said, "For one's life does not consist in the abundance of the things he possesses."

In God's eyes, the bottom line isn't your bottom line! In God's eyes, the richness of *being* is much more critical than having.

We're constantly at a crossroads of, is my life's goal to enjoy things or to be deployed for God's plans?

We must be willing to walk away from comfort to get up and change our lives.

Exit Plans?

God was giving Moses an exit plan that involved a whole new life. Everyone should always have an exit in mind when they go anywhere. I have a lot of weddings and funerals, and I always have an exit plan in mind. After the graveside, I am heading for the car. The wake is for the family.

Weddings: I have done thousands! I used to say they are my favorite. They are happy, lust, and love, gazing lovingly into each other's eyes. But now I realize at many weddings I conduct, the couple is so gaga with lust and kissy kissy, and let's get to the honeymoon; I don't think they are listening to the syllabus I am reciting! Let's hope they hear it on the video. They paid to get it done, right?

At funerals, *people are listening*. There's nothing like the death of a loved one to wake you up to the reality that life is abrupt. At funerals, there's brokenness and quietness. It's like now there's an opening, and all of a sudden, life stops, and we are forced to read the syllabus.

When I do a wedding, I have an exit plan. I am going to make sure I get your names right. I will have you write a love letter to each other that you will read at the altar and every year on your anniversary, so it's your words to each other, and I will sign the license! But that's enough; I don't need to see you on your honeymoon. That's just between you and your spouse. I don't want to throw birdseed at you. I don't want to hold a sparkler or blow bubbles while singing sappy love songs from Air Supply's greatest hits! I'm already thinking, even as I'm shifting into, "*Do you take so-and-so to be your so?*" about how quickly I can get to bed. A good time is 8:30 in bed with a heating pad and a book!

When people say when going somewhere, "Hey, do you want to ride together?" I'm trying to size you up. How long are you going to linger? Let's take separate cars, or can

I get an Uber? People talk about Taylor Swift concerts. She made over a billion dollars this year on tour; a billion, and I can't name a song. After hearing about her security, I could never go to a Taylor Swift concert. They lock you in there. You can't leave. Standing up for hours, people in the front rows are wearing diapers. If I need a diaper to see Taylor, I am not even going!

Following God involves knowing how to exit. The evil one will want you to stay vague and fuzzy. He doesn't want you to read the syllabus. He doesn't want you to be clear on your purpose, your identity!

Jesus modeled clarity of identity in John chapter 6 when he became very popular after feeding the 5,000, and everybody was super pumped on all the Krispy Kreme donuts they were eating that day. *Everyone wanted a piece of him. Everyone wanted an autograph. Everyone wanted a selfie.* Everyone wanted something. It says in John 6:15 (NIV), "Jesus, knowing that they intended to come and make him king by force, he withdrew again to a mountain by himself."

What does that tell you? **That tells you that even if you take the steps to better yourself, there can be lonely moments in your life. Sometimes you'll feel lonely. But that loneliness for Jesus was not a liability. It was an asset. It was there that he was refueled. It was there that he was strengthened. It was there he kindled the divine spark within his soul.**

Jesus made sure his fires didn't burn too low.

He wouldn't let them take him by force to make him a king. He went to be alone with the Father, who was able to remind him, *you already are a king.* You see, many people, if you give in to their plans for your life, will try to get you to leave what you have to get, which is already yours and can't be taken away. But they'll try to give you an imitation substitute version of it that's always less than. Never let anyone but God defines who you are and will be! They can't take it away if they don't give you your medal. They can't take away your identity if they don't give you your identity.

Identity determines activity, and proper identity determines your destiny.

Some people let destiny and life determine identity, but that's getting it backward.

One of Shakespeare's tragic heroes puts it like this:

> Tomorrow, and tomorrow, and tomorrow,
> Creeps in this petty pace from day to day,
> To the last syllable of recorded time;
> And all our yesterdays have lighted fools.
> The way to dusty death. Out, out, brief candle!
> Life's but a walking shadow, a poor player

That struts and frets his hour upon the stage

And then is heard no more. It is a tale.

Told by an idiot, full of sound and fury

Signifying nothing.[41]

If, in the end, life signifies nothing, why bother doing anything?

Thom Yorke, the frontman of the band Radiohead, gives a blunt but resounding answer: "It's filling the hole…that's all anyone does."

Asked by his interviewer what happened to the hole, Yorke replied, "It's still there."

It's a sobering thought. My Philosophy teachers taught me this in school; they were militantly atheistic, and the conclusion was: Everything we do—all the holidays, the conversations, the achievements, falling in love, choosing where to live and who to marry and what to wear and what to eat and how to bring up the children—is an unloved magazine in a doctor's waiting room. It's nothing more than an empty distraction until our name is called, and we receive the news we've been dreading all along: Time's up. *Prince or pavement-sleeper. It doesn't matter.*

We all spend our days trying to fill up the ravenous hole inside us, and then, in a cosmic irony we could laugh about, if we were not inconveniently dead, we end up taking up space, filling a hole in the ground four and a half feet under. Trust me, it's four and a half feet, not six.

Before you reach for another bottle of Prozac, stay with me here. I don't believe Shakespeare is right. I don't believe my Philosophy teachers are right. I don't think we are destined to fill a hole six feet under. Why? Because I lived with these questions for years, wrestled with them, and have heard my Creator speak to them. I have read the Creator's syllabus. I have listened to the burning bush talk to my heart. In a dream I had my senior year when I was stuck wondering what to do with my life, I heard God speak to me. Have you ever heard God talk to you or your life? Sometimes God doesn't sound anything like Morgan Freeman. Sometimes God speaks in a whisper, a dream, a song, what seemed like a throwaway line from your mom, but it's an answer to a deep question. So, I pondered what and who could overcome this hole in my life, the hole in my heart, that nagging sense of emptiness. And it was looking at one of my friend's lives in college that I realized he had something different. His questions were answered, and he spoke to me and said, "I follow the only one who overcame the hole in the ground, the only one who tells you and me you were born for this."

I follow the one whom the grave could not hold: Jesus.

Ephesians 1:4 (NIV) says, "For He chose us in him before the creation of the world to be holy and blameless in his sight."

41 Shakespeare, W. (n.d.). *Speech: "Tomorrow, and Tomorrow, and Tomorrow" by...* Poetry Foundation. https://www.poetryfoundation.org/poems/56964/speech-tomorrow-and-tomorrow-and-tomorrow

This verse says you have been set apart to do God's work before the beginning of time. In other words, instead of complaining about your life, what if you thought, *I was born for this moment. God wanted me in this time in history to make a difference?* What would it mean in your life, as you look at your life and say to yourself about your challenges, problems, and things that make you question whether you are big enough for this moment to hear and to read: You were born for this? This moment in time, this moment in history is an amazing day to be alive because God has put you here for this moment.

Will you meet it, or will you run from it?

Can you believe: Before God said let there be light, he said let there be you. That is the only conclusion to Ephesians 1:4.

He set you apart and picked this moment in history for you to be alive, so what are you doing for history? What in the world are you doing here? Hopefully, not to fill a hole in the ground…but to make up there come down here, God's kingdom to come.

For me, I am a hope dealer. It's all I have to give, but I live to give it. I grew up with a narcissistic "it's all about your soul," escape-based view of Christianity. But I think I was lied to. It's all about having a "personal" relationship with Jesus—that's what they said! Think about it… It's still around in a lot of churches today. The Christianity I grew up with was hyperfocused on accepting Jesus into your heart and having a personal relationship with Jesus. It said, "Here are the minimum requirements to get your passport into heaven, to make sure you have a ticket on the plane that is leaving earth!" But where in the Bible does Jesus say that? It's all about me and *escaping* this earth. The goal of my faith growing up was "beam me up, Scotty!" The goal of my faith growing up was to get out of here before God "torches" this place in a moment of judgment!

Are we reading the same Bible? Yet…and it's a big yet…*I have studied the Bible over the past thirty-five years, and what I read about Jesus is totally different than what I was taught growing up.* The Christianity of the Bible says, "Follow Jesus; live and walk and love as he did on earth, making up there come down here, bringing heaven to earth." When you make up there come down here, it's not for you, it's for others. You are letting people know that there is a God who is with *us*, a God of El Roi, a God who sees you. A God who knows you. The Christmas story is not a story of escape; it's a story of invasion. It is a story of God coming to earth to be Immanuel, to be with us. It's not all about you going to heaven. It's all about you bringing heaven to earth.

A person can say few more powerful words to himself than these, "I was born for this." The sheer force of believing such a thing, the galvanizing strength it brings to all the currents of life, makes it a certainty we should settle for ourselves once and for all. *It is primarily a spiritual belief, existential, of course.* Believing that we were born for a moment in time and a given purpose requires believing in a *God who decides such things.* It means recognizing that we aren't accidents and that our lives aren't ruled by chance alone. We accept that there was a determination before we were born. *We rec-*

ognize the work of a Chooser. We acknowledge the writer of the syllabus. We recognize God can set a bush on fire and set a fire in our hearts.

You are deciding that this is true, and this changes everything.

We look at our otherwise terrifying world, and though we might be daunted by it, we need not fear or cower from it. We were born for the challenges we face this year and beyond. If you believe this, then when you think of your past failures, you might grieve over them, but they will not destroy you. You get better, not bitter. You rise anyway. You choose joy despite the circumstances. You never quit fighting for the right, the good. You are a child of God, and act like one! You were born for this. This is your true identity. This is the name tag you can't ever take off. You think about your obstacles and enemies and are sobered up, but you are also aware that overcoming them isn't up to you alone.

God is with us.

God is helping us.

Guiding you.

Strengthening you.

Shepherding you.

Empowering you.

We were born for this. Someone is with us. It is a belief that inspires greatness. Churchill believed it. He once said, **"Over me beat unseen wings."**

Read that last sentence again.

Do you believe that over you, beat unseen wings? I do. The greatest realities are unseen. Faith is a telescope that allows us to see what the naked eye cannot! Churchill told the British people they were destined for victory. They believed him because they were. Dr. King believed it. The Apostle Paul, Augustine, Alfred the Great, Martin Luther, Elizabeth I, John Wesley, William Wilberforce, George Washington, Abigail Adams, Sojourner Truth, Abraham Lincoln, Booker T. Washington, Theodore Roosevelt, Golda Meir—in short, millions since and before, have believed it. It is why we know their names. It is why they lived exceptional lives. We are tempted in our angry, swirling age to wish we lived at some other time, like before nuclear proliferation. We are tempted to live in a pleasure bubble called our comfort zone. But not children of God. Not if you can believe, "I was born for this." Not if you think that over you, beat unseen wings. Those words, that faith, completely realign us to our world and even to our God. They make victories possible. What do you believe? Are you here to try and fill a hole in the ground? Or were you born for this?

Only read the syllabus that God gives to you!

Jesus didn't need to go with the people who would try to make him a king because he was already a king. A king not meant to wear a crown of gold, but one who was sent to wear a crown of thorns. A king who would not sit, at least on the first coming, on a golden throne. But *a king who would be stretched out as a suffering servant upon a wooden cross.* By remembering who God said he was, he could combat the propensity to give in to who people wanted him to be. You cannot receive a wake-up call; you can't take back your life if you live for the approval and pleasure of other people.

Living to please people will keep you from pleasing God.

So don't give in. This means that if you want to live a life you've never lived, you must do things you've never done! To kick butt, you must first lift your foot!

How about Paul the Apostle in Acts chapter 21? Let me paraphrase. He had been doing ministry in Ephesus. He ministered in Ephesus longer than any other place. They have this epistle called the Ephesians that's just full of love. You see, his heart is just full of love for this church. He loved them, he loved them, he loved them. He's their pastor; it's his church. And his ministry there went gangbusters. And yet the Holy Spirit began to call him to leave where he was and to go somewhere different. He was supposed to leave Ephesus. And a man prophetically told Paul that if you go to Jerusalem from Ephesus, you will end up in prison. You're going to end up in chains. Even death could happen. So, the church at Ephesus said, well, obviously, God's not in all that. He doesn't want you to go, so don't go, Paul! Stay here!

Paul's struggle was basically "I love you wholeheartedly, but God's Spirit says to go somewhere else!" God's syllabus told him to leave to do ministry elsewhere! People were pleading with Paul not to go to another church, and Acts 21:12–14 (NIV) says: "When we heard this, we and the people there pleaded with Paul not to go up to Jerusalem. Then Paul answered, 'Why are you weeping and breaking my heart? I am ready not only to be bound, but also to die in Jerusalem for the name of the Lord Jesus.' When he would not be dissuaded, we gave up and said, 'The Lord's be done!'"

Paul knew what you need to know, that *good* is the enemy of *best*. The best is God's will.

He's preaching at Ephesus; that's a good thing. Saving marriages touching hearts it was good work. But the good is the enemy of the best, and the best is God's will.

People who read the syllabus constantly have to figure out how to exit on good things so that we may lay hold of the best things.

There's nothing better than knowing you are walking in the will of the Lord at that moment, doing what he called you to do! How do you know? You listen to your burning bush. You read the syllabus.

Some of you, though, are trying to do too much.

God can't bless your yes until you grow your no.

Do you start crowding your life with so many things that you don't have the free bandwidth emotionally, mentally, spiritually, and financially to give yourself over to God's unique will for your life and stop letting other people tell you how to follow your calling?

Moses is famous for many things. Manna comes to mind. Sticks that turn into snakes come to mind. Ten Commandments come to mind. Moses is most famous, though, for a departure. He's most famous for exiting. The Book of the Bible that, in summary form, we are reading about here is called Exodus. Exodus means out of the way into somewhere else or a departure; *It's an exit sign.*

It comes to a point in Moses's life where he walks into the court of the Pharoah, a.k.a. his grandfather, and now he's walking in there on behalf of the Hebrews he identifies with! Now, he has thrown off his assumed identity as Egyptian and refuses to be called the son of Pharaoh's daughter or the grandson of Pharaoh. And he strolls in one day and says four famous words, *let my people go.*

Moses had to solve the identity crisis before following God's lead. Am I an Egyptian? Am I Hebrew? Am I a child of God called by God to lead His people? You've got to follow God's lead. *Sometimes He calls you to walk away from things because you're enslaved to them. Other times, He causes you to walk away from things because they are just scaffolding, preparing you for what's coming. Scaffolding doesn't go up to stay up forever. Scaffolding goes up so you can build the actual thing. Can you identify things in your life that were scaffolding that prepared you for the next season in your life?*

Then, the other C word besides comfort, that we must surrender, that Moses had to surrender, is *control.* Why is this so hard for us? I like to follow the leader as long as I am the leader. I would be good with college if I got to write the syllabus. But you are not in charge of the burning bushes God places in your life. *We must be willing to give up control, for if you follow God's plans for your life, you will be put into situations where you feel so out of control.*

Like what? I don't know, like being told to walk through the Red Sea with an enormous army coming behind you, trying to kill you, and your only strategy is going to involve a stick. Welcome to ministry. *We will be out of control, but that's a good thing because it puts you in a place where you can be under HIS control.*

We walk by faith and not by sight.

I think it's important to remember that whatever victory came before was meant to feed your faith in your next one so that you don't always have to doubt God! He's going to be faithful here. Right? We could speak; I've seen enough. I'm not going to get quaky and shaky with every new hiccup. I've seen enough. I've seen God work. He was faithful there; he's going to be faithful here. If He got me out, He's going to bring me through.

He didn't bring me out of Egypt to kill me in the Red Sea. We're going to let go of control.

And then another C. This is like my report card from high school, all C's and *credit*! We're going to exit credit, needing to receive credit for every little thing, needing people to see what we did and know our contribution, needing that finder's fee for that introduction you made in good faith. But now, they went on to do this, and I didn't get compensated for what I did.

I recently had a lady leave my church because "I didn't thank her publicly enough for all she was doing!" If you work in the Kingdom of God to get recognition, you are doing it wrong. Do you think Moses got to have a Volunteer Appreciation dinner one day with him as the guest of honor? No.

To always be wanting "atta-boys" is immature and silly. You are grown. Act like it. Once, an employee asked me to thank him publicly in front of the staff. I said do you get paid? Did your check get directly deposited? I need to thank people better, but that's another chapter!

But to live seeking credit, to live that way, you will be miserable. No one's going to want to be around you. It's like being in a black hole. Did Moses seek credit? No! When your burning bush is so grandiose and amazing that everyone knows you could not have done it, and only God could have done it, God gets the glory.

Imagine how big your world would get if you just became smaller.

Matthew 6:4 (NKJV) says, "Your Father, who sees in secret, will Himself reward you openly." How does the phrase go: *There is no end to what you can accomplish if you don't care who gets the credit?*

Moses said, "Pharaoh, let my people go." Comfort. Let my people go. Control. Let my people go. Credit. Let my people go. God is our Lord, not things like riches and living like royalty! We're going to exit them. We're not going to hold on to them any longer.

Rules to remember as you read your exit syllabus:

Number One – Don't leave for the wrong reason.

Don't leave for the wrong reason regarding your job, marriage, relationship with your kids, friends, and place in the world. Most times, the character is not built by quitting. "Pain is temporary. Quitting lasts forever." When they give up right now some people give up on all situations when they get tough. Most of the time, falling in love and growing in love with the same person must happen many times in one's lifetime.

What is the wrong reason?

The wrong reason would be that I'm not getting validated there. I'm not getting noticed. I'm not getting the opportunity. It's hard here. I'm tired here. I feel unappreciated. That's not God leading you. That's God developing you. That's grace.

This is David. I've been anointed king, but I'm not crowned king. In between, I will be living in some dark, uncomfortable caves.

Imagine the president of the US winning an election, and fifteen years later, s/he steps into office. That's a long season. This is David's season: fifteen years he spent in caves on the run from King Saul, whom he knew he would replace. Fifteen years later, he was fighting for his life. He could have ended Saul's life on several occasions, but he always took the longer and the higher road. He would not short-circuit on that and take matters into his own hands. He was willing to persevere and persist and honor what God had put him into, and knowing in due season, he would come through it. We're not going to leave for the wrong reason.

Make sure you are not just running from something because it's hard, but you have something you are running to, something you have been called to!

Number two – Don't resent your current season.

Don't resent your current season. What you're in, God is using currently, even if it feels insignificant! God might invite you to a grander story in your minor, insignificant season. Your burning bush has not yet been set on fire. The syllabus has not been handed out yet, or you are in a scaffolding season.

Derek Sivers taught me this. He started a company called CD Baby back in the day. It was a massive deal before iTunes to allow a band that doesn't have a record label to put CDs out into the world and their music out into the world. Does anyone reading this remember CDs? I used to collect them, loved them, and bought them. Now, it's all digital streaming. Derek talks in an interview about how he started the company. He said, "Well, it all started at a pig show!" Of course, all major CD recording artists get their start at pig shows, right? Wrong.

A pig show? "Yeah, I love music. I wanted to play music but couldn't get opportunities. An agent called, 'Will you play at a pig show? Pays $75.'" He had to pay $58 for the bus ticket, but he did it and made $17. He played his heart out. He got back. The agent said, "Derek, you did well. They were happy. Can I send you to the opening of this art museum?" Absolutely. The pay is $75. Awesome. The bus ticket was $60. Crap. He was going backward. He lost that $2. Now, he only earned fifteen dollars. But he did it with his whole heart. Another call came next week: "Hey, would you be willing to play at a circus?" He's like, that's not what I became a rock and roll star for, playing in the circus. But he said. They said, "This one's steady work. Three shows a week: Friday, Saturday, and Sunday. Seventy-five dollars a show, but you're on set." He said, "Are you kidding me? Now, I'm a professional musician. I've got a steady gig." And he took it. And he did it with so much enthusiasm, so much heart. The circus blew up, and how he would do this was a big deal. Pretty soon, he was making $300 per show. He said that money allowed him, as he continued at the circus for ten years, wanting to be a rock star but playing at the circus like a clown, to buy his first house. While at the circus, he started this little side thing because he said it's so hard for musicians to get their songs out there. After all, Nashville's got this big kind of evil empire. He thought—let's democratize it and make it available for any garage band to get their music out there. So he started this thing called CD Baby. He sold it for $22 million and donated it to charity. He just had it in his heart to do something big and crazy and be faithful to small stuff.[42]

I wonder if some of us feel stuck at the pig show today and are tempted to resent our current season. What if God will be using it to open up new doors of opportunity if you're faithful where you are?

Number Three – Don't cling to a previous season.

How many people have been held back and hamstrung from entering some milk and honey territory because they're just moping about how good the onions and leeks were back in Egypt? We had fajitas Moses back in slavery. The good old days were so good. Can't we go back?

Nope. The good old days weren't always that good. Today can be better. Oh, man, it was so good back there. Yeah. So how do we do that? How do we not cling to the previous season?

This is where about 1,200 marbles suddenly become relevant.

Marbles? What marbles?

Has Pastor John lost his marbles? Don't say Amen. Remember the 80's. I love the 80's! Journey, Bryan Adams, Madonna, Rush, and Bruce Springsteen ruled the radio! We played outside from sun up to sun down, and our parents had no idea what we were doing! We had Sony Walkman's! There were no cell phones and no social media. Remember, oh, it was so great, Pastor John! Admittedly, there were some great times. I remember this. I remember that. I remember, but what are you doing? You're looking back. You can't run forward looking backward. You'll need a chiropractor to deal with that issue that it will create in your neck and spinal situation.

Don't cling to the former things. God's doing a new thing.

So how do we do that? It involves marbles. For you old folks, let me suggest that each of you buy about *1,000 marbles. Yo*u might say, "Pastor, how do I know if I am old?" Okay, simple test. Everyone, be as quiet as you can. Shhhh. Now stand up and now sit back down. Did your body make noise? Did your knees sound like Rice Krispies? Snap, crackle, pop. Yes? You are old. If you are old, you know it. If your body made no noise,

42 Ferriss, T. (2015, December 14). Derek Sivers on Developing Confidence, Finding Happiness, and Saying No to Millions . *The Tim Ferriss Show*. other.

if your body still has a quiet mode in operation, you are young. For you, young folks, maybe buy about 2,000 marbles.

Either way, I am dead serious; you should buy some marbles. I bought mine on Amazon.

Anyhow, this hit me on birthday number 53! I was lying in bed thinking, *53 years, where have they gone?* Then I thought, *Wait, how many Saturdays is that? How many Saturdays do I get if I live to be 75?* When I added up the number of Saturdays an average person who lives to 75 has approximately 3,900 Saturdays. I did this by multiplying 75 by 52. Trust me, I used a calculator in the slowwww math class. Unfortunately, I added up how many Saturdays were gone by. I figured out I had already spent 2,756 Saturdays with 1,144 left if I was lucky enough to live to 75! So, I have bought 1,200 marbles and now dwindled them down to 1,144 and placed them in a transparent container. Ever since then, I have been taking away one marble every Saturday. As the marbles diminish, I see *visually* how short life is, forcing *you* to get *your* priorities right. Watching these marbles diminish helps me see how brief life can be. I know these marbles will eventually all be gone. Some of you oldies, you are already on bonus marbles! If I run out of marbles, every other Saturday after that will be a bonus! How do you feel about the idea of dying? Is it something you think about often? Or does it make you feel anxious? Generally, death is a taboo subject.

We're taught that death is something we should shy away from and try to forget about. If we start contemplating our mortality—so this traditional wisdom goes—we'll become anxious and depressed. It's quite the opposite.

Whereas our ancestors would have regularly watched people die and seen dead bodies, we're shielded from death by modern medical practices. When was the last time you saw someone die or held their hand as they took their last breath? I have done this over one hundred times. It changes you, trust me. You start focusing on your last breath and what that could look like.

You don't want it to be a breath of regret, fear, or if I had only…

People usually die in hospitals rather than at home, and soon after death, their bodies are taken to funeral homes, where we usually must make an appointment to see them. But one thing I have consistently found in counseling folks is that surviving an encounter with death—or even just seriously contemplating death—can have a powerful positive effect. This is why you should survive and overcome cancer rather than survive and overcome winning the lottery. Something happens to us when we focus on our last day. We begin to live even fuller lives today. We begin to see, "I only get to do this once!"

"I only get this moment one time!"

I've found that people who survive accidents, serious illnesses, cancer, and other close brushes with mortality look at the world *with new eyes*. They no longer take life and the people in their lives for granted. They have a new ability to live in the present, with a new appreciation for small and simple things, such as being in nature, looking at the sky and the stars, and spending time with family. They also have a broader sense of perspective, so worries that had oppressed them before no longer seem important. They become less materialistic and more altruistic. Their relationships become more intimate and authentic.

Their shadow self dies, and the accurate truth of who God made them to be starts living.

For some people, an encounter with cancer, death, or a terrible car crash or life-threatening illness is their burning bush. It wakes them up and helps them realize what is and is not important in life. In many cases, these effects don't disappear. Although they may become slightly less intense over time, they become established as permanent traits. They have a habit of waking up and saying: *"Don't let the gift of this day be stolen by the ghosts of yesterday!"*

Encounters with death indeed can sometimes wake us up to truly live.

They snap us out of a trance-like state in which we are indifferent to life and unaware of the blessings in our lives. It's the weirdest thing.

Marcus Aurelius put it like this: "Think of yourself as dead. You have lived your life. Now take what's left and live it properly!"[43]

Contemplating your death can help you live a happier life today!

Text your friends and neighbors and tell them, "You are losing your marbles." Go ahead! It's ok. Let my people go. Don't cling to your former season. Don't long for the onions of Egypt. If God called you out of it, it's for a purpose. Let's face the future. Come on, who's ready to leave Egypt? It would help if you went from wanting to change your life to deciding to change your life. Let's pack our bags. Let's leave these former things and move forward, with all our hearts, into what God has for us. Come on, I don't want to turn it into salt like Lot's wife. I'm not looking back to Sodom. I'm going ahead. I'm moving forward. I got my call. I got my marching orders. I've read the syllabus, stopped, turned aside, and got my burning bush! I know who I am. I know who I belong to.

I know what my life is about. It's changing yours by filling it up with hope!

I've got my eyes on the prize. I'm ready to run with all my heart for the upward call. Make a decision today to let go of the god of comfort. Let go of trying to relive the past. Let go of control. Let go of always needing credit and buy some marbles! Let's decide for God as Moses did. Let's leave the promised land of self for God's Promised Land.

---

43 Aurelius, M. (n.d.). *A Quote from Meditations*. Goodreads.
https://www.goodreads.com/quotes/293726-think-of-yourself-as-dead-you-have-lived-your-life

CHAPTER TEN

GET BIG BY THINKING SMALL

We are all what we repeatedly do.

—Aristotle

YOU CAN GET BIG BY thinking small. You can get big by living small. I got this concept from one of my favorite books by Charles Duhigg titled, *The Power of Habit*. He talks about how little habits, keystone habits, can unlock enormous change in our lives. A couple of my favorite examples from the book are that he correlates the positive discipline of going to the gym, even as infrequently as once a week, with a lower rate of credit card spending. If you can find self-discipline and willpower in one area, it spreads to other places. He also shows a strong connection between sitting down as a family at the dinner table and eating dinner just a couple times a week, with kids getting better grades in school and having higher self-confidence. We worry about: "How do I help my kids, you know, in school?" We think about: "Do I need to get a tutor?" Maybe the answer is that the TV is off, phones are not on the table or at the restaurant, and sitting at the dinner table, just talking. Right? Like, that can't work? It's too simple. Maybe. Maybe the answer lies in the small things we easily overlook, right?

Here's my personal favorite. He points in the book that a study was done that found that if you make your bed in the morning (all the mothers in the house said "Yes!") as soon as you get up, check this out, those who do so are found to be able to stick to a budget better than those who do not. So make your bed. Sometimes Renee, my wife, gets in such a hurry to make the bed that she makes it with me! My wife's been telling me this: I feel like if I can have a victory before I even leave the bedroom, then I'm already on the right start. My day's rolling in the right direction.

Start with one victory before you leave the bedroom, and you are on your way to more victories throughout the day.

Get big by thinking small.

Ever get tempted to make the wrong choice? Last week, I was walking our dog, Lexy. While we were on our walk, Lexy did what dogs do. I always carry this little blue bag with me while walking Lexy. Then this thought came into my head, *It's 6:30 a.m. It's dark. I don't have to pick that up. I could leave it there. Probably nobody will notice. I probably won't get in trouble.* Then these other thoughts will go with an idea like that, *You don't have to live by the rules everybody else has to live by. You can be special. You can be entitled.* Now, where does a temptation like that come from? From me and my brain, of course! Of course, I have much darker temptations than that. I have many more riveting temptations like that. Would you like to hear some of those? No! Sorry. Too bad. I can't write that book yet; I am still employed! Sometimes, when it comes to silly temptations and stuff like this, Renee will say to me, "John, you can only be young once, but you can always be immature!" She will also ask me this question: "Why do you do what you do?"

Have *you* ever been asked that? It's a good one. Percentage-wise, how many of you can say that you like about 84.5 percent of what you do and who you are? I dare you to ask your good friends or spouse, "How much, percentage-wise, do you think I need to change?"

Some of you are like, "One hundred percent—a complete makeover!"

One of the underlying fundamental truths of this book is a straightforward point: **You are only one small decision from a different life.** You are only one new small habit from a bigger life.

It's true, but what's also true is that your life tends to keep moving in the direction it's already moving. So, I hope you like where your life is heading. Otherwise, you need to make a decisive decision to change, but it can be just one small change, one small habit at a time. Think about adding three small new habits each month for one year. You will have thirty-six new habits; your life will be much different.

When I was growing up, my dad asked me this question: "Where do you want to be five years from now, John? What do you want to be doing five years from now, John?" One of the rules I tend to live by is that the greatest indicator of someone's future behavior is their past behavior. Most people know this intuitively, so when you tell people I am going to change, they usually think—change, yeah, this won't last through the afternoon. But if you are going to change your future behavior and life, it begins with a decision to change the way you have been living.

Let me tell you what research shows, and this is challenging, depending upon whether or not you like yourself or need to change yourself. **You are only one decision away from changing your life—but do you need to make that decision?**

It depends. Research shows that, in most cases, *the future you is simply an exaggerated version of the current you.* You know, we think about the future sometimes rather romantically. It's this mysterious thing: Who will I be when I grow up? You're going to be exactly like you, just exaggerated. If you want to know what you'll look like in five years, ten years after, and twenty years after, look at yourself with more miles on the odometer.

What do I mean? If you're kind today, you'll be kinder in the future because these things deepen. These things mature. If you're generous today, you'll be more generous. Picture a more generous person who looks somewhat like you, who just has a little bit leatherier complexion. Your kind face will look a bit harder, but still kind. You'll be a kinder, more generous person. If you are cruel today, you will still be crueler. You will be harsher still. Those things will deepen as they break into the cracks of who you are and strengthen your character. The ways you let in become the ways you are set in. Which is why Jesus says I stand at the door of your life and knock. Will you let me in? Why was Jesus's first miracle at a wedding? Because he was invited to a wedding, and they needed more wine. Have you invited Jesus to your wedding? Could it be, on some level, that simple? Yes. Because once you invite him into your heart and life, like any house guest, he rearranges your schedule, what you do, and your activities.

Your decisions today will determine who you are five years from now. If you are disciplined today, you will still be more disciplined. This makes the selection of a spouse so important. Most people are looking for the wrong things. They're looking at the flower, being fooled by the grass, and let's face it, beauty fades, but character is forever. Let's not be fooled by the outside of a person and forget the most important part of anyone is unseen.

The things that get better with time are the invisible attributes etched on the inside of the soul. The most beautiful part of a person you can't see, so look for what lies underneath all the veneer and wrapping paper. But this isn't a chapter on swiping, right? This is a chapter on deciding who we want to be and decision-making.

Time doesn't change who you are. It reveals who you are and makes you more of who you are. Time isn't going to change you. Oh, I'm going to be different in the future. No, you'll be making choices then like you are today; you'll be more set in those ways.

For the religious folks in the pool, you might say: I will need a Scripture verse for that. Proverbs 11:27 (NKJV) puts it this way: "He who earnestly seeks good finds favor, but trouble will come to him who seeks *evil*." If you seek good, look for good in people, look for the good in situations, look for the good in life, and live with faith-filled optimism. Guess what? You're going to find it and favor. But if you're seeking trouble and evil, if you're the first to find the problem in any situation, the first to see the faults in everybody, you will find that! How would we know that's true of you? Oh, we would just read anything you write—the comments, the statements, the emails, the text messages, the quips, the retorts, the things you snicker at. If you're looking for evil, you're going to find trouble. *Are you a part-time archaeologist—you know that person who* looks for the bad in everyone, digging up their past failures, reminding them of how they were drunk? They will always be intoxicated, and you are calling for a full forecast of a life full of drunkenness?

Or, are you looking for what is sweet in someone, loving in someone, seeing what they could be, a glorious flower, revealing the one who created them as an excellent loving God? Do you see beyond the obvious to what could be? Do you call for a forecast of goodness and love in a person's life?

Every day, a hummingbird gets up and flies around to find flowers, beautiful, sweet, and colorful, full of nectar to feed on. Everyday hummingbirds find what they are looking for. Likewise, every day a vulture gets up and flies around looking for dead crap and finds what? Dead crap, dead animals, ugly, rotting, bloated animals that are dead. Every day, vultures find what they are looking for.

Which do you tend to be more like today: Hummingbird or Vulture?

It takes just as much energy to find the good in a person as it does the bad, so you might as well find the good. One of the greatest changes in our faith walk with God is eyesight—the vision of how we see ourselves, our role, and the truth about others.

The Bible says, "See what great love the Father has lavished on us, that we should be called children of God! And that is what we are!" (1 John 3:1, NIV).

See, I see you as a child of God, treat you as a child of God, and then adjust the crown on your head until your head grows into it. Is it not true that the best teachers saw what we could be but were not yet? Is it not true that is how Jesus sees each of us and calls us to see each other?

I have a pilot friend, and he says if you are flying west to east and it's a straight shot, you better aim for 30 degrees north of your destination. You better aim so you will hit your target landing site. Why? Inevitably, there is usually a strong headwind, called life, gravitational forces, and such, a strong southern wind blowing in the middle of where you are, and you will end up way south of where you were going. Why? Because the wind will fight you and take you south. So, always head north of where you are supposed to land, and you will always land where you need to be. So it is true of people. Always see someone better than they are by at least 30 degrees; when you land, you will see they have grown into the person you wanted them to be.

Didn't Jesus do this by seeing who someone could be, should be, and eventually will be in history, not just what they were now? It was Johann Wolfgang von Goethe who said words that changed my vision of others:

"If I accept you as you are, I will make you worse; however, if I treat you as though you are what you are capable of becoming, I help you become that."[44]

44 von Goethe, J. W. (n.d.). *A quote by Johann Wolfgang von Goethe*. Goodreads. https://www.goodreads.com/quotes/424596-if-i-accept-you-as-you-are-i-will-make

How can someone's vision of what you could be…help you become better than you are?

I can't help but think of my mom and my dad, my English teacher, Mrs. Linda Swanson, and another high school teacher, Donald Zook. They had this sort of vision and understanding. Once you get it, you will never need glasses when you look at others.

Jimmy Buffet said it this way: *It takes no more time to see the good side of life than it takes to see the bad.*[45] It's always good to quote Mr. Margaritaville, stop the overly religious readers from continuing, and clear the pool! Your life's direction is moving now and will likely continue unless you decide to change. Sometimes it takes someone to see in you what you can't see yourself. Sometimes we are blind to our hidden giftedness.

So, the importance of this chapter is for you to consider your ways. This is the most popular phrase in the book of Haggi: Consider your ways. Sometimes we don't like how we look in the mirror.

The Bible says it this way when talking about rolling a stone.

"Whoever digs a pit [for another man's feet] will fall into it, and he who rolls a stone [up a hill to do mischief], it will come back on him" (Proverbs 26:27, AMP).

If you have a critical nature, a wounded spirit, that kind of critical spirit will boomerang back on you. *Dig a pit of condemnation for someone, and you usually fall into it!*

You are what you eat. You become like what you watch. You reap what you sow. So, future you? It's not so mysterious. It's current you, exaggerated.

That means, though, good news: if you don't like what you're getting, you can change what you're doing, because you are one decision away from changing your life.

Let me tell you who will be one of our Presidents one day. Her name is Mari Copeny. Why do I think she's going to be President one day? Because of what she did years ago. Remember in 2016 when everyone became aware of the problems with the water supply of Flint, Michigan? Residents were becoming sick and dying, and something had to be done. Do you know how that story broke and became national news? Amazingly, at eight years old Mari Copeny got the federal government's attention to the water crisis with a letter to President Obama in 2016. When the president visited Flint after reading her letter, the spunky kid donned her beauty pageant sash for the meeting, earning her the nickname "Little Miss Flint." The visit resulted in federal aid to help the crisis but Copeny's advocacy didn't end there. She funded over $500,000 for Flint and enabled her community first by handing out bottled water and more environmentally friendly water filters. She was eight years old and raised half a million dollars. What is her next goal? To run for president herself. She's got my vote![46]

---

45 Buffett, J. (n.d.). *Jimmy Buffett - It Takes No More Time to See the Good Side...* BrainyQuote. https://www.brainyquote.com/quotes/jimmy_buffett_425230

46 Harrison, L. (2024, February 2). *Black History Month Clean Water Champion: Mari Copeny*. Clean Water Action. https://cleanwater.org/2024/02/02/black-history-month-clean-water-champion-mari-copeny

Because what's true from five years ago is more accurate of her today! Do you like the direction of your life today? Do you want an exaggerated version of who you are today in five years? If you don't like what you've been getting, you must change your actions. It would help if you made some different decisions. It would help if you valued some other things. It would help if you watched out for what ways you're letting in because the ways you let into your life are the ways you get set in. Your ways—the habits, thoughts, and choices you let in are the ways you get set in!

Levi Lusko once said: "The evening of life is determined by the morning of it."

If you are still living in the morning of life (you are young), you can make decisions before the evening comes. And if we're living in the evening of life (you are old), we can make decisions before that dawn breaks out. It's never too late to do the right thing.

Also, when deciding what to do with your life, there's an important axiom always at work: Ongoing consistency is much more important than short-term intensity. An ongoing consistency, every time, trumps short-term, flared-up intensity. Have you ever worked out for an hour and a half for the first time in two months and wondered why you didn't lose forty pounds? I ate one salad for breakfast today. Why don't I look better?

It's like people who come to church on Christmas Eve and Easter. They are "Submarine Christians" who rise to the surface twice a year. How spiritually fit would you be if you only went to church twice a year? Imagine joining a gym and using it twice a year. How physically fit are you going to be? Consistency, not intensity, is the key to changing your life.

Consistency in the little things leads to victory in the big things! The problem for many of us is that nobody has time for consistency. I want to diet one day a month. I want to work out once a year! We're just discouraged. Why? We want to go from the before picture to the after picture in one day!

"Do not despise these small beginnings, for the Lord rejoices to see the work begin" (Zechariah 4:10, NLT). We despise the day of small things. I am on the elliptical, Miss Elliptical, the other woman in my life, and I am huffing and puffing like Thomas the Big Fat-A## Train. I look down, and it's been twenty-five minutes, and I have burned 150 calories. That's it? That's a coke. That's half a protein bar, which I ate twice before getting on the elliptical. I have to do this elliptical every day, or Full-Face John (as my wife calls me) shows up, or Fluffy-Face John. I do despise Miss Elliptical, but I like what she does for me. I fit in my pants. But I have to do the elliptical consistently.

Why does God tell us not to despise the day of small things because these small things add up? *A very big God ordains small things.* Don't despise the small things of prayer, which God uses to change people's hearts. Don't despise the small things like making your bed. Don't despise the small things like saying three words: I love you, every day to your loved ones. Don't despise the small habits of letting go of grudges. It doesn't change the past, but it sure enlarges the future. Don't despise the small things like writing these words, by which God is glorified and people encouraged.

The small things done consistently add to life change and start with one decision to change. *I read several Bible verses, Pastor, and I didn't turn into a man of God overnight.* It's so frustrating, Pastor! Is there a pill for loneliness? *Isn't there something I can buy on Amazon? Why can't I be a great husband?* Is there a marriage conference I could go to? You have to do the dishes and quit being a jerk. I know, but I tried that once, and it didn't work out. And I don't understand. You can't jump from the before picture to the after picture without going through *consistent decision-making*. Decisions every day consistently make you who you want to be!

A study was done in Australia about the effects of sunscreen on aging. They split 900 people, with an average age of 39, into groups. One group was told to wear a high-powered sunscreen and wait for it whenever it's sunny. If you're going to the beach, if you're going to be out in the sun, man, throw some sunscreen on it. That's probably our strategy for many of us, like SPF 50. It's sunny. I need that on. The other group of people were told to wear SPF fifteen. What's that even going to do? Fifteen, are you kidding me? But I want you to wear it *every day*. In Alaska? Wear it. Are you not going outside all day? Wear it. You're going to be in a dark environment for a whole week?

Wear sunscreen SPF fifteen every morning as a part of your routine. Five years passed, and they studied both groups' before and after pictures. And the group that was told to put the higher SPF on only when it was sunny when comparing the photos, they, everyone who looked at it, and the scientists who did the study, could not deny there was aging that had happened in a short period of five years. There was aging. Man, that blemish wasn't there. That wasn't there. This person looks older. It's only been five years but look how much older they are. Would you believe that the group that put only SPF fifteen on every single day had no visible signs of aging? And in five years, their pictures looked virtually identical. It turns out that slow, ongoing, consistent, steady beats flared up. Oh, it's sunny. I got to get the sunscreen out, especially the intensity, quickly. It was the day of the small things with sunscreen, and that daily habit changed those five years.[47]

What's true of your skin is also true of your soul.

It was just one small habit, sunscreen every day, but it showed up significantly!

What are you doing daily for your soul, heart, and relationships? We spend so much money and time on the outside and so little looking at the inside.

What if you spent just as much time on the inside of your heart and life as you did on the outside every day? Would your heart and soul look a little different?

47 Sunscreens, E. G. to. (2023, May 23). *Skin cancer: EWG's guide to sunscreens.* Skin cancer | EWG's Guide to Sunscreens.
https://www.ewg.org/sunscreen/skin-cancer-on-the-rise/

Don't underestimate the power of a grain of sand or a pebble in your shoe to cause significant changes in your life. It's why Solomon said it's the little foxes that can ruin our love. The little things can become big things in a marriage or a relationship, for better or worse.

One of my jobs at the church where I work is to oversee and run a school with 200 kids. We have chapel time at the school, and once a year, we have grandparents come in and sit with their grandkids and have a donut. "Grab a donut with Granny," I think it's called! A four-year-old girl was sitting on her grandmother's lap two weeks ago. I was walking by and had this amazing moment. As the little girl moved her hand across the older woman's face, she said, "Granny, what are all these lines?" Grandma says, "Those are my wrinkles. They mean that I'm getting older." The little girl asked a great question:

"Do wrinkles hurt?"

What a loaded question! We are going to get them eventually, even you Botox-happy folks. Live long enough, and you will find yourself wrinkled! Everybody must address that question if one lives long enough: *Is it fun to get old?* You get to decide how you age. My friend who is a Life Coach, Dane Boyle, always says: *Age with Awesomeness!* I love that spirit. You will age regardless, but how you do it is up to you! His title speaks to the importance of your agency, your existential choice to do it with a spirit of awesomeness!

Speaking of grandmothers, one of my favorites is Esther Schmidt. She makes the best peanut brittle on this side of heaven. She just called me the day before my birthday. Now, she lives in a nursing home but is as sharp as a tack. She said, "Happy Birthday, John." I said, "I am still 52. My birthday is tomorrow, Esther!" She said, "I am sorry, John. I guess I am losing it. I am 97!" I said, "Wow, 97, that's awesome!" She says: "No, I don't want to be 97. I wish I were 95 again. I felt good at 95!"

Should we look forward to getting older or dread it? Should we apologize for it or brag about it? Do wrinkles hurt? I think wrinkles are proof you lived, you laughed, you loved, you cried! Speaking of wrinkles, have you ever made an ugly face at someone, and your mom said, watch it, your face will get frozen like that?

What is the face you get stuck with? What is the life you get stuck with?

Well, it's like when your mom told you when you were young, and you were making faces at each other: "Don't keep making that face, or it'll stick that way." There's science behind that. You can grow a smile or wrinkle lines depending on your routine. The life you get stuck with is the life you make. *Why not make it a good one?*

Good news: You are only one small daily decision from a different life.

Let's jump into one very important decision we all make every day:

How do we use our time?

How many of you would say:

I wish there were more time to do something important to you.

When I ask this question in church, virtually every hand goes up. Everybody says I wish I had more time to rest, read, spend time with my kids, date my spouse, garden, fish, surf on my phone, or surf in the ocean! I wish I had more time to do something really important to me. But if you're like most people, you say, I've got the yard to mow, dishes to do, chores to complete, a work project, bills to pay, kids to raise, and I've got to get the Instagram caption just right.

I don't know if you've noticed this, but whenever I ask people, "How are you doing?" I've seen the most common response is: I'm…let's say it all together….sooooo busy? How are you doing? Busy. I'm busy, busy. I don't think I've ever asked anybody how they were doing, and they said, "I'm relaxed, I'm just chilling. Life is easy. I'm having quality time with my kids. I don't have much going on."

If the devil can't make you bad, he'll make you busy. He'll make you busy doing things that may not matter. How are you doing? I'm busy. This is why I never say I wish I had more time!

I never say I don't have enough time to…

Why?

I have time for what I choose to have time for.

You have just as much time as Taylor Swift, Beyoncé, or any other of your heroes who accomplish a lot!

We all have time for what we choose to have time for.

Anytime I say *I wish I had time to do something else.* The problem is I'm choosing *something over something else.* Therefore, I will never say I don't have time for something!

I choose what I have time for.

Who's in charge of your calendar? You!

We all have time for what we choose to have time for. If you don't have boundaries around your time, other people will. I choose, you choose, she chooses, he chooses, it's our decision:

I choose the important over the urgent.

With God's help, he'll empower me to choose the most important over the most urgent.

What? Pastor, I thought that urgent things are always important. I want to distinguish between important and urgent a little bit. Because urgent things are not always important, there is a difference, and I'll give you a few examples.

For example, if you're a business owner with an upset, angry customer, dealing with that customer is urgent, right? But creating systems to keep customers from getting upset *is important.* 2 different things are urgent and important.

If your car engine needs repair because you didn't change the oil on it, getting it repaired is urgent, but what is changing the engine oil? What is that? It's important, right? It's important.

You're sick because you didn't take care of yourself or sleep. You're overwhelmed; you're doing too much. Going to the doctor to get treatment for being sick is urgent, but taking care of your body so you don't get sick is important. I'll only choose the important over just the urgent. It's easy to get swept up, to fight fire after fire. *But what if, rather than fighting fire after fire, we figured out how to prevent the fire from happening in the first place?* That's important.

Fires are urgent.

Preventing fires is essential.

If you choose what is important, you won't deal with as many urgent things.

If you choose what is essential, you won't deal with as many urgent things, but the opposite is never true. If you're only deciding what is urgent, you won't be faced with more important things, so that we will pick the important over the urgent.

Luke chapter 10 is a story about two sisters named Mary and Martha. It almost sounds like a sitcom, *Mary and Martha.* Martha does what so many of us do. She is so overwhelmed by the urgency that she misses the most important thing. We'll pick up the text in Luke chapter 10, verse thirty-eight, and how Luke described this story. He said as Jesus and his disciples were on their way, he came to a village where a woman named Martha opened her home to him. She had a sister called Mary, and we'll see Mary choose what's most important.

"Mary sat at the Lord's feet listening to what he said" (Luke 10:39, NIRV). Mary chose what was important. Martha did what many of us do; she surrendered to the urgent.

Martha got all wigged out, wanting everything to be just right, and I don't blame her because Jesus is in the house. Now, be honest; how many of you would go into frenzy mode cleaning up your home if you found out someone you respect was coming over? Does anybody do that? We do it at our house all the time. Someone's coming over, and it's like, everybody, now—throw stuff under the bed, in the closet, light the expensive candle, the one we've saved for company, and put on worship music because they're coming to Pastor John's house and there needs to be worship music. It's got to be just right. Panic, panic, get it all together. This is just for a regular person. If Jesus is coming, you can imagine what's going on. The forty-five-throw pillows on the couch and the bed must be in perfect little rows, and the potpourri has to match the shower curtains! I mean, it's Jesus, the Son of God, the King of Kings, the Lord, the Prince of Peace, and the Great I Am coming into the house.

Martha freaks out, as many of us would, and misses what's important. In verse forty, it says: Martha was distracted by all the preparations that were…what? *That had to be made.* I don't know about you. I'm getting more and more distracted all the time. I was looking for my keys in my office for probably three minutes. Where are my keys? Where are my keys? They were in my mouth the whole time I was looking for them. The next day I was looking for my Airpods and you know where they were, don't you? I don't know why I'm writing this, but it's cheaper than therapy. I'm trying to work these issues out. Martha was distracted by all the preparations that had to be made. I love that phrase—*I have to do this.* This is so important; I have to get this done. She came to Jesus. What did she do? She tattled on her sister. She tattled and said, "Lord, don't you care? My sister has left me to do all the work by myself. Tell her to help me out." Martha is wigging out, throwing a fit. "Jesus, tell her to help me out." She was distracted by all the preparations that had to be made.

I wonder how many of us, including me, have been faithfully pursuing the urgent and neglecting that which is most important?

A big question to ask is this: What is the most important thing you've been distracted from pursuing?

What is the most important thing when you think about your life?

What is the most important thing you've been distracted from doing? I hope you'll take a moment just to let this settle in. What is the most important thing? Stop reading and write it down. Is it a goal? A relationship? Your health? What is your purpose in life? Write it down. You are much more likely to take it seriously if you write it down! Then, take one step toward your most important thing.

Start living ready, aim, fire, rather than fire, ready, aim.

Some of you, honestly those of you who are Jesus followers, would say I've been distracted from spending time with Jesus. I haven't put him first. I haven't had intimate time feeding on his word. I haven't aligned my heart with him. I have been distracted from this.

Some of you would say I'm so busy doing things for my children I haven't enjoyed my kids. I haven't made a real investment in them. Some of you, if you're sincere, would say you've become child-centered parents. Your whole life revolves around your kids. What have you neglected? You've neglected the marriage, which is the rock that should hold the family together. Because you're so busy doing things for your kids, you've neglected what would strengthen and nourish your kids spiritually. The best thing a marriage can do for your kids is to have a great marriage. By your example, they watch and learn about roles, expectations, forgiveness, conflict, and love. You've neglected your relationship with each other. *Remember, the kids are meant to go; the marriage is intended to stay.* Don't let the kids become such a buffer that you wake up one day and look over at a stranger when they are gone. God first, spouse second, children third. The healthiest thing you can do for your kids is model a healthy, loving, unified marriage.

Some would say I've neglected my physical body. There is so much going on and many urgent things, so I haven't had time to eat better. Fast food is convenient, but who has time to work out? There are so many other things going on that I can't exercise. I'd love to walk three days a week; I can't get to it. Some of you think it would be something more internal. There is an addiction, a habit, or a reoccurring sin that you need to deal with. You need to confess and get help, but you've neglected it. It's really important, but you haven't dealt with it. Why? Look at the text: Martha is distracted. In verse forty-one, Jesus answers her: He says Martha, you're worried and upset about many things.

Some of you, if you had a life verse, that might be your life verse.

Think about it. You're freaked out all the time, all the time. Aah, I'm not going to get it all done, aah, diapers, kids, husband, underwear on the ground, got to get… You're worried and upset about so many things. Jesus said that few things are needed, or indeed, only one. Then what does he say? He says Mary has done what?

Mary has chosen what is better, which will not be taken away from her.

What has Mary done? She has chosen what is better. She made a choice. Martha surrendered to the urgent. Mary chose what was important. Listen, if we're not intentional about this, I promise you, the urgent will crowd out the important, and this happens all the time. We have a choice. We make choices. We have time for what we choose to have time for.

Practical Tools:

First Practical Tool – Create artificial deadlines.

You may ask, what in the world is an artificial deadline? An artificial deadline is an artificial deadline.

That's what it is. It's a fake deadline. It's artificial. It's not real. I'll give you an example. When is my Sunday message due? When is it technically due? Technically, it's due on Sunday at 9 a.m. or 11 a.m. Central Daylight Time because that's when I start talking. That's when it's due technically. But I think it's due earlier because I have an artificial deadline. My artificial deadline is a week before Monday at three p.m. For twenty years now, I've made a deadline, and my message is done Monday at three. The reason is that it's an incredibly important part of what I do.

Why would I leave something important up until the last minute?

I also have a lot of other important things that I do, like leading the church and being a dad, so putting an artificial deadline frees me of important tasks so I can devote my energy and mind to other important things. If all the important things are hanging, weighing in the balance, I'm never 100 percent focused on anything. I'm always divided so that I will finish by this artificial deadline. We will create artificial deadlines, which frees us up to do that, which is so much more important.

Second Practical Tool – Be ruthlessly selective in your "yeses!"

Be incredibly careful and prayerful about what you say yes to. Everyone is so busy; they are too busy.

Today, the barrier to a meaningful life is not a lack of commitment *but over-commitment.*

For most people today, the barrier to a meaningful life is not that you're not committed; you're way overcommitted and doing *way, way, way, way too much.*

How have you been? Busy, busy, overwhelmed, busy, busy.

Understand this: busyness does not necessarily equal productivity. *Busyness* does not equal *meaning.* Busyness does not necessarily equal fulfillment in life.

Most people, instead of adding to your to-do list, you should start a to-don't list—like I no longer do these things. The most successful people are strategic and always say no to good opportunities. Why? So they can say yes to the best. No to the good, yes to the best. The best leaders do not do more; they do more of what matters most. The best moms don't do more; the best do more of what matters most. The best teachers don't do more; they invest their energy in more of what matters most. The best and most effective followers of Jesus don't do more and more, more, more; they do more of what brings glory to God.

Third Practical Tool – We are going to do what matters most first!

Mark Twain said, "If it's your job to eat a frog, it's best to do it first thing in the morning. And if it's your job to eat two frogs, it's best to eat the biggest first."[48] Matthew 6:33 basically says: First seek God's kingdom and righteousness, and then everything else will be added. Get the top button on the dress shirt, and all the other buttons line right up naturally.

The problem with us is that we're all seeking everything else first and wondering why we don't have a life that matters.

We seek him first. I've got my reading plan every morning. I read while walking. I pray and devote my whole body to God. I pray this every morning on my walk, "God, give me the mind of Christ that I may think on things to honor you. Give me eyes to see only what is pure. Give me ears to hear your spirit speaking. May my mouth be an encouragement to everyone. May I speak the truth. My heart is deceitful above all things. God, give me a heart so I may serve you. Use my hands today to bring glory to your kingdom.

---

48 Twain, M. (n.d.). *Mark Twain - if it's your job to eat a frog, it's best…* BrainyQuote. https://www.brainyquote.com/quotes/mark_twain_414009

REV. JOHN W. ROBERTS

Direct the steps of my feet that I will go where you want me to go." Every day is a realignment. If we want to seek and honor God, we seek him first. Help me to be so full of hope; when life squeezes me, hope is the only thing that comes out! When I frame my day with that prayer on my morning walk, guess what? Great things happen. When I frame my day waking up consumed with all I have to do, great things do not happen. Worry and anxiety occur.

We do first what matters most.

Sometimes people ask me, "How do you have time to prayer journal? How do you have time to work out? How do you have time for dinner five nights with your wife? How do you have a date night every Friday night?" Because these things go on the calendar first. You've got to be so busy drinking out of the well of your life you are not trying to drink someone else's well. Set your boundaries, or other people will: *I won't respond to what everyone else wants me to do until I've done what God wants me to do.*

You are only one decision from a different life.

Carl Allamby grew up on welfare for most of his life. He recalls many days spent in his childhood home in Cleveland, Ohio, without lights, water, or utilities. He barely graduated from high school and took many menial jobs until he landed as an auto mechanic. He worked for several years for an auto shop until he opened up his successful auto shop. He had a dream as a child not to be an auto mechanic but to go from motors to medicine and to be a doctor. Allamby added, "I remember having a desire at a young age to become a doctor—but my life circumstances led me to a much different place. From my experience, it isn't easy to focus on your education when your mind is filled with challenges outside the school's walls. Food insecurity, safely making it to and from school, affording decent clothing and basic school supplies, or just trying to fit in took precedence over studying and getting good grades." He said his parents "always taught us the value of working hard for what we wanted and never giving up on your dreams, no matter how improbable."[49]

He first enrolled at Ursuline College in Pepper Pike, Ohio, starting in 2006 when he was thirty-four and was fascinated by a biology course. He finished that degree and realized his calling from God was to be a doctor. So he went to medical school, graduated at age forty-seven, and finally, now at age fifty-one, he's Dr. Carl Allamby, an ER doctor. Listen to the parallels he says about being an auto mechanic and doctor: "Every day is different," he said, "and just as with a car, my work in the emergency room has the potential to go from 0 to 60 in seconds."[50]

You are only one decision from a different life.

49 Association of American Medical Colleges. (n.d.). *Carl Allamby*. Students & Residents. https://students-residents.aamc.org/career-changers/carl-allamby

50 Sudhakar, S. (2022, September 19). *Cleveland Auto Mechanic becomes doctor at age 51, inspires others to pursue their dreams*. Fox News. https://www.foxnews.com/lifestyle/cleveland-auto-mechanic-becomes-doctor-inspires-others-pursue-dreams

Let me tell you about baby doll, Renee, my wife. She doesn't love hosting and entertaining like I do. My idea of a good time is for twenty of you to be in my living room. The more people at our house, the happier I am! Not so for Renee. Her idea of a good time is reading a book on the couch, with no one else around, not even the dog! The tension between Renee and me is not about having people over but about what the house looks like. Last semester, my son Zach had four roommates—a five-bedroom apartment, four guys, including him, and a female roommate. I said, "Zach, are you getting along with your roommates?" He said, "Yeah, except for the girl, Dad." I asked, "Why is that, son?" He replied, "Well, Dad, let's just say her idea of a clean apartment and our idea of a clean apartment are two different worlds. She wanted to start charging me for cleaning up the common area." I told him you probably should start paying, which is not bad, then asked him, "What's the best thing about your classes at UT?" He said, "When they are over!" Ha! Academics—he loves it. I also said, "This will never go away for you, son. Your wife's idea of cleaning one day and your idea of cleaning will always be worlds apart."

Over the years, Renee and I have always had this tension where I wanted to host thirty people, but Renee wanted the house to be just right, so every week before people came over, it was like a panic zone, and we'd fight. I know you don't think we'd fight, but she can fight. And as her dad warned me, she may be small, but she always wins! Like a hummingbird versus a gorilla, and the hummingbird wins every time! She can fight, so we're fighting about the house. The house has got to be correct, and it's like massive stress. We want to host, but there is so much pressure to get the house right. I will never forget when Renee came in one day; she had this relief. This joy was beyond what I had seen in a while, and she said, "Got an idea." I said, "What is it?" She said, "What if we choose people over perfection?"

I think that will preach, but I'm unsure what it means. She said, "What if we just choose people? For example, when people come over, do we choose and administer to them, love them, and have a relationship with them over perfection? In other words, the house doesn't have to be just right; we can just be ourselves, and if they don't like us, then that's okay, but we're just going to be ourselves, and we're going to choose relationships over image. We're going to choose people over perfection."

I was like, "Yeah, that makes total sense." So now, come on in if you come over to our house. There may be Captain Crunch on the tile, and there may not be worship music playing, and an expensive candle may not be burning because we can't find it anywhere in our house. But I can tell you there will be some drinks in the refrigerator and we will sit down and enjoy one another. Why? Because people are so much more important than things, we will choose the important over the urgent.

It has changed our lives. I'm telling you, we have people over all the time.

You are only one decision from a different life. Do you like who you are now? Because chances are, unless you change your daily habits and start putting on sunscreen, you will be more exaggerated five years from now. If you don't start choosing the important over the urgent now, you will let the tyranny of urgency run your lives.

Create artificial deadlines. Be very selective about what you say yes to. Start a "to-don't" list. Design your life. Build routines, not to-do lists! Examine your daily habits. Seek first the Kingdom of God. Get your calendar right because you have time for what you make time for. Set up your life so the fires don't happen, and you don't have to put out the fire! Live prepared so you don't have to prepare. If you choose actions like these, these are the actions of restoration; these are the voices that help, not hurt, the future you!

What is one small step you can take right now that will lead to a bigger life?

CHAPTER ELEVEN

LESSONS FROM A SPLINTER: SIX STEPS TO HEAL YOUR WOUNDS

There is always tension between the possibilities we aspire to and our wounded memories and past mistakes.

—Sean Brady

AT THE HEART OF MANY of your problems is your offended heart.

Let me tell how God revealed this to me, *because only God can speak through a splinter.* I have a wooden fence in my backyard, and one of the boards got loose, so Renee told me I need you to go *pray over* that board; the screws have come loose. That's the preacher's wife's code for adding it to the honey-do list. I was out doing what I always do: working with tools (smile, I still have my Handy Andy Junior Tool Set) and trying to fix this board. I mishandled the board and ended up getting some splinters in my hand.

Have you ever got a splinter in your hand?

Have you ever been hurt in life?

It happened on a Saturday. I could not get the splinters out of my hand. They had gone further down under my skin, so I went to church on Sunday, and I want you to know *those people offended me.*

Do you know who those people are?

Every one of you that shook my hand hurt me.

People squeezed my hand, said hello, and shook my hand, which hurt me!

They didn't mean to hurt me; they didn't know they were hurting me, but they hurt me nonetheless.

They didn't know they were offending me, but I did. I kept track of all of them and wrote their names down.

Those people will not be getting any more Christmas cards from me!

They hurt me, and now my heart has a bunch of splinters in it. Instead of removing those splinters, I will let them fester and get infected, and pretty soon, I am not healthy. I am wounded, I am hurt, I can't love, and my heart can't beat without hurting.

Have you ever shaken someone's hand with a splinter?

Why would you leave a splinter in your hand?

You don't.

Have you ever got a splinter in your heart?

Why would you leave a splinter in your heart?

People do.

They let wounds fester and get infected and become much worse over time.

Time does not heal all wounds. Intensity wanes over time, but healing does not automatically occur. You have to work on your vineyard to remove the weeds. You and God heal wounds, not time. Quit telling people it takes time. Time does not heal all wounds. Pulling the splinters out of your heart and giving them to God does. This is why God's Word says in Ephesians 4:26 (NIV): "*Do not let the sun go down while you are still angry.*" Take the splinter out, and don't let it fester. If you get a splinter in your hand, stop and remove it. Otherwise, you are choosing to live wounded, like a victim. This verse says—*The day of your hurt should also be the day of your healing*. The day you get a splinter is the day you remove the splinter unless you want an infection or to live like a wounded bird. The same day someone offends you should be the day that, as a follower of Jesus, you're working to bring reconciliation into that relationship.

But what do we do?

We fail to caringly confront them (carefrontation) and tell them you are hurting me when you shake my hand. We fail to tell them their actions are hurting me, please stop. We let the wound fester. We nurture it. We take our wounds, and we have a pity party. We show our friends and say, "Can you believe this splinter she gave me? Can you believe how wounded and hurt it is now?" It's been in my hand for three days, and I want to nurse it, curse it, and rehearse it. Someone says, "Why don't you talk to them and have them remove the splinter?" Oh no, no. See, this splinter has become my identity. It's who I am. I don't know how to be and live in this world as a victor, but I do know and claim identity as a victim. In fact, from now on, please call me "Splinter!" Splinty for short.

Have you ever met someone like this where all they want to do is tell you how wounded they are? Here's the reality: The longer you play the victim, the more you remain the victim. If you play the victim, you stay the victim. Your woundedness then becomes your identity!

When Shadrach, Meshach, and Abednego went into the fire for "failing to worship the King," Jesus was the fourth man in the fire and protected them. The Bible says in Daniel 3:27 (NIV): "They saw that the fire had not harmed their bodies, nor was a hair of their heads singed; their robes were not scorched, and there was no smell of fire on them." They went into the furnace, and they came out and they didn't even smell like smoke! They came out of the fire that was supposed to consume them and didn't smell like smoke. I can't grill a hot dog on my outdoor grill without smelling like smoke. (smile) In other words, they didn't let that wounding experience define them. Don't let the fires of life make you smell like smoke. Don't let an ugly moment ruin your pretty. We all have an excuse from our past for why we are the way we are. Or we all have a story of how we overcame our past and why we are the way we are.

Story or excuse? One or the other. Can't have both.

I want to live my life around people who took the splinter out, not people who went around showing everyone their splinter! What if you lived in this world with a heart of love as God intended? The same day you get the splinter, remove the splinter.

Honestly, this principle has helped my marriage of over 30 years be strong in the way it is. And I give my bride Renee credit for this because early on in our marriage, she said, "We're not going to go to sleep mad, ever." I didn't say, "We're not going to go to bed mad because we'll go to bed mad, but she won't let us go to sleep mad, like ever." And it can be annoying, like, "Let's just sleep. We'll deal with this tomorrow." She says, "No." And this has helped. Renee has taught me to take the splinter out now.

I don't know how this is possible, but those of you who are married will know it's true: No one ever trains you in the rules of warfare. You don't learn it in a premarital class, but the moment you fight in bed, there are unwritten rules that you all intuitively know and live by. There are ways that you gain points, and there are ways that you lose points when you and your spouse are fighting. You earn points by being back-to-back. You have to be back-to-back. You gain a point by huffing. You gain a point by throwing your shoulder violently away from the other person. You gain an extra half point by bringing the covers with them. You lose points if your feet drift into enemy territory. You ain't touching my toe! You ain't getting toe for the rest of your life. And then you lose if you do something Godly like talk first, right?

These are the rules. How do we know them? I don't know, but you intuitively know them when you get married. We had been married for three months when we got into our first fight, and it was a big, big fight. Everyone had splinters all over the place, and Renee said, "We're not gonna go to sleep until we settle this." We got in a fight on Sunday, and we didn't sleep till Thursday. I'm just exaggerating a little, but not by much.

How different do you think our friendships, our families, and the body of Christ would be if, on the day that I offended you, I owned it and apologized and said, "Would you please forgive me?"

Or the day you offended me, I had the grace as I've been so often forgiving to choose to forgive you. Or the day we had a misunderstanding, an agreement, or a hurt, we both said, "Hey, let's just let that thing go."

Let's remove this splinter. Sometimes you need two people to remove a splinter. Sometimes you need God to help you remove the splinter.

It's hard to shake hands or walk through life with splinters in your feet, hands, and heart. How different do you think the world would be if we worked toward healing on the same day of the hurt as followers of Jesus?

Don't let the sun go down while you're still angry because you don't want to give the devil access to divide, distract, or discredit you from being who God is calling you to be.

The experience will be painful. It hurts to remove the splinter. You have to deal with the offense. The splinter must be removed. Until the offense is resolved, it will be impossible to maintain close relationships.

Here's the real rub. If someone decides to let the splinter stay in their heart, it's like cancer. It grows and takes over their heart.

The Bible talks about the danger of living with an offended heart three thousand two hundred years ago. It's found in Proverbs 18:19 (NLT): "An offended friend is harder to win back than a fortified city. Arguments separate friends like a gate locked with bars!"

According to the above verse, we have a greater likelihood of conquering a well-guarded city than we do of regaining the trust of an offended brother when they won't, and we won't remove the splinter.

Anyone can allow you to become offended, but you get to choose if you will live offended! People are rough. They will give you splinters, but you can let the splinter remain!

Essentially, Jesus said in Mathew 11:6 (ESV): "Blessed is the one who is not offended…"

Proverbs 19:11(ESV) says, "Good sense makes one slow to anger, and it is his glory to overlook an offense!"

It's your glory to overlook an offense, to take out the splinter.

Someone said, "We are like beasts when we kill. We are like men when we judge. We are like God when we forgive."

Five steps for leading an unoffending life:

Step 1 – Look in the mirror. Recognize you have a splinter or two!

When we judge an offender, we feel morally superior, while at the same time, we fail to recognize our moral shortcomings. This is called fundamental attribution error. It's an erroneous way of looking at life. This is when we make a mistake, we blame circumstances. When someone else makes a mistake, we blame their character. If you've ever chastised a "lazy employee" for being late to a meeting and then proceeded to make an excuse for being late yourself, you've made the fundamental attribution error. This tendency is to cut yourself some slack and not blame your character but hold everyone else's character to blame. We are very good lawyers when we give others splinters and very good judges when we see someone living with a splinter.

Pastors are not immune to this problem. Before blaming others, we should take a close look at ourselves. We are all human and are prone to making mistakes. We will occasionally be disappointed by broken people in a broken world. Ecclesiastes 7:21–22 (NIV) says, "Do not pay attention to every word people say, or you may hear your servant cursing you—for you know in your heart that many times you yourself have cursed others." I love this verse. It's saying look in the mirror before you judge anyone else. Quit taking everything personal, quit taking everything to heart, all the things that people say. What if we made this a habit of not taking things personally?

Step 2 – Decide you are not going to *live* offended anymore.

I didn't say never get offended anymore. That's going to happen. Splinters will happen, but it's your choice to live with or without the splinter.

I got called over to a family's house the other day, and the parents told me about their 22-year-old daughter, who was currently locked in the bathroom upstairs, having broken up with her boyfriend and losing her job on the same day. The parents were afraid that she might be so down and out she might be suicidal. So, I began to knock on the bathroom door, and I ended up having most of the conversation through the bathroom door. Have they ever been there with a loved one?

I knocked on the door and told her who I was. Then I asked her the best question I have learned to ask people when they are going through a difficult time, "How can I help you? What can I do to help you in this moment?"

Let them tell you what would be most helpful, right?

I will never forget her response. She asked me for something I could not give.

Ever been there?

She yelled through the door, "Just go out and get me yesterday and most of today. I want them back."

I told her I couldn't do that, but I did say Jesus could. He can't give us back our yesterday. He can do better than that. He can forgive the sins of yesterday. He can forgive the splinters we give ourselves or to others. He can heal the pain of yesterday. He can restore the energy wasted in the selfish pursuits of yesterday. He can restore the relation-ships you severed yesterday in your sin, selfishness, and pride. Christ does for us not only what we can't do for ourselves but also what others can't do for us.

It was a struggle, but eventually, the bathroom door swung open, and healing had begun.

I have never forgotten those words, "Go get me yesterday and most of today." What if you could relive one day from your past? Which day would you choose? We all have a day or two, don't we? I love to ask what-if questions.

We don't ask enough what-if questions.

What if your dog could suddenly talk, and it told your most embarrassing secrets? What if God created an entrance exam to reach heaven? Would you pass the test? What if you could never sleep and remain healthy? What would you do with your extra time? What if you could become invisible? What would you like to do? What if you could insert a magical chip into your kid's brain so they can become a genius? How many of you would do that? What if you could become all your mom hoped and prayed for when she held you as a child? One of my favorite pictures is of my mom, who is 57 years old, holding our son, Jacob, and loving him as his nana. It's magic in my mind because Jacob is nine months old. He's just so full of promise, potential, and what-ifs. I remember when Renee and I went to our first doctor's visit two months into Renee's pregnancy, and they had done some bloodwork. There were a bunch of what-ifs, but most of them were not good. What if your baby has Down syndrome or spina bifida? The doctor gave us a horrible list of what-ifs. What if your baby is born with all these problems? So you might think about an abortion! I asked myself: What if *it doesn't have to be this way*? Doctors practice medicine, but they don't always get it right.

It takes just as much energy to ask Godly, positive, good what-if questions as it does gloom and doom what-if questions.

I will never forget when the doctor returned to the exam room and said to Renee and me, "So, after giving you all a chance to visit, what do you think you two want to do?" Renee and I were like, "Well, what we are going to do is get a crib!"

What if we trust God with our baby and love this baby no matter what happens?

I remember praying over Renee and touching her belly: What if God had special plans for this baby? What if this baby, Jacob, would one day become a doctor who would save lives? What if he helped cure some cancer? What if this baby changed the world? Jacob is now going to medical school!

Can you picture God holding you as a baby and asking, "What if over your life?

What were the dreams and hopes God whispered over your soul when God made you in the secret place, when God wove you together in the depths of the earth, when you were fearfully and wonderfully made?

What if you are not just "smart mud" with khakis on? If you are just smart mud, why do you have these thoughts at two in the morning about what happens to you when you die? Why do you long to make a difference in this world? Why do you long to have something you do outlive you? Why do you long to help others? Why do you get a helper's high (God designed your body to release feel-good hormones) when you help someone else? This is where secular humanists will fail you. Evolution doesn't explain these longings.

What if you lived today like this was the last day of your life? If you do that every day, one day, you will be right.

Why aren't you living out the life God intended for you to live? Because of the splinters others put in your heart and life.

Because you have let some of life's wounds harm your heart and soul irreparable.

I don't want to live that way, jaded, cynical, like a wounded bird.

Wounded birds, wound birds. Hurt people, hurt people.

My mom had a phrase she would always say to me—John, make sure you watch out for and she would always whisper it to me—*those people.*

I want to talk to you about those people. Now, just for fun, say Amen out loud if you think you might know who I'm talking about when I say, "Those people!"

Yeah, if you are reading this in a coffee shop, don't point at them because they are crazy, and they're everywhere.

Those people can be challenging. Those people are often critical. They can be controlling. They're often incredibly arrogant at times. Those people can be mean.

They always live as a victim complaining about what they could turn about.

Those people know everything about everything, and they're going to tell everybody every chance they get. You'll see them shouting up a storm in the airport: "You can't cancel my flight. Don't you know who I am?"

Why yes? You are one of those people.

You will see them airing their messy lives on social media, violating what social media is all about: *Show the best and hide the rest.*

You'll see them spreading the rumors at the office. There's almost always one now at every big family gathering. It's almost like a spiritual principle. You get all the relatives in there, and one of those people will be in the house. And if you say there's not one of those people in your family, it's probably you. They're everywhere.

A couple of years ago, I did a sermon called "Those People," and it's a true story. A lady just went off, upset, furious, and ticked. She was offended and felt compelled to tell me so. She came to see me the following week. I thought she was scheduling time to have coffee and join the church. Ha! She starts the conversation like this: "What are you doing, preacher, talking about those people? That's not a Christian thing to do. Who are those people? What do you mean by those people? You're supposed to be a man of God. A man of God wouldn't talk about those people. I don't want to hear and talk about those people. Who are those people anyway? You shouldn't talk about those people." And I just looked on and smiled and thought, "You're going to be a sermon illustration one day. You are so those people."

If you follow Jesus, this will mean more to you than if you are not. As followers of Jesus, we know that we're called to love. We're called to love everybody, and we're called to love those people. We say it this way at my church: We welcome everyone who welcomes everyone.

Some of those people are a little more difficult to love!

The word of God in Ephesians 4:26–27 (NIV) says, "In your anger do not sin. Do not let the sun go down while you are still angry, and do not give the devil a foothold."

Ephesians 4:29: "Do not let any unwholesome talk come out of your mouths, but only what is helpful for building others up according to their needs, that it may benefit those who listen."

Ephesians 4:31: "Get rid of all bitterness, rage and anger, brawling and slander, along with every form of malice."

"In your anger do not sin," which tells us *it is not a sin to be angry.* The Bible says that God is slow to anger but gets angry.

We have to be careful with anger; it's like fire. Fire in the fireplace warms the house. A fire in the living room burns a house down. It's not that I should never feel angry. It's what I do with this feeling of anger. Again, feelings are temporary; facts are forever, so make sure you deal with the temporary wisely. Then, ask: What does God get angry about? What did Jesus get offended at?

I learned this from Bridgette in Honduras on my mission trip. Through Good Works Honduras and HNI Charities, I went on a weeklong mission trip to some remote villages in the mountains of Honduras along with doctors and nurses to join them in administering medicine and annual physicals to people who never get to see doctors or dentists.

I met Bridgette. She was in fifth grade. She spent all day with me as I played with the kids and was able to help install clean water systems in their homes. She spoke perfect English and perfect Spanish. Do you know how heartbreaking it was to meet her parents and all four of us go to her brother's grave? He was four years old and had died from parasites and chronic diarrhea due to unclean drinking water. I asked Bridgette how she had learned such good English. It turns out she was born in America. Her parents "illegally" came to the US, had her on American soil in Texas, and then got deported after many years. Most kids in Honduras didn't know they were poor. They had dirt floors and sheets for windows in the hovels they called homes. Bridgette knew better. *She had tasted poverty in America, richer than any poverty in Honduras.* She asked me at the end of the day, "Will you adopt me, Padricito Juan (Father John)? Will you take me back to America?" She knew I could give her a life she would never know in Honduras. So, when I returned to the United States and heard about how people offended me, I began to feel nauseated.

Are you offended because McDonald's took too long and got your order wrong?

Are you offended because the Pastor's sermon was over twenty minutes long?

Are you offended because your groceries cost more this year than last year?

You're offended because your doctor, whom you can see as many times as you need, took thirty extra minutes to call you back for your exam?

Are you offended because the hot water in your shower takes thirty seconds to heat up?

These are very minor splinters, my friend—hassles at best. Don't make them into heart-aches. When you go on a mission trip and see how blessed you are in the US, you realize the difference between hassle and heartache. Imagine living with dirt floors, towels for windows, no electricity, no running water, and chronic diarrhea because you don't have clean drinking water. This is their life. Tell me again why you are upset.

Was Jesus offended when the thief on the cross asked for forgiveness?

Did Jesus say you can live your life any way you want and then ask for eternal blessings during the two-minute warning?

Did Jesus tell Peter after he denied him three times, Pete—I am so wounded, I don't think I can let you be my disciple anymore?

Was Jesus offended when a prostitute poured perfume on his feet and wiped his feet with her hair?

A whore touching a rabbi?

How offensive it was for some!

Was Jesus offended by sinners? Did he ever say to God—I was going to do the cross, but those people, they are so mean, they tore off my clothes, gave me a crown of thorns, and they want to crucify me?

Who did Jesus most get offended by?

Are you ready for this?

Religious people. Jesus got offended by what offended religious people in his day. I am not sure he's still offended by religious judgmental people.

He got offended by the religious people who wanted to stone the woman caught in adultery.

He got offended by the religious people charging high prices and ripping people off when they came to the temple to worship, turning worshipping God into a financial boom for them.

Jesus did get offended when religious people got angry at the wrong things.

Jesus did get offended when he would do a miracle on the sabbath, heal a man with a withered hand, and all the religious people could do was ignore the miracle of the healing and focus on the fact that it was on the Sabbath that Jesus broke a "rule!"

We are not supposed to work or heal on the Sabbath!

I believe everyone is fundamental about something. We are all religious fundamentalists to some degree, and for me, the only thing I want to be fundamental about is what Jesus was fundamental about: **Indiscriminate love.**

Love God, love your neighbor. If everyone were fundamental about this, the world would be better.

What if you were to stop living offended about things that don't matter? Start getting offended about things that do matter. Living offended, living like a victim always, is a sin.

Let's call it what it is. Stop getting offended about petty, first-world problems. It takes just as much time to find the good as the bad. It's all about where you look.

It's a choice. To repeat this previous point: A vulture looks for dead stuff all day and finds it. A hummingbird looks for flowers all day and finds them. What are you looking for all day? I bet you find it.

Quit staring at your belly button and start looking around at who you can help.

We are so privileged.

We have so much.

Everyone who reads this book is rich by the world's standards.

I will bet everyone who reads this book makes at least 30k a year. If you do, you make more than 90 percent of the world.

The average person in Honduras lives on $1.50 a day. The average person in America lives on 155 dollars a day. There's no one reading this book who will wonder if you can afford your next meal or if your water might have a parasite.

You might wonder when your next cup of Starbucks is on its way.

What if you lived in gratitude rather than greed? No one reading this book is going to wonder if your children or grandchildren will die today from chronic diarrhea.

You are flat-out rich.

But are you rich toward God and others?

You might be overextended in debt, but who's choice was that?

Does anyone here ever play Frisbee or Frisbee golf? John Bowes, chairman of the parent company of Wham-O and the maker of Frisbees, once participated in a charity effort. He sent thousands of the plastic flying discs to an orphanage in Angola, Africa. He thought the children there would enjoy playing with them. Several months later, a representative of Bowes' company visited the orphanage. One of the nuns thanked him for the beautiful "plates" his company had sent them. She told him the children were eating off the Frisbees, carrying water, and catching fish. When the representative explained how the Frisbees were intended to be used, the nun was even more delighted that the children could enjoy them as toys.[51] On one level, that story is rather amusing. On another, it is very sad. Some people would prize even our cast-off items, who would be grateful to eat what we throw away.

It matters to Christians that there are people in need, not just because we are nice people, but because there was a time when we were in need.

We are the recipients of grace. God loved us when we were helpless and undeserving. Not one of you has been given abundant life or salvation because of who you are but because of who God is. Don't tell me you earned everything in your walk-in closet.

Knowing this, we should look around for others who are helpless and perhaps even undeserving so that we may pass on the love we have received.

They are not hard to find.

We gather every week in our Grace Presbyterian sanctuary, or what the kids at the school call Chapel Time. We gather in the "Grace Chapel" to remember God's salvation and calling over our lives. Have you ever thought about the word chapel? The word "*chapel*" comes from the Latin CAPELLA, which means "cloak." The word originated from St. Martin, a Roman soldier who gave his cloak to a beggar dying of cold. St. Martin's cloak became a relic and was kept in a building that soon took on the cloak's name, CAPELLA. The word became CHAPELLE in France, and in England, it was CHAPEL. However you pronounce it, a chapel is a cloak of God for poor beggars such as us.

We are all beggars at the foot of the cross.

We are all beggars when it comes to God's forgiveness.

We are all beggars when it comes to our blessings because we know ourselves to be beggars where the grace of God is concerned; we do not shun the beggars of this world.

51 Burkey, R. (2005, May 19). *Sharing Jesus in Practical Ways*. Sermon Central.
https://www.sermoncentral.com/sermons/
sharing-jesus-in-practical-ways-richard-burkey-sermon-on-evangelism-how-to-79253?page=2&wc=800

Have you ever begged for a second chance, wisdom, or love?

Have you ever dimmed your light to please someone, begging for approval?

Our church has a group called the *BOC or Beyond Our Congregation.* The very name screams we are looking beyond our collective belly buttons! Is there anyone here really proud of your belly button? Beside Britney Spears? *Don't look down and complain. I don't like how my belly button looks, either, especially after my hernia surgery.*

BOC is the outreach arm and legs of the Church. We want to do things to bless those who can never bless us. We want to give to those who are helpless because we once were helpless and received God's grace.

Today, 3,800 people will die due to unclean drinking water, most of them children.

Someone's child, someone's cousin, someone's daughter, someone's son, some grand-mother's prayers will go unanswered because they are drinking dirty water.

So tell me again, what are you so upset over?

I didn't text you back quickly enough.

I didn't email you back within twenty-four hours.

I haven't thanked you enough or patted you on the back.

I didn't say hi to you at the coffee hour.

Tell me again, what made you so mad, and do you think God is mad about this too?

Does it involve a preventable death?

Like most things in life, we can complain and remain or change and not remain. It's up to *you*!

Through HNI Charities and Good Works Honduras and our church, the best week of my life this year was spent in Honduras, where I could go, along with nurses like Deborah Houlihan, and deliver medicine and water treatment systems to families in Honduras and hope. That's all I got, hope. I am a hope dealer, and everyone deals with something.

You can give a family of four clean, lifesaving water for over a hundred bucks for ten years.

Have you wasted a hundred bucks lately?

I am proud to be a part of a church that recognizes we should and can do something as simple as giving a cup of cold water so that next year, I don't have to talk to parents who have buried their four-year-old!

Do you know how petty some of your concerns sound when I am standing at the grave of a four-year-old?

Get some perspective broader than your backyard.

It sounds ridiculous; your voice in my ear about how you are so offended when I'm still dealing with the echo of the cries from parents who just buried their kids because of parasites in the water?

Seriously.

I am not writing this to be offensive!

How ironic if you got offended at this chapter rather than being offended that we live in a world *where we shame ourselves by letting people die, ignoring Christ's calling on our hearts.*

If you choose to get angry, let's get offended and angry about the things in life that Jesus got offended and angry about!

I have been reminding myself over and over and over again that there is no win in being and living offended.

There's no win. I've never found my life to become more joyful when I'm ticked off about what somebody said to me. My marriage has never gotten better when I'm angry at some injustice in this world. I've never gotten closer to God; I've never had more intimate conversations when I've walked around with ongoing unforgiveness toward someone who hurt me in my life.

I need to remember that there is no win in living offended, but I'm likely to be offended, so what do I do? Well, I tell myself this:

Being offended is inevitable, but living offended is a choice.

Being offended is going to happen. I'll probably offend you. Someone else is going to offend you. You probably won't get out of the parking lot on Sunday morning from church without some other Christian offending you with their driving.

Being offended is inevitable, but living offended is a choice. It will happen, but you can still choose how you respond to an offense.

That is one of the reasons the apostle Paul tells us that you've got to be careful. Because if you hold on to anger, and if you're constantly nurturing an offense, and if you're rehearsing the hurts, what you're doing is you're giving the devil, you're giving Satan the father of lies and the prince of darkness, you're giving him what Scripture calls a foothold in your life.

I always thought of a foothold, like if you're walking into a room with a door, and you put your foot in the door, and that keeps your foot in the door. Or maybe if you're rock climbing, a foothold might be when you throw your foot up and put it in a little crevice. The word in Greek is different. The Greek word for this is Topos, which means a place or a room.

In other words, If you go on and live in your anger, you're giving the devil a place in your heart or giving him room to work in your life.

I don't know about you, but I don't want to give the devil any access to anything that matters to me. I don't want my anger or my offense to give the devil access to attack anything close to me. I don't want to give him access to my marriage, to Renee. I don't want him to attack the intimacy that we have. I don't want to provide the devil with the ability to attack my children and come into their lives and maybe even divide us. I don't want to give the enemy the ability to attack my friends, the people that I do life with, and I don't want to give the devil access to my church. *If I live in anger and harbor bitterness and live easily offended, scripture says you're giving your spiritual enemy access to your life.*

What if you decided not to live any longer with an *offended heart?*

Step 3 – Practice mercy. Mercy is the act of giving to others what they do not deserve.

Did you deserve Jesus dying from your sins?

Jesus loved and died for the person you hate too!

The extent to which we show mercy is the extent to which we will be shown mercy.

In Matthew 6:14–15 (NIV), Jesus said, "For if you forgive other people when they sin against you, your heavenly Father will also forgive you. But if you do not forgive others their sins, your Father will not forgive your sins."

If you forgive others when they put a few splinters in your heart, God will forgive the times you put splinters in the hearts of others!

James 2:13 (NLT) says it even more strongly. "There will be no mercy for those who have not shown mercy to others. But if you have been merciful, God will be merciful when he judges you." It means what it says!

Step 4 – Lower your expectations.

Ever put up a fence? One side is smooth, and the other side is rough. People are the same. Everyone has a smooth side, and everyone has a rough side.

Sometimes you are going to rub into someone's rough side. People are sometimes placed on pedestals, and we are scandalized when they cannot walk on water. People will disappoint us.

2 Timothy 3:1–5 (MSG) states: "Don't be naive. There are difficult times ahead. As the end approaches, people are going to be self-absorbed, money-hungry, self-promoting, stuck-up, profane, contemptuous of parents, crude, coarse, dog-eat-dog, unbending, slanderers, impulsively wild, savage, cynical, treacherous, ruthless, bloated windbags, addicted to lust, and allergic to God. They'll make a show of religion, but behind the scenes they're animals. Stay clear of these people."

If you want a Biblical verse telling you to stay away from *those people,* here it is!

People will fail us.

The greatest joy we will ever receive is from those close to us.

The greatest wounds we will ever receive are from those close to us.

We must learn to recognize this is how life is and forgive them.

Step 5 – Lose the detailed logbook.

Healing requires that we not only confront our issues (remove the splinter) but also avoid reliving, rehearsing, and rehashing our past pain, as this can negatively impact our relationships. Once you have stewarded your pain and learned from it (wear some gloves in the future), quit reliving it!

If you are the one in the relationship who keeps bringing up what the other person did a week ago, two years ago, or ten years ago, you are doing it wrong. Some of you are blaming people who are dead. How can they change anything? They are dead! *Quit dusting off yesterday and placing them in your today!* Quit taking the past mistakes fossilized in your memories and reliving them today.

The past is good to learn from but a horrible place to live.

You can't live today if you keep tripping on the past. We cannot move forward if we are anchored in the past.

I can't shake hands with you today and not be hurt if I have not removed the splinter I got from you yesterday.

Remove the splinter, don't nurture it. Don't nurture your wounds; heal them!

It is time to give our logbook to Jesus!

In Isaiah 43:25 (NLT), God says: "I—yes, I alone—will blot out your sins for my own sake and will never think of them again!"

Some of you need to memorize this verse.

God does what we cannot do. God forgives what we cannot forget.

God will never think of your sins and splinters again, so why are you rehearsing them in your head and letting them prevent you from living today?

You are not a failure just because you failed.

Your name does not need to be "Splinter."

To accuse us, the evil one keeps a detailed logbook in which he records everything we do.

The Bible calls him the *accuser of the saints.*

When we go to that wooden cross, and we see the body of Jesus, we see he is bleeding from our splinters, from our sins, our mistakes. Yet the blood of Jesus is enough to remove all our splinters, and they are remembered no more.

God has lost your logbook of splinters. Why don't you lose it too?

Step 6 -Try to understand the offender.

I believe that some offenses are not a result of what occurred but instead of what the individual thinks transpired or how the individual perceives the person's attitude toward them.

Therefore, it is imperative to listen carefully to gain a complete understanding of the facts.

I am taking the time to reflect on the situation and comprehend the individual's viewpoint.

Sometimes people will tell us a story. But it isn't the story they are telling that we should heed, but the story remains untold.

We will be unable to hear it if we are not paying attention.

James 1:19 (NLT) says this: "You must all be quick to listen, slow to speak, and slow to get angry."

"We are to be quick to hear but slow to speak." Rather than "quick to speak and slow to listen!"

Try to understand what's under the thing and where they are coming from.

Appeal to their smooth side and recognize that everyone, including you, has a rough side.

People with splinters in their hands never join hands.

People with splinters in their hearts never join their hearts.

If you have a splinter in your heart, remember your heart doesn't have to be this way. It can be healed; you don't have to smell like the smoke of the fire you have been through.

CHAPTER TWELVE

DON'T FAKE IT, YOU WON'T MAKE IT

To anyone who faked it, did you make it, yet?

—Victoria Cooke

I HAVE HAD TWO MOMENTS IN ministry when people got my name right but my title wrong.

Titles are hard to fake, names not so much.

The initial one was my first thirty seconds in my office at First Congregational Church in Escondido, California. I was thirty years old, worn out from an eighteen-hour drive out of Texas, and carried my first sermon book box into my office. I sat down in my big pretentious faux leather chair, the type you get at Office Depot for a solid ninety-nine bucks. In walks Jack, an unknown older church member who was kind of like a Walter Matthau-type guy *or the grumpy old man.* As I am sitting on the chair, he throws a bag of oranges onto my lap and says welcome to the church.

Now, if you know me, I love fruit, so I immediately, out of politeness, try to start peeling one of the oranges because I love fruit. I had never seen an orange like this before, but they don't peel like the "regular" orange you buy in the grocery store. The orange starts falling apart, juice is getting everywhere, and it's not going well. *Cleanup on the new faux leather chair, right?* Jack looks at me and says, and I quote, "Geez, those are juice oranges, you *jackass.* You don't peel them, you juice them!"

I look up, and this is my first thirty seconds with one of the holy church members of my new church for whom I have just uprooted my entire family from Texas, and I say, "It's *Reverend* Jackass to you!"

You can't fake knowledge about juice oranges, can you?

For the next six years, that's precisely what he called me, *The Most Holy and Reverend Jackass John Roberts.* It didn't matter if my parents were visiting or it was Christmas

Eve; it was Rev. Jackass! It always made me laugh. I had a name tag made but never had the guts to wear it much! I mean, honestly, I've been called worse. It also reminds me there is a whole story in the Bible about a prophet named Balaam who has a talking donkey. The donkey talks back to the prophet and helps him see what he could not see. The conclusion of that Biblical story has always been: *If God can speak through a donkey, he can certainly speak through any jackass like me!* See Numbers 22:21–39 (NIV) for those who don't believe me! It's in the Bible. God can speak through any jackass God chooses. I don't mind being insulted, but I have a ninety-hour, four-year master's degree from Southern Methodist University that gave me the title of Reverend, and I intend to use it! It's funny—titles and what they convey; how we label people, jackass or not. No one is just a jackass. No one is just a jerk. We are all a bit of a mixed bag at the end of the day.

This story leads me to another funny story about a more serious time when my title as Reverend was mixed up with another Holy Surname. It was a typical Friday funeral service—show up at 11:30, service at noon, and graveside at 1:00, no problem. I have done a thousand funerals, so I was not worried. I had already met with the family, so I knew how they wanted to honor their loved ones. Yet, on Wednesday, the funeral director called and asked me if I could pray with just the family on Thursday night at the viewing! Ok, a little bit unusual for a Presbyterian Pastor, but I have done that once or twice. Can you be there around 6:45, Pastor? Sure, no problem. Again, it's slightly off since the viewing was from six to nine p.m., but grief makes people do funny things. Believe me, I know. When I pulled up to the funeral home and saw about two hundred cars, I thought, wow, this is a big family. I might want to add some thoughts to my thirty-second prayer! Upon entering the viewing room, I realized the casket was front and center, and two hundred people sat down. I thought, "Is the service tonight?" My Catholic readers know where this is going! I walked into the room at 6:45, and some grandma, some abuela, grabbed my arm and said, "Thank you, Father, for being here tonight for the Rosary. Where is your parish?"

Parish? That's a Catholic deal. My parish is now called: "O God Help Me Now!" Have you ever been a member of that parish? I have a congregation, not a parish. Father? It's Reverend, or Reverend Jackass, to those who know me, or John. I quickly slipped off my wedding ring, quickly ordained myself "Father Faker," and prepared to conduct the Rosary! Well, if God can speak through a donkey…but the big challenge: I had no idea how to perform a Rosary. I just knew it involved a lot of Hail Marys, and right about now, I was saying my own Hail Mary! At this point in my life, I had been to one Rosary, and it was a distant memory. All I remember was that there was a tremendous amount of repetition!

I quickly retreated into the men's room and will never forget it. I looked down at my watch: 6:52. I had eight minutes to Google, learn, and spit out a proper Rosary

Service—no time to call and yell at the funeral director. I was here and would have to try to fake it until I make it.

At 7 p.m., I walked out, and the most different un-Catholic Rosary began. "Good evening, Father Clueless here. Let's begin…"

It started poorly and got worse from there. I read it word for word right off the good old internet. Don't believe everything you read on the internet. Some people still believe the earth is flat, and they built websites dedicated to telling you so! I know I was making mistakes; you should have seen their faces. From looks of consternation to what was going on to eventually down-right pity, I did find out that every time I got quizzical faces, if you made the sign of the cross, that seemed to reset everything and allow folks to forgive me.

Have you ever wanted a reset button on a day, a comment you made, or a relationship?

I must have made the sign of the cross enough to make the Virgin Mary proud. My favorite comment was from one lady who said, "Father, I have never been to a Rosary quite like that. Where did you go to Seminary to learn to be a priest?" Or another comment was, "Are you a second-career, brand-new priest?"

Paging Rev. Jackass. Well, it wasn't Notre Dame…and, ma'am, you probably will never be to another Rosary quite like that. But what was I doing? I was going to fake it until I made it.

Such bad advice and a bad slogan—*faking it till you make it* is disingenuous. Have you ever seen people try to fake it till they make it financially? They try to show they are making it, living in cars, houses, and clothes they can't afford today. They promised to pay them tomorrow via the credit lines. Eventually, the creditors win. You can't fake cash flow. Have you ever seen a couple faking love? Have you ever seen a deaf person faking that they can hear, reading lips, or anyone else?

Looking back, I should have been honest with that crowd. I should have told them, "Look, I am a Presbyterian pastor ill-equipped to lead this Rosary. But I thought I would fake it till I made it." I am sure people were polite and discussed how bad it was when I was gone! I did call the funeral director and tell him never again! It wasn't my best because there are some things you can't fake, like love, rosaries, finances, and the condition of your heart. If I had a second chance, I would not have removed my wedding band and pretended I had a parish down in the valley, a small one you never heard about: Our Lady of Perpetual Money! (smile)

We fake it and try to make it when tired, burned out, and spiritually dry.

Integrity means we are honest and don't try to fake it…*even when we're tired*. After Christmas, Renee and I drove up from Corpus Christi, Texas, to Bryan, Texas, to visit her dad and sister. After opening gifts and lunch, Renee and I drove five hours, and I went to get checked into a hotel. Now, I had a bunch of paper in some binders of my second book, and Renee was editing it in the car. And I was tired because we had put a lot of miles in. I just wanted to get horizontal immediately. At the front desk, the girl says, "Well, what brings you to Bryan, Texas." And I said, "Family." And as I tried to put my manuscript down, the binder with my paper broke open, and papers flew all over the desk and the floor. Then she said, "What's with all the paper?" I told her, "Oh, I am writing a book!" She said, "What's the book about?"

I wanted to go to bed. *Just give me my hotel key card, woman,* you know? I stopped, and I chose to engage. Because you can look at customer service people and engage or treat them like they're robots or treat them like they're a piece of furniture, you can be on your phone not even looking or looking at them almost like they're just a hurdle to you getting to what you want. But I engaged for a second. I just said, "My book's about how to get through impossible circumstances in your life. How to make it through tough stuff you face. It's about how it's not always: 'It is what it is…'" She said, "That sounds like a book I need." And so we talked for a bit. I gave her a card with Grace church, the website, and the YouTube channel, and I gave her a copy of my first book. Well, check this out. I found out about her via the email she sent me. She had just lost her mother and just moved from Oklahoma to Bryan, Texas and was struggling. In her own words, she had been looking for a church, and so she was able to find one. Two days later, she sent me an email. She has already watched the month of December services on our YouTube channel. Why? Because she invited me to speak into her life, to give her some hope. How often do people invite us to speak hope into their lives? Do we listen?

I extended my faith, beliefs, and values into a life where I was invited! Jesus worked the same. Jesus is polite. He stands at the door of your heart and knocks. Jesus doesn't kick doors down. God can't save anyone against their will.

When I was in college, I worked at Mr. Gatti's. Does anyone remember that place? I was a busboy. It taught me the discipline of hard work and the power of being a servant. I would clear tables. The servers would pre-bus the tables, get rid of the meals as soon as they ate, and I would come in when the customer left and knock out all the remaining cups. And if the waiters and waitresses were lazy, I'd get the plates too. And I just said, if I'm here, I'm not just going to sit in the back, you know, drinking Coke like some busboys would. I'm just going to go out there and work.

Soon, I had this reputation among the waitstaff, as if I were bussing your tables, and it would always be clean. They'd have more customers and more money from the night. So, I started getting requests; they wanted me to work their tables and shifts more. And I had this one general manager who was a raunchy guy. Anytime I overheard him talking behind the line, it was always filthy. It was always about some girl in the bar. So it was just not an awesome encounter. But I remember having my first interview with him, and I told him I needed Sundays off because I was attending church. I went to the Methodist Campus Ministry because they had a cute girl named Renee there and Jesus! I wanted both! I never shared the gospel with the guy. I would come home smelling like pizza dough. Thankfully, Renee loved the smell of pizza! So I remember one day, he grabbed me by the shoulder and said, "Hey, John-boy, you got any other Christian buddies at that church of yours?" And I said, "Yes, sir. I think I do. Why?" And he replied, "Because you know what? If they all work as hard as you, I'd hire only Christians in this store." What a great thing. Come on. I'm telling you: **The quality of your work can cause the volume of your life to get louder!**

It's called integrity, and integrity demands that we be who we claim to be, titles and all!

One way to check for this is to ask yourself: Does what comes from your lips match what you're living in your life? Because if your story lacks integrity, there's no validity to it. Don't be the real jackass who is *living a lie betraying what you're preaching with your mouth*. It's called hypocrisy, one of the most damaging things to the gospel. I mean, you've encountered it. I have experienced it. And I'd like to say I'm sorry for the times I have lived hypocritically. Because we've all had bad days, and we've all done it. It can be used as a scapegoat, and it can be used as just a catchall so we don't have to come to church. People say, *Well, the church is all just full of hypocrites. Well, to some degree, yes. And we have room for one more, so please join us.* But to another extent, We do want to be walking the line. We do want to be walking the talk. None of us are going to do it perfectly, but listen to the power of integrity, the power of clean living, the power of purity, the power of being faithful to our spouses, the power of being good moms and good dads, and living out at home what we're talking about in church. It's great to gather in church on Sundays, but as I have said, if what happens on the weekend doesn't impact what's happening during the mid-week, then what happens on the weekend doesn't work. What good is it to raise our hands to God on a Sunday but then, throughout the week, treat people harshly, have a reputation for being dishonest and unethical, cutting corners, telling lies, not being kind, and not being generous? Do you see what I'm saying? If we want our lives to be lives of love, stability, and consistency, we must live out what we're preaching: trust Jesus, honor Jesus, live for Him, and let our lives be authentic based on what we say we believe.

David said in Psalm 25:21 (NIV), "May integrity and uprightness [right living with God and others] protect me, because my hope, Lord, is in you." Now you hear that and think that's not very encouraging because I'm not an awesome Christian.

I'm not writing this chapter and asking you to be! I wrote this chapter because:

I'm asking you to be an authentic Christian.

I'm just asking you not to say something with your mouth that's not true about your life.

Well, I've got a whole part of my life that's a mess. I don't want to tell him that.

No, no, do tell everyone that.

Tell them exactly that. That's what I am doing in this book and in my messages every Sunday!

Tell them that's why you're so happy you have a great Savior. Tell them you're glad that the pit you fell into of sin was deep, and you're not proud of it, but you're thankful that God's got a big ladder. And God let down a big rope. **Your righteousness doesn't come from everything you've done. It comes from everything Jesus did. Where you fell, own the failure. That was wrong, but God is good. I'm going to praise Him for what I once was.**

Paul said I was a blasphemer. Paul said I was a persecutor. Paul said I put Stephen to death. But I thank God that He saved me and that He cleansed me. I'm telling you something. My purity doesn't come from me. It comes from him. And my integrity doesn't come from me; it comes from him.

Jesus is the superhero. We're the damsel in distress. Let's not pretend we are the ones who got nailed to the cross.

I have had lots of failures in my life. I had to learn how to love someone way different than me in my marriage after getting married because that is what happens when a gorilla marries a turtle. I don't recommend learning how to fly a helicopter once you are in it. Learn to fly it before you get in one. Learn to love and about love before you grow in love. Any idiot can fall in love; falling down is easy. *It's growing in love that takes work.* It's staying in love that takes work. It takes work to grow in love many times with the same person over fifty years. So I reveal my brokenness and my dark moments not because I am proud but again to say that if God can work through someone broken like me, God can work through you! Jesus said, "Blessed are the poor in spirit" (Matthew 5:3, NIV).

Contrary to what we would expect, brokenness is the pathway to blessing! There are no alternative routes; there are no shortcuts. The very thing we dread and are tempted to resist is the means to God's greatest blessings in our lives.

My brokenness is a better bridge for people to God than my pretend wholeness ever was!

When I fake wholeness, people see it. No one believes you know about a juice orange when you try and peel it. No one believes you are a "Father" when you fake a Rosary. No one believes you are Christian when you can't love! No one believes you when you are a Christian who lacks integrity.

I've been doing ministry for thirty years now and have one goal: to break the hard-hearted and heal the brokenhearted. I don't need proud people in my life. Proud people are the ones who fake it and try to make it. Proud people focus on the failures of others and can readily point out those faults! Broken people are more conscious of their spiritual needs than anyone else's. Proud people keep others at arm's length. Broken people are willing to take the risks of getting close to others! Give me a church of broken people who recognize they need help! Ultimately, we were all humans…drunk on the idea that love, only love, only God, getting involved in our lives could heal our brokenness! The deepest cuts are healed by faith. God will mend a broken heart if you give Him all the pieces. Leave the broken, irreversible past in God's hands and enter the invincible future with Him. God uses broken things. It takes broken soil to produce a crop, broken clouds to give rain, broken grain to give bread, broken bread to give strength. It is the broken alabaster box that gives forth perfume. Peter, weeping bitterly, returns to a greater power than ever.

"Fake it till you make it" is bad advice.

Have you ever tried to fake good blood pressure?

Have you ever tried to fake intimacy?

Have you ever tried faking a full head of hair when you are bald? Comb-over anyone?

Have you ever tried to fake a good marriage?

Have you ever tried to fake a growing, loving relationship with your kids?

Have you ever tried to fake spirituality?

Have you ever tried to fake a Rosary?

Have you ever tried to microwave brisket? It won't taste good, nor will your life if you fake it.

One time, I conducted a funeral with a prominent pastor who had a bad toupee; it was terrible. He wasn't faking it till he made it. He came in late for the funeral, fifteen minutes late, and met me in the narthex of the church, and his toupee was sideways. It wasn't right, and I should not have said it, but it just came flying out of my mouth, word vomit, word diarrhea. Have you ever been there?

I said, *"Before you go into the service, go to the bathroom and fix that squirrel you got on your head!"*

Paging Rev. Jackass.

Faking it till you make it is analogous to a bald guy wearing a toupee. Why do that? They have hair transplants today and medicine today. They look amazing, so amazing, you can't tell. My dad had hair transplants done and had more hair in his eighties than in his forties! I remember people asking my dad, "Why do you tell people you got hair transplants, and why would you spend money to do that?" I loved his response. He said, "Well, if you have a missing front tooth, you go to the dentist, and they can fix it. Likewise, if the front of your hair is missing, go to a surgeon. They can fix that." No one goes around lying about going to the dentist.

If you have a broken arm and a cast is on it, you don't go around and pretend your arm works and try and use it. You tell others, and it's getting healed. It takes time. Sometimes people sign the cast to say hey, heal up, friend!

When someone is depressed or has an anxiety problem, don't tell them to fake it till they make it. That leads to suicide. That leads to death. That leads to more anxiety and mask-wearing.

Why do we try to hide a broken and depressed spirit when we don't try to hide a broken arm? Brokenness is brokenness. It looks and manifests differently in people's lives, but there is no gain in trying to fake it. Faking your happiness leads to more anxiety and shame.

Why do people say: Fake it till you make it? I get it—you want to project confidence. There's nothing sexier than confidence. I always tell the ladies that I counsel the sexiest part of a woman is not her lips, eyelashes, boobs, or butt! It's her confidence, the way she carries herself. But for confidence, to be honest, it has to be real, not faked. There has to be a sense of what you are confident about and what you are confident in. It will eventually hurt you if you keep stretching the truth about yourself. Stretch marks always show up. Unfortunately, faking it till you make it can add to that *impostor syndrome feeling.* Faking your confidence or abilities to do something can be more damaging than productive. You may end up feeling more fraudulent than you were in the beginning. It can lead to avoiding people and your problems too. Instead of asking for help for your anxiety, you are busy covering it with a happy mask or staring at your *digital pacifier* (phone) for four to ten hours a day, which research shows leads to more depression. Hiding and faking till we make it is catering to what we think others want. We can't try to cater to what we think others want. They want a father who knows the Rosary or someone who knows what a juice orange is because we have no idea how to do that or precisely what they want. We think we know what others want us to be, but do we? It's ironic that we only think we know what they are thinking, but you are not inside their head.

What if we were just honest? What if we were just unsexy? What if we were opportunistic and savvy in seizing chances to demonstrate who we are, being unapologetic and confident, even if that means sharing our confidence with people, battling insecurities, and working at changing our lives?

Faking it until you make it doesn't work: It's stressful. Faking a Rosary was stressful. Today, it's sort of funny, and it makes for an excellent true story in this book, but I would have been more relaxed had I just been authentic.

Living authentically at all times is called integrity.

When you are free to be fired from your job because you are doing it as authentically as possible, you are free to go to work truly! Better to say, folks, I am sorry. I will do my best, but I barely know the difference between a juice orange and a regular old orange, but I will give it my best! You can learn. You can grow. You can be proud of progress, not perfection. It reminds me of when I was doing a funeral, and the director came in with the body in a closed casket made from wood, some fancy pine, or something. About halfway through, while one of the family directors spoke, the funeral director approached me and said, "Hey, we got the wrong body here. That's not Mabel in the casket. That's Gertrude. Gertrude is in the bronze casket in the viewing room. In between now and taking this body to the graveside, we have to switch them!" What would you do? Funerals are overrated, but you get some stories if you do them for thirty years! They didn't have a class for this in Seminary. How do you tell the family, "Well, if Jesus can turn water into wine, he can turn wood into bronze?"

Fake it till you make it? No, I told the family what happened, and they laughed about it and they said it was definitely their loved one because they were late to their own funeral!

If you always fake it, you will repel people. Better to be authentically broken and struggling with your faith than pretending you always believe, you never have doubts, and you are the next bishop!

Show me someone who acts like they always have it all together all the time about everything, and you will find people walking in the opposite direction.

We should always "hang A lantern" on our weaknesses!

This phrase comes down to us from generations ago when you walked from the farmhouse to the barn, for example, and you hung your lantern on a peg so you could milk the cow or saddle the horse. To "hang a lantern" means to shine a light, to illuminate. So, I'm urging you to shine a light on your weaknesses in front of those you love and interact with. Let one of your boundaries become transparency and authenticity. Be willing to admit you live into things in life. You are not faking it because people see the truth. We live in an age of constant brand management. We usually try to hide whatever is weak or unsightly about us. "Put your best face forward," we are told. You take forty-one selfies for everyone that gets posted after 37 AI filters. Trust me, I could have written a better book than this if I had just let someone like Tyndale Publishers or AI write for me. But how inauthentic is that?

Very.

When I wrote my first book, Tyndale Publishers, one of the leading Christian Book Distributors in the whole country, said they would publish my book. They read my first chapter, edited it, and sent it back. I read that first chapter and said, "Wow, this is good. Way better than what I submitted!" One glaring problem, however, was you could tell I didn't write the book. Renee, my wife, read the redacted version, and she said, "Oh man, this is good. It's way better than your first draft. I think you should go for it." Tyndale

Publishing could have distributed my book much broader than Amazon. It could have an international impact. But here's the rub: the first time one of my church members read the book, or anyone who knows me would have said, "Great book, so great, it's obvious you didn't write this, Pastor John. So ahh, who wrote it?"

Thanks to my new ghostwriters, I lay in bed that night with visions of becoming the next Stephen King of the Christian writing world. I could fake it till I make it. But then God whispered in my ear, and I believe he whispers it to you as well:

"You have to write the book that I have placed in your heart!" You can't lip-synch your way through faith. You can't lip-synch your walk with God or with your spouse or with anyone. At some point you have to sing the song God has placed in your heart. Quit comparing yourself to others and wanting to be like them. At some point, you have to be something you have never seen before. When David went to check on his brothers and heard Goliath insulting God and Israel, he was ready to fight. At first, he said, "Give me whatever a man wears to fight." He tried on Saul's armor, but when he didn't fit in it, he couldn't fake it with Saul's armor. He had to be something he had never seen before, a twelve-year-old warrior with a slingshot who knew that Goliath was too big to miss.

You have to be something you have never seen before—you. Authentically you.

God places you and your gifts in your heart, no one else's! *No one else can write your book or your story! You can't wear someone else's armor to fight your battles.* At least not with integrity and authenticity. Hang a lantern on your book; hang a lantern on your life. People can see who you are anyway. *You can only be fully loved when you are fully known.* If I go around wearing a mask, and you love the mask, I know that deep down inside, if I take off the mask, you may not love the real me because you have never seen the real me. Take off the mask and live with authenticity. At least then, you know that people genuinely love you for you, making you *you*! If you try to fake it and not hang that lantern, here's the problem: People usually see what is wrong with us. They want to know if we do.

Are we blind to our flaws?

Are we deceptive about them?

Can we be trusted with such things?

God, I hang a lantern on my weakness. Let them see my brokenness, but also let them see how you healed me. *Hurt people hurt people, but healed people heal people as well!* If you can see what's wrong with your friends, open your phone and text them to say: It's so obvious! I guarantee this will get the conversation started toward honesty. It's good to be willing to show people where I am weak. It shows strength.

Don't hang a lantern on something you are "faking," do you?

How many of you can see a problem with me that I have been hanging a lantern on?

My weakness is I am a control freak. I got more than one, but I can't write forever here. So I pray to God, help me see my need to control and surrender everything to you.

See, because sometimes I can be quite needy, like Needy Ned! God, help me see my need to control, manipulate, and surrender everything to you because, in this teaching, it will be easy to get zeroed in on "Those other people." We have to remember all of the time every day, that in one way or another, we are *Those people* in life! I can't speak on your behalf, but I can tell you about me, and that is: I have a deep and ungodly desire to control everything. I can say this: God loves you, and I have a wonderful plan for your life! I want you to do what I want you to do! I mean, that's true in my marriage. I want Renee to do what I want. I want my children to do what I want them to do. I want our church to do what I want our church to do. I want my schedule to go the way I want it. I want my finances to do what I want, and if something breaks, I don't want that! And the bottom line is that I like to be in control for two reasons: 1. Because I'm afraid of sur-rendering to someone or something else. 2. Deep down, I hate this, but if I'm just dead honest, I believe I make a better God than God. I want to be in control. And if you want to be in control, chances are pretty good because you're afraid of letting go. You believe you make a better God than God. And guess what? I don't make a good God, and you don't make a good God because you don't know the whole picture and you don't have that much power.

Yet, we try to control and manipulate, and we will never have a relationship that does what God wants when one has power in an ungodly way rather than mutual submission. Now, there is a difference between leading well. I should lead my children, not control them, not manipulate them. And I've had to come to where this has been a massive point of spiritual development in my life in the last three years. And those close to me can tell you that I have tried to take and name those things that I want to control and say, God, I cannot control these. They're yours, and by faith, I give them to you.

God, I give you this church because it is not mine. It's yours. I can't do anything with this church, but with you, and through you, this church can grow and thrive!

I give you my family. Oh, dear God, I've got two kids driving, two kids in college right now! Help me, Jesus! Okay, I know many of you have been through that, and you've warned me. Nobody prays like a parent with teenagers just now going out on the road. And I can't control that; they're His, and I trust Him.

I've got my schedule just so insanely out of control. How can I get it under control? God, I trust you to be enough in me. I trust you to be enough.

I don't know what it is for you, but I can guarantee that many of you are those people who are trying to control someone else. You've got your thumb down on your kids and just hanging out. You're not leading them. You're controlling them; they resent it and want out. Or you've got a marriage where you're passively aggressively giving jabs and threats and fear, and listen, and you'll never have what God wants. Or it could even be your health. God's got to do this, and if God doesn't do that…! Listen, God is God and will be glorified through whatever He chooses to do. So you take what you want to control; that's what you want. You've got the death grip on it, and you say, God, you know what? This isn't mine. God, it's all been yours since the beginning of time. And I, by faith, open up, and I surrender this to you. And here's what Scripture says in Isaiah 26:3 (NIV): "You will be kept in perfect peace…" I don't know a lot of people in perfect peace. I know people in perfect turmoil and fear and anxiety, but you will be kept in perfect peace …all who trust in you, God, all whose thoughts are fixed on you!

When you surrender instead of faking it, you start making it.

The other key to not faking until you make it is curiosity. Live curiously. Ask questions of your heart, of your life, of your marriage. Be curious. Be more explorer than expert. Be more Dora the Explorer than I know everything about everything.

Did you know Jesus asked?

In the Gospels, Jesus asks many more questions than he answers. To be precise, Jesus asks 307 questions. He is asked 183 questions, of which he only answers three.

Asking questions was central to Jesus's life and teachings. Jesus was curious, not an expert. He was only fundamental about love.

When you hear the name Albert Einstein, what do you think of it? Does anyone think you are not much of a student? That was his reputation, which is hard to believe when you think that Einstein is now in the dictionary as a synonym for genius. But apparently, there was a day when his teachers were worried about him and thought perhaps he was "slow."

They called Einstein slow.

They were wrong.

They put me in the slow math class, and they were right.

Einstein was just bored with what teachers were trying to teach him! He was already a few clicks above where the experts were. He famously said that the number one thing that got in the way of his learning was his education. Ugh! Yikes. Because look, readers are leaders, and leaders are readers, right? Yet, not everybody learns as Einstein did. He was very much a self-learner and a self-feeder. Albert Einstein was an insatiable learner and someone who never dialed down the childlike curiosity that Jesus wanted to be a part of every day of your life. Jesus said that you should have faith like a child, for such is the Kingdom of Heaven, never to stop asking why, never to stop pondering, and never to stop imagining. Einstein set out to figure out *how God speaks regarding math*. But in his later years, he pointed back to his childhood, specifically, a gift he received from his father, as one of the big things that set him off on this life of curiosity, imagination, and asking questions.

As the story goes, he was sick one day and couldn't attend school. And his father came home to visit him. I watched Mutual of Omaha's Wild Kingdom and Captain Kangaroo when I was sick from school. Remember those shows? Anyhow, Einstein and his family were living in Munich at the time. And his father brought him a gift, and the gift was a compass, just a simple ordinary compass. As a five-year-old, Albert did what all of us would do. He sat there looking at it and tried to figure it out.

His father wisely didn't tell him all about it, how it works, and what to do with it. He didn't say to fake it till you make it. He wanted his son to be curious! He just gave it to him and let the compass do the talking. Albert said that he would stay up all night, literally, up all night with chills running up and down his spine, spinning back and forth in his bed, watching the compass needle move, trying to figure it out and trick it. But he realized that no matter what he did, the needle found its way back north every time. And he said, speaking about this moment in his life later on, "That experience (the compass) made a deep and lasting impression on me. Because something had to be behind hidden things."[52]

Here's the trick of the compass: When you close it and put it away, you are still surrounded by whatever was causing that needle to move. The compass makes what was already there, just invisible, observable.

Think about that briefly as it applies to your life and faith. Right now, I can see the effects of the magnetic forces, but if I put the compass away, they're still there. The gift of a compass helped him know what couldn't be seen with the naked eye. And that's the gift of faith. It helps us see beyond what we can see with the naked eye!

Einstein began asking, if those forces were there, which I didn't know about, what other forces might be there? He asked questions when he looked up at the stars.

Who made the stars? Why am I here on earth? What or who moves the needle on the compass?

Have you ever asked that? Who moves the needle on the compass of your life?

What forces are at work in your life?

What points you true north?

Curiosity can lead you to discover science and self-discovery!

Einstein asked those questions. Einstein said, "I want to write an equation that should be small, little, less than an inch long. But I want that simple equation to explain the universe's rules." Einstein came up with:

$E = MC^2$

52 Einstein, A. (1999). *Autobiographical Notes*. Open Court.

That energy can become mass, and mass can become energy, explaining how the stars shine. In less than an inch, a little equation explained the rules that govern the universe.

Of course, he also came up with his theory of relativity, which is to say that the faster you move through space, the slower you move through time. How many of you suddenly feel like you are now with me in the slow math class? Have you seen the movie Interstellar? It will make your head hurt! Someone said you could explain the theory of relativity to me in a way that I can understand! He said, put your finger on a stove, and a second will become an hour. Spend an hour with a pretty girl; an hour will feel like a second. Ha! I love that. That is the theory of relativity for dummies like me. In case you're wondering, Einstein was a hit with the ladies, mainly because of his violin. Yep, he would just really kill them. He'd woo them by playing some Bach, playing some Mozart on that violin. Einstein, you classical playing dog, you!

But I want to bring you back to Einstein's bed as a five-year-old, as he sat there, almost tortured by the question, What is moving the needle? And that's the same question I want to ask you:

What moves the needle in your life?

Is there a force that points you in the same direction over and over, the direction of love and not hate, true north, the way of generosity and not greed, integrity and character and not lies and deceit?

What keeps you going when life is tough?

It's tough to fake this, and why would you want to?

It's tough to make it in life if you don't have this. It's hard to fake it if you don't have this. No matter what Einstein did, running around, closing it up, spinning it, and pointing it in one direction, the needle on the compass always pointed true north.

What keeps you going when life is tough?

The answer in Einstein's day was the molten iron within the Earth's core. But that's not the explanation for what's moving the needle inside of us because the truth is, no matter where you live, no matter what your name is, no matter what kind of music you listen to, we all experience the same phenomenon. And that is the universal sensation *that there's something more.*

There's something out there. It's not just eating. And it's not just having a good job. And it's not just watching the football game and seeing my Steelers or Cowboys win. It's not just sex. It's not just work and success and money.

Haven't you felt it, that universal sensation that, hold on a second?

Hold on a second: There's something more.

Maybe it's what led you to pick up this book. There's something more than paying your bills, having a fat 401K, and ending up in a nice nursing home.

I have felt it moving throw pillows. I didn't know that was a thing when I first got married. I had one pillow on my bed, on a twin mattress. I had one pillow on my bed when I got married. Then Renee came along, and we got a queen size bed. I figured out two pillows. I came home on the first day of marriage asking, "What's with all these new seventeen-and-a-half throw pillows doing here? What are all these things? They're not functional. They go on the bed."

Why?

So you can take them off before you go to sleep? And then what? You put them back on the following day. I thought, hold on a second. I haven't lived on this earth for very long. How much of my time am I spending on this? I started calculating: How much of my life will I spend on these throw pillows?

I think we've all pondered life's meaning in ways small and large. And if we're just the product of chance, and if we're just smart mud, and if it's all just a biological lottery winning that causes us to be here on this earth, why should we care about meaning? If Earth is in the Goldilocks zone, and we are just the right distance from the sun to support life, and it's all random chance, why bother?

If it's true that you don't have a soul, and if it's true that when you're dead, it's just lights out, game over, thanks for playing, is it fair? Does it matter? Natural selection, survival of the fittest, dog-eat-dog, weak being preyed on by the strong: if that's true, then:

Why, why, why do we ask questions about immortality? Why do we long for greatness? Why do we not want to die the second death, the death of being forgotten? Why do we want to do something that outlives us? Why do we ask: Is there a God? Does he know my address? What keeps us going in difficulty?

Here's a question I wrestle with, and I should not, if I am just smart mud or a monkey with pants on:

Is God good when life is not?

That's the question of theodicy. Is the heart of life good, bad, or indifferent? Is it something I assign meaning to?

Sam Cooke had one of the most amazing male voices ever. Besides Steve Perry, or George Michael, maybe one of the best. He once sang that there are times when life seems good; it was a song called "Summertime."

> It's summertime, and living is easy.
> Fish are jumping and the cotton is high.
> Your daddy's rich, and your mama's good-looking.

Hush baby

Don't you cry

Hmmmm…

One of these mornings, you're going to rise singing.

You spread your wings and take to the sky.

But until that morning, there is nothing that can harm you…

With your daddy and mommy standing by

They are standing by.

Hmmmm…

Cotton is high, Daddy's rich, and Mama's good-looking; life is going well. There are times I have felt life is that good. There have been moments when the cotton was very high indeed! There are also times when I felt life can be very challenging and not good.

Is the heart of life good, bad, or neutral?

Do we get to assign meaning to this world, or does it lean toward good or bad? This question was one of the main reasons I went to Seminary. It's called the question of theodicy: Theodicy is a noun that means "the vindication of divine goodness and providence given the existence of evil." The vindication of divine goodness is saying that sometimes stuff happens in life where we view God on trial, his very character being questioned. But we must also remember that not everything comes from God. Some things are from the father of lies or what the Bible calls the accuser of saints. When I make this argument, most people say, Ok, God is not the author of evil, but he allowed it. Again, allowing something to be in the scope of possibilities and authoring evil in your life are two different worlds. I think the best way to view challenging things is to say that life, the evil one, or pernicious circumstances put us into *a situation, but God is the one who calls us and enables our way out of those situations. What do you base your identity on more?*

Moses was put through a lot, including a crocodile-infested river at birth in a basket. What does his name mean? Drawn out of water. God drew him out of that situation, and Moses would go on to pull his people out of slavery and bondage to the Promised Land. But the point of this section is to ask: Have you been there? Life doesn't feel very good, but rather evil. Live long enough, and you will feel it. I have. I have been there with the parents of the 19-year-old kid I buried one time from a drug overdose, grieving with the parents of a five-year-old kid I buried from cancer, or burying my mom, who was doing nothing but serving God faithfully with all her time! What do you do when faced with inconsolable sadness? What, if anything, can be made of the prayers we've whispered in the middle of the night, restless with fear and the threat of loss, prayers that have had no apparent answer?

At the end of life, every single human being has a reason to believe God is not good.

But the opposite is also true.

At the end of every life, there is evidence of God's goodness in every breath we've been given.

Isn't that faith, I once was blind but now I see?

Isn't that faith a great prescription for your eyesight?

This is the importance of the Christian season of Christmas!

What if Christmas says that God is good when life is not? Christmas is not a compliment. God didn't send his son because we were doing so good. Christmas is God lighting a candle into a very dark world! You don't light a candle in the middle of a sunshiny summer day. You light a candle in the darkness. Our world, and this world, without the candle, is dark. That first Christmas, God came into a very dark world. Herod was busy killing every baby under two years old, trying to kill baby Jesus. Jesus's family had to become immigrants and flee to Egypt. The Magi had to return to their old lives but go in another direction to avoid Herod.

How do we say that God is good when life is not?

What if the answer is Christmas, Easter, and God's promise to always be with us, especially when life is not good?

It is tempting to want clean answers, to be able to point to healings and miracles.

But clean answers have never helped the one who is suffering. How do we say that God is good when life is not? There are no easy answers. You can't fake it till you make it with this stuff. But we have to keep showing up and seeking those answers. Why did Mary Magdalene become the first to see the Risen Jesus rise from the tombs? Why was Mary Magdalene the first person Jesus entrusted with the message of his Resurrection— even though Jesus, for sure, knew the Jewish culture considered a woman's word and testimony worthless? Because she showed up with all her struggles and fears and took them to God.

Because she showed up.

She brought all her questions, doubts, and tears to the tomb, and it was there that God met her. Perhaps hope grows the most when we take all our fears, questions, and doubts to the one who created us.

It's where God always meets us in the middle of life on earth.

Isn't that the point of the incarnation of this whole God with us?

We limp our way through this question, sometimes full of faith and confidence that the character of God is ultimately good, sometimes shaking our heads, saying: "Lord, I believe, help my unbelief."

You can't fake belief, can you?

But I believe the fact that Jesus knew about suffering and suffered so that I might have abundant life and eternal life proves that the heart of life is good. Sometimes you must search for it, but we tend to find what we look for just as a bee tends to find the pollen in the flowers! What is this inherent longing within us to live forever? Why do we care about things like forgiveness? Why do we care about things like guilt? Why do we all have this awareness, whether we like it or not, admit it or not, that there is such a thing as right, and there is such a thing as wrong, and there is a difference? Ecclesiastes basically tells us that what is moving the needle in our lives is God and God's pull on our life… This entire chapter tells us there's more to life than meets the naked eye. The greatest realities are unseen: "God has made everything beautiful for its own time" (Ecclesiastes 3:11, NLT). Notice this, "He has also set eternity in the human heart; yet no one can fathom what God has done from beginning to end" (Ecclesiastes 3:11, NIV). The needle in our hearts keeps pointing back to eternity, keeps pointing back to immortality, keeps pointing back to transcendence.

Like Einstein, we might try to trick it. We might try and medicate it. We might try and numb it. We might try to write off those feelings we have. We might eventually eliminate the guilt by saying there's no God because if there's no God, there's no guilt. Regardless of what we try, the needle still moves. What's moving the needle? His name is Jesus. And you were made to live in a relationship with Him. You were made to make up there, come down here, God's kingdom to come, God's will to be done. And until those two things click into place, you will always be haunted by the idea that there should be something more.

Sometimes, though, our needle gets confused by other things—like fear, anxiety, and worry, and we get distracted. True story: Larry Waters had a healthy fear of ice. He'd been around it and lived near it long enough to know that it wasn't anything to play around with. That's why he parked at the lake's edge, unloaded his four-wheeler, and decided to take that across, not the heavier vehicle. With his wife Chrissie on the back, he cautiously began the journey across the lake, noticing that in the layer of snow that covered the surface, there were tracks from cars that had gone through it relatively recently. And so he assumed if the heavier car or truck could make it across, he could too on the much smaller, lighter vehicle. He was whizzing across, and at the halfway mark, he heard and felt the ice cracking and the vehicle jolting. And then it pitched forward and, in his words, before he knew it, had stopped, dropped, and rolled straight into the icy waters below the lake.

The vehicle sank to the bottom like a stone, but he and his wife Chrissie were floundering in that hole. And both of them instinctively made their way to the edge and sought to do what all of us would do at the edge of a pool. That is, of course, to push yourself out. But they couldn't grasp the frozen edge, the ice, and his hands. No matter how they tried, they couldn't escape this hole. And soon, their hands were numb. He said they were clawing at the edge and couldn't do the one thing they told their hands to do: pull them out. They were also full of water, with their wet clothes and feet filling their shoes. They were heavier than usual. They just began to realize, and it dawned on them they were going to die there today. Larry swam over to his wife Chrissie, and with his few moments of life remaining, he kissed her and told her he loved her. They accepted that they were going to die cold, afraid, and alone.

You can't fake out death, can you?

Those words the couple experienced that day have rung true for me many days. I've laid in bed, lurched from a dead sleep, and found myself completely unable to do the only thing that I wanted to do: rest peacefully. But my mind was on fire; frayed, worried, my wheels spinning 1,000 miles an hour. Anxious thoughts, fear-filled thoughts, thoughts of self-harm, and harm coming to those that I love. Have you ever been there? See, other things in my head move the needle!

President Teddy Roosevelt and his rough riders went into the battle of San Juan Hill, where he came across some barbwire. He had to cross the barbwire and fight in a battle! He went from the idea of being a soldier to being a soldier. He overcame fear, and when he did, he felt the power of the wolf rise in his heart![53] If you accept God's calling on your life, power, like a wolf, can increase in your heart. Some of you are thinking, *We are not supposed to be wolves, are we?* We thought they were bad: three little pigs, the big bad wolf, and all that huffy and puffy, so I researched it. The Bible describes evening wolves. The first book of Habakkuk describes an enemy coming against the nation of Israel that's hasty, bitter, terrible, and dreadful. "Swifter than leopards and more fierce than evening wolves" (Habakkuk 1:6–8, KJV).

Charles Spurgeon described these evening wolves as being the things that come against you by night. There are good wolves and bad wolves! The attack, the assault, comes for you when the sun goes down. Ever notice how the worst worries and fears come at night? I'm convinced that I don't think the devil takes much time off during the day, but I know the devil works the night shift! I mean, I'm just convinced of it. There's just something about two a.m. and three a.m. where things seem worse. Things seem darker. You have to fight against these evening wolves that come your way actively, or they can move the needle in your life.

At three in the morning, I suddenly felt like Larry Waters drowning in a lake of ice water! It's hard to fake swim when you are drowning and freezing in fear and anxiety. All of a

---

53 Morris, E. (2001). *The Rise of Theodore Roosevelt: Revised edition.* Random House.

sudden, I was having these horrible, bombarding, invading, unwelcome thoughts in my mind, trying to smother me, trying to pull me below the ice, into the icy waters of fear and desperation. People today are drowning in anxiousness, worry, and anxiety.

Anxiety seems to be in our day the new normal, and worry is just a part of everyday life for so many people.

And depression: this dark cloud that oftentimes has such a stigma attached to it. When it's inside the head, the stigma of unholiness is often attached. As though it were somehow a betrayal of your love for God to say I'm hurting in this way.

But don't fake wellness when you are hurting. Tell people, "I am hurting." Will you sit with me? Will you encourage me? Will you love me until I am whole? People want you to pray and be better. People say, "Have you ever thought about not struggling with that anymore?" These are unhelpful things. But then there are also things we do that cause these things to be more and more prevalent and can even, at times, cause them to come into being where they were not. Here's why. You're giving your mind over to anxiety, as we can choose to. We can choose to worry. If you know how to worry, you know how to pray. Give those worries to God and turn them into prayers.

We can choose to do these things because Jesus said not to worry. And if he said not to worry, it can also be a choice.

Think about it. The horsepower in your engine can't be going forward and backward simultaneously. Rivers only run forward, not in reverse! According to the book *Emotional Intelligence* by Daniel Goleman, *the cognitive horsepower in your mind can't be allocated to worry and to worship simultaneously.* According to the book, self-management and emotional intelligence are some of the keys to overcoming depression. The number of worries people report while taking a test predicts how poorly they will do. If you've ever thought while you're taking a test, I wonder if I will fail. I think I'm going to fail. I'm afraid I might fail. I don't think I know the answer. Anything you're worrying about is horsepower. This is not focused on the test. So listen to me very carefully.

Worrying makes you worse.

You do worse anytime you're worrying. So anytime you're choosing to worry, think I'm allocating and dedicating necessary, precious, finite horsepower in my mind cognitively that I could be choosing to put over here, that I could be choosing to put over there. Now that you know that, how many of you are worried about that?

I'm saying these wolves come, and we give them more than we should. We give them more space than we should. They put their foot in, and we let them in the door, provide them with a moose, and give them a muffin. Don't give pigs parties. Don't give mice cookies. I'm telling you something: you give yourself away. And now, in our day, what's happening? *We've collectively chosen as a culture to accept worrying as the new normal, as though we had nothing to do about it!*

The CDC says that suicide is one of the leading causes of death in the United States. For many of us, in just your lifetime and mine, the suicide rate has shot up by 25 percent. Many say those numbers and estimates are probably too low. Why? Because so many people try to make their suicides look like accidents, especially men who want to have their families provided for by insurance policies. They do everything they can to try and not nullify the policy by making sure no one knows what they did was an act of taking their life. And here's where we're at, where we're dealing with these wolves, and it's a problem. So, I have this needle in my soul, and it moves. Sometimes it moves because it's pointing me toward God, and sometimes it moves because I've got fears and worries…so I turn to God's Word. What does God say about me? About you? Who are you? What moves your needle? I found this verse: "For you are all children of the light and of the day; we don't belong to darkness and night" (1 Thessalonians 5:5, NLT). You can stop and take a big breath in because that's awesome!

You are sons of light.

If you're a Jesus follower,

What does God think about you? He believes you're a son of light and a daughter of the day.

That is to say that you are not your pain.

You are not your past.

You are not guilty.

You are not your shame.

You are not your family of origin.

You are not your dysfunction.

You are not your overeating tendencies.

You're not your obsessive-compulsive nature that drives people away from you.

You are…who are you?

A son of the light and a daughter of the day.

You don't have to fake any other identity.

You can cling to what the one who made you claims about you.

How did the song go: "You are my sunshine, my only sunshine." That's who you are. And yet when the enemy can get us to identify ourselves as our mistakes, he can keep us crippled in a loop and a downward spiral of disorder. But when we hold on, stop for a second, and say, I am who God says I am. It flips the script and changes the game.

Your daily activity should come from your new identity.

What you choose to do tomorrow, what you choose to do with the precious minutes and hours you get living this life of faith, this new life, should come from your day-to-day activity. It should come from your brand-new identity.

It will move the needle.

Let's return to someone who got in touch with who he was as a son of the light!

When Teddy Roosevelt died at sixty, the sitting vice president said this about him. I love this so much. He said, *"Death had to take Roosevelt sleeping, for if he had been awake, there would have been a fight."*[54]

And he's right.

The guy was a stone-cold killer. Not only was he a rough rider and their leader, but he was also the original barbwire crosser. He was just so many things. He wrote twenty-six books. Having written a thousand sermons, I can't imagine writing twenty-six books. One time, he took down pirates. Pirates, yeah. The pirates stole his boat. He was so mad that he got two of his friends and hunted them down for eight days. He snuck up on them and arrested them. He couldn't put them in handcuffs because it was so cold their hands and feet would have fallen off in the night. If they were handcuffed, they couldn't move them to keep warm. So he took their boots away, and he just sat there with a gun for eight days. Don't you steal my boat!

You're wondering how tough Teddy Roosevelt was? He was campaigning to be president a second time. Because the first time he was president, it was because the guy who had the office was assassinated. So he's just an innocent, instant president. So, he had a campaign to be the president for the second time. And he was crisscrossing the country on a train, just going back and forth, stomping everywhere. He gets up one time to give a speech. Theodore Roosevelt's opening line was hardly remarkable for a presidential campaign speech: "Friends, I shall ask you to be as quiet as possible." His second line, however, was a bombshell. "I don't know whether you fully understand that I have just been shot." The horrified audience in the Milwaukee Auditorium on October 14, 1912, gasped as the former president unbuttoned his vest to reveal his bloodstained shirt. "It takes more than that to kill a bull moose," the wounded candidate assured them. He reached into his coat pocket and pulled out a bullet-riddled, fifty-page speech. Holding up his prepared remarks, which had two big holes blown through each page, Roosevelt continued. "Fortunately, I had my manuscript, so you see, I was going to make a long speech, and there is a bullet—there is where the bullet went through—and it probably saved me from it going into my heart. The bullet is in me now so that I cannot make a very long speech, but I will try my best."[55]

54 Glass, A. (2018, February 9). *Congress eulogizes Theodore Roosevelt, Feb. 9, 1919 - Politico*. Politico. https://www.politico.com/story/2018/02/09/congress-eulogizes-theodore-roosevelt-feb-9-1919-391633

55 Klein, C. (2012, October 12). *When Teddy Roosevelt Was Shot in 1912, a Speech May Have Saved His Life*. History. com.
https://www.history.com/news/shot-in-the-chest-100-years-ago-teddy-roosevelt-kept-on-talking

If you think I write long-winded chapters, say Amen! Well, he gave fifty-page speeches—and the thickness of the speech saved his life. It pays to be wordy. He spoke for ninety minutes before he was taken to the hospital. He lost that election, by the way! Maybe he was crazy, I don't know.

The guy was a fighter, and you need to be too. If you let God into your heart and life and invite Jesus into your soul, some fire will move the needle! Don't let your fires burn too low! A fire in your spirit must exist because this life is not a playground. It's a battleground, the stakes are high, and there are people everywhere we need to reach. It would help if you had a different mentality; once you've declared war, your mentality shifts. Once you realize, oh my gosh, these are not peace conditions. We are at war, which means we must also live that way. One of the keys to living right is preparing for life every day. Jesus did this all the time. He was always spending time alone with the Father. That helped him. During prayer time, he helped move his needle. See, the truth is, when it came to Jesus, he always had a game before the game. When it comes to Jesus, the game before the game was when he accepted the mission. The game before the game was where he suited up in the locker room and was willing to walk out onto that court and face the bright light. I'm telling you, *it was the game before the game.* It was at Gethsemane that he was sweating blood. *At Calvary, he was walking in peace because he had got himself straight in Gethsemane on his knees. Because you can't rise up like a wolf if you don't bow down like a lamb.*

In Gethsemane, Jesus got on his face on the ground. And so here's what's impressive. He did something I've never noticed between the Last Supper and Gethsemane. We talk about the last supper, the bread, and the cup. And we talk about Gethsemane; sweat drops like blood. And we know, then, that it leads to Calvary and Easter Sunday when he rose out of that grave. That's the end of that story. So, in the end, he wins, and we're on the winning team. Never forget that. *When the enemy reminds you of your past, you remind him of his future, right?*

So, between the Last Supper and Gethsemane, there's a detail. It's just one little footnote in Matthew 26:30 (NIV): "When they had sung a hymn, they went out to the Mount of Olives."

Hold on a second, when they had sung a hymn? The Last Supper is over; the whole deal is done. But we are not heading to the Mount of Olives yet. Well, we have to go, we have to go, we have to get there. No, no, no, no, stop. Let's sing together. Stop. Let's sing together. They sang a hymn. And then they went on to the Mount of Olives. And that is so powerful. Why? If Jesus knew that, before the greatest battle of his life was here, he needed time to prepare himself by singing, how much more do we need it?

Why?

Because with this battle looming, he understood what we needed to know. Worship is a weapon against darkness. But it's not just a weapon. It's the whole war. Listen to me carefully.

Worship is not just a weapon that wins the war.

You can't fake authentic worship.

People say: Did you go to church today? Did you go to worship? You worship every day. You worship something every day with how you spend your time.

Worship is the war.

It's the war of: What will you honor the most?

What are you seeking after?

What's the master passion of your life?

Is it you?

Is it your money, your number of sex partners, your fame?

Even suicide is an act of worshipping yourself. It's, I'm going to take myself out. It's ignoring God's glory. It's ignoring God's plan. It's ignoring what he wants to do. It's taking your life into your hands. It's not honoring him, and trusting him, and saying, thy will be done. It's an act that says, my will be done.

I'm not saying that all depression is a choice, but we can still choose what we do amid the depression, right? Some people will need medication. Some people will need to see a therapist. I'm not saying any of that is not valid. But still, in the midst of that, you have to choose who or what you will worship. Who or what is at the center of the glory of your story? And what we need to do is do what Jesus did. We lift our voices, sing songs, and worship when facing a battle. Tell our problems to God. Lift our voice and praise him! Lift our voices! Come on, sing to him, and shout to him in triumph! Now, worship is more than singing. But it's not less. Worship is more than singing. There's a lot of aspects to it. Giving is worship. Obeying is worship. Bible study is worship. All of that's worship. But it's not less than singing. Meaning that every time we see a picture of prayer, it involves singing. It consists of this idea. Why? Because there's something that shifts inside of you when you sing. There's something that alters your mood when you choose to sing. So it's so important that you raise your voice, not just to God, but also to his people. And that means, sometimes, you pick up the phone and call someone and say, I'm hurting, I'm scared, and I'm alone. I'm thinking about doing something bad. I need help. I need encouragement.

You got to fight.

You got to fight.

You've got to keep fighting.

And then, after that, here's what you do.

Keep showing up. Don't fake it.

Keep showing up.

And that is the fight.

Keep showing up.

Just keep showing up.

Keep showing up another day. One of my favorite stories I've heard in recent history is the story of the company Leatherman. This is a simple pocketknife that has pliers in it. I recently bought my son a Leatherman pocketknife and told him this story.

You could take for granted a pocketknife and pliers. Well, it didn't exist till it did. Tim Leatherman was on a European trip with his wife right after college in Portland, Oregon! He and his wife had a car, a Fiat 600, that kept breaking down. He had a Boy Scout knife and a pair of pliers with which he kept working on the car. And he asked himself if they had only one that was the same: pocketknife and pliers. That would be amazing because then I don't have to change hands. And he wrote it down—things to do with my life, make a pocketknife with pliers. He got home from the trip and decided to do it. But it was easier said than done. Two years into the project, he broke down weeping in his brother-in-law's garage on his birthday because he couldn't get the pliers and pocketknife to behave. But he said the following day, he got up, showed up, and continued. In the third year, the patent was issued for what we know today as a Leatherman. Only then it was called Mr. Crunch. He called it Mr. Crunch, my pocketknife and pliers combination. And then, at this point, we would say he made it and lived happily ever after! But that's not how it went. Even though he had successfully made one and got it patented, he, for five years, couldn't get anyone to buy one. Every store, every hardware store, every company rejected it, turned it down, said there's no market for that. The company, Stanley, that makes the thermoses, wrote him a letter saying no one will ever want this. So we will not purchase it from you. He was distraught. In year 7, he said he almost gave up. But a friend encouraged him to keep going. This is before Kick-start and Shark Tank, ok? His friend said, "I'll work with you. Maybe there are some things you haven't thought of yet." So they kept going. In year eight, a little-known company called Cabela's said, "We'll buy 500 of them."

Five hundred of what they had the sense, by this point, to call a Leatherman, not Mr. Crunch. And Tim Leatherman sent 500 Mr. Crunches to Cabela's. And they, in return, got $12,000 for it. And the rest, as they say, is history. The company, which is headquartered in Portland, employs over 400 people. Over thirty models of the Leatherman have been issued.[56] It's a tale as old as time, the success story of this company, and there

---

56 Leatherman. (2018, July 16). *Made of Mettle: The Leatherman Documentary.* YouTube. https://www.youtube.com/watch?v=rvCgGgokH_E

are probably many people reading this who have one in their pocket even now. They're passed down from father to son and generation to generation. And you think about what it took for him to keep showing up for eight years when experts told him it would never work. And that war, doubt, and the wolves attacking him at night, said—it's a waste of time. Can you see him alone in that garage on his birthday, weeping, wanting to give up, wanting to quit? How many times did he wake up at three a.m. with the voices of doubt saying you can't do it—and those voices of fear and insecurity that moved his needle in the wrong direction? Can some of you relate? Winston Churchill once said, "Success consists of going from failure to failure without a loss of enthusiasm."[57] And I wonder, where are you on that journey? What are you thinking about quitting?

You can't fake quitting, can you?

What do you think about giving up?

What dream are you beginning to lose faith in?

And where are you on that journey? Don't let those other voices move your needle. Remember, you are a son of the light and the king's daughter.

Live out your identity.

Fight for what is right as a child of God.

Because I'm saying to you that a fight is not just one round, and it's over. It's not just—well, there, I fought. I tried to control my thoughts. I tried to speak differently. I tried to start a company. I tried to write the sermon. I tried to start a business. I tried to work on the marriage. That's not a fight!

A fight is bloody round after bloody round!

A fight is getting knocked down and getting back up again!

A fight is spitting your tooth out in the sink!

A fight consists of going from failure to failure, to failure, to failure without loss of enthusiasm.

I want to speak life over your tomorrow as any good hope dealer would.

I want to tell you that God loves you, plans for you, and wants to do more through you than you would ever know!

But you've got to fight!

What about Larry?

We left Larry and Chrissy drowning in the hole.

---

57 Curtain, M. (2017, October 24). *Winston Churchill's 12-Word Definition of Success May Just Change Your Life*. Inc. com.
https://www.inc.com/melanie-curtin/in-just-12-words-winston-churchill-gives-
us-a-definition-of-success-that-could-outlast-them-all.html

He kissed his wife goodbye. But he said, just before he began to sink, he reached down and felt a Leatherman in his pocket. And God only knows why or how he thought of it. But he opened it up, and using the pliers, he said he could dagger the ice's edge and pull himself up and out.[58] And he said he immediately pivoted around and was able to pull his wife to safety. And here's what I want to leave you with in this chapter.

Yes, you are fighting a difficult, bloody battle.

You are trying to win the war within.

There is a needle within you that points to God, but other magnetic forces want to pull you in different directions!

But you are not the only one.

There are people all around you—people in your family, people in your life, people you don't even know their names yet, and they're trying to win it too.

If you give up, how will God ever use you to reach them?

---

58 Leatherman. (2017, April 18). *Tool Tales: Ice Breaker*. YouTube.
https://www.youtube.com/watch?v=U_1cLoBIMK4&t=60s

CHAPTER THIRTEEN

DON'T CRY BECAUSE IT'S OVER, SMILE BECAUSE IT HAPPENED!

*If your heart is broken, you'll find God right there; if you're
kicked in the gut, he'll help you catch your breath.*

—Psalm 34:18 (MSG)

I WENT TO THE AT&T STORE last Saturday night, trading my iPhone 10 for the iPhone 15. I walked into the store and greeted the AT&T guy, a young guy about thirty. He got my new phone, and I traded my old phone and transferred my data. So while we were setting that up, in walked a seventy-five-year-old woman and her daughter and then this super tall Black guy, like a seven-footer, and his wife. I am not sure if he played for the Spurs, but he was an athlete. The AT&T guy was helping all three groups at once and bouncing back and forth between us. So, with my loudmouth, I am looking at how long it will take to transfer all my old photos and data from my old phone to the new phone. I say, "An hour? I will pray over this phone and see if I can make this go faster."

At that point, the seventy-five-year-old woman said, "You pray?"

I said, "Madam, not only do I pray, but I am also a professional prayer."

Her daughter was like, "You get paid to pray?"

Renee interjected, "He's a pastor."

Joking, I said, "Yes, I climb the mountain of prayer daily and sit and go, "OMMMM."

Have you ever been joking around and suddenly someone says something and you know it's not a joke? The seventy-five-year-old woman said, "I need prayer," as serious as she could be. She started crying and said, "I just lost my son, Andy. He was forty-nine. Cancer. He went in three weeks."

The dam of her soul just broke open right in that AT&T store. She started wailing and crying loudly, then yelling, "No mom should have to bury their child…and my son's dead, and I have been left for dead!"

Have you ever been left for dead?

Have you ever looked at your dreams and thought they were left for dead?

Have you ever looked at your body in the mirror and thought, there's little hope?

Have you ever looked at your marriage or partner and thought there's little hope?

Have you been so overcome with grief that you feel as if you have been left for dead?

Now, I realize maybe 50 percent of the readers won't know what I'm talking about, so I have to write to the other 50 percent.

Have you ever had anybody do anything to you to take you out, and they thought you were dead? And they thought you'd never be back? And they thought you'd never get up? And they thought you would never change? I have had the abused woman on the couch of my office telling me about how her abusive husband said she will be stuck in a single wide trailer if she ever leaves him, so you know, get used to the abuse! You will never quit doing what you are doing. And they suppose you'd never be anything? Has anybody ever told you, "You can't be anything without me?"

Do they suppose you to be dead?

They left you in trouble?

They left you in debt?

They left you with the kids?

They left you with the bills?

They laugh, and they go on to the strip club, and they suppose you to be dead?

Have you ever had somebody leave you and think you can't cook, you can't clean, you can't iron, you can't wash, you can't make it without me?

I'm going to expose what a bum you are, and they suppose you to be dead?

Well, this is a resurrection book! I am a resurrection author, a dealer of hope!

We are reading words about resurrections here!

God is a God of resurrections, and what happens then can happen again today.

Sometimes you just lie there and let them think they've won. Sometimes you've got to stop fighting and stop kicking and stop fussing and stop cussing and stop calling and stop yelling and stop texting and stop writing and display real steel and act like you've got me and just lay there with blood running down your forehead and act like, I'm harmless. I don't have any more power. I can't get up, so they can go somewhere else because they will leave you alone as soon as you shut up. Your mouth is fueling the fight. If you still know God is God, God will fight your battles. You don't have to defend yourself because the battle belongs to God. But how can God fight your battles if you keep grabbing the sword out of his hand? If you just be still and lay there, they will leave you for dead. *But just because they left you for dead does not mean that you are dead.*

Stop reading and look at somebody and say, *It ain't over.*

I may be broke, but it ain't over.

I may be sick, but it ain't over.

I may be down, but it isn't over.

My business might close, but it isn't over.

I may have lost my loved one, but that doesn't mean I have to die too!

As soon as you all get out of my way, I'm getting back up again.

Come on.

If God can raise Jesus from the dead, everything else is easy for God to do!

So there she is, this sad and grieving mom, pouring out her heart and soul to a group of strangers in the AT&T store. I threw my arms around her and started hugging her, and she was crying on my shoulder so hard that my shirt was getting wet! I didn't know this lady but was trying to communicate God's love. Next thing I know, the daughter was hugging me and her mom and she was crying. Renee looked at me like, *What's going on? I can't even get a hug from my German husband at home, and here he is hugging these two strangers, but I see that God is working!* Now, the Black couple was leaning in, watching all this, and so was the AT&T worker. The mom, Carol, was her name, said, "I just want to know my son's okay. I want to know he's in heaven. I want to see him again. Can you pray?"

So I looked at her and said, "Ma'am, it's no accident that I am standing right before you and you opened up to me. It's no accident because God wanted me to be in front of you right now to tell you there is only one verse you need to know. The Bible says: "It's gates will never be closed at the end of the day, because there is no night there!" (Revelation 21:25, NLT). Do you see that? The sun never sets in heaven. No nighttime in heaven? No darkness to rule the night or day? *The gates are always open!* You will see Andy again and embrace Andy again. He is in heaven, not because of what he's done or didn't do in forty-nine years but because of what Jesus has done. He died on the cross for Andy and rose from the dead. They left Jesus for dead too, but he rose for you and Andy so that the gates of heaven would always be open!"

Like God's arms, Heaven's gates are always open for us!

We started to pray and tears began to fall. I mean the floodgates opened up, and as I was praying, I was pausing, because I was searching my heart for healing words and I heard this deep bass voice say, "Help him, Lord, help him." And I looked up and the Black couple had completed the circle. Everyone in the AT&T store, minus the AT&T worker, was in a circle holding hands, all praying for Carol and her daughter. We were having church in the AT&T store on a Friday night! As I ended the prayer with an empathetic Amen, I heard this deep baritone, Barry White-ish guy start singing, "Amazing Grace, How Sweet the Sound, that saved a wretch like me…I once was lost, but now am found, was blind but now I see…"

Now the door was buzzing as strangers walked into the store and saw us all grouped up in a prayer circle and their faces were like, *What? What is going on? Is this a new plan being released here? Like what?* One guy darted in and then right back out, saying, "Oh, okay, I will head over to Verizon!"

This was the Friday before Easter. Listen, friends, before I celebrated Easter service on Easter morning in church, I had a very special Easter service in the AT&T store with Carol and her daughter and a few other precious souls. We didn't get religious and take up an offering, but we did get deeply spiritual and there was healing that night!

Carol looked at me and said, "All day, I have been praying, *God show me a sign that you are here. Show me a sign that you love Andy*, and here God showed up today through you, a real-life pastor at the AT&T store! I thought God had left me for dead, but God showed up, held my hand, and sang a hymn over my heart!"

Come on readers, if this event doesn't get your fire lit, your wood is wet!

I walked up to the AT&T worker, and he said, "I haven't been to church in a while, but I never had church show up at work!"

Why wouldn't God show up where we work? He's always with us. What's lacking is our awareness!

Friends, it's a great feeling when you see God show up in your life, but it's the greatest feeling in the world when God shows up through you *for someone else*!

When I was young, I wanted a miracle—the winning lottery numbers. I prayed to God like he was some sort of cosmic vending machine.

I used to pray, "Come on, God, bless me."

Now I pray, "Come on, God, use me to bless others."

Blessings for you or blessings for others through you. It's called faith that has spent some time in the oak barrels. They don't make great Scotch in eighteen days; they make it in eighteen years. Nothing good in life comes in a hurry: Not transferring your data off your old phone to a new phone, not food, not a great marriage, not the growth of a tree, not a great friendship, not your relationship with God, not grieving or loving someone.

Quit trying to microwave the frozen turkey. God is not found in the drive-through. God is found in the sit-down restaurant. Have you ever gone to grieve with someone and told them to hurry up? Have you ever started to fall in love with someone and tried to "Amazon Prime" the relationship and make it more than it is, putting twenty years of love on top of a 2-week-old relationship?

Everything good in life is like building a campfire. You must start with the little twigs, and the shavings of wood, get that started, and then add bigger twigs. You can't just throw the big old 3-foot-wide oak log on top of the match and wonder where the fire is.

It takes unhurried time with God and loved ones.

It takes unhurried love with God and loved ones.

It takes unhurried grieving with God and loved ones.

I also shared with Carol another passage from Psalm 23 (NKJV), the line where David says, "My cup runs over."

What does that mean? Let me ask it this way. Have you ever had someone stay too long at your house, or stay too long after the meal and the dessert, and the apple pie and the coffee? What do we do when a guest stays too long at our table? We say things like, "Well it's getting late," or "I have to work early tomorrow morning. I best start cleaning up." Or even, "Look at the time," or "Get out!"

They were a bit more subtle in Biblical culture. In Biblical times, when you were having a meal with someone and you wanted to communicate to your guest that it was time to go after the meal, you as the host, only filled up their glass halfway. This meant after the meal, please leave. I have to work tomorrow, right? But if you wanted to communicate to them that they were welcome to stay, you filled up their glass all the way. That meant you were welcome to stay as long as you liked. I don't have to get up early tomorrow.

The point is, David said God invites us all to the table, every one of us, (it's Joy to the Whole World, not the select few who look like you) and our cups are running over. That means God is saying: You are always welcome at the heavenly table. You have a cup that overflows with the mercy, grace, and love of Jesus.

I told Carol that Andy has that cup and it's overflowing as he has a place at God's table. Carol gave me a long hug and I gave her my card. We met the next day for coffee and it was there we discussed how I knew Andy was alive and in heaven. She asked me what others ask: Show me in the Bible where it says Andy is ok. Now everyone wants a two-hour movie from the Bible's perspective on heaven and it's not there. We get a thirty-second preview. We are told there is no handicapped parking in heaven, no need for doctor's visits, asthma inhalers, global warming, rape or violence or war or incest, or death, and we are given new bodies. We are told there is no more death or crying in heaven because God wipes the tears from our eyes! But as I told Carol, John 11 is where you should go if you've been left for dead. In John 11, Jesus is showing up in a city called Bethany after a friend of his named Lazarus has died. We know that Lazarus was one of Jesus's closest friends. Jesus is showing up not while Lazarus is in the intensive care unit, not while he's breathing his last, and not while he's just died. He's not showing up for the funeral. Jesus is showing up after he's already dead. He's already buried, and most of the casseroles from the wake have already been eaten.

John 11:17–25 (NKJV) says, "So when Jesus came, He found that he had already been in the tomb four days. Now Bethany was near Jerusalem, about two miles away, and many of the Jews [*notice it says many of the Jews*] had joined the women around Martha and Mary, to comfort them concerning their brother. Then Martha, as soon as she heard that Jesus was coming, went and met Him, but Mary was sitting in the house. Now Martha said to Jesus, 'Lord, if You had been here, my brother would not have died. But even now I know that whatever you ask of God, God will give you.' Jesus said to her, 'Your brother will rise again.' Martha said to Him, 'I know that he will rise again in the resurrection at the last day.' Jesus said to her, 'I am the resurrection and the life. He who believes in Me, though he may die, he shall live. And whoever lives and believes in Me shall never die. Do you believe this?'"

Spoiler alert, Jesus goes on to raise Lazarus from the dead that day.

Carol could relate to Martha at this moment. Some of us relate to Martha.

We have questions for you, God. Why weren't you there for this? And why did this happen? And if you're so loving, what about that? And if you cared for my brother, why did this happen?

If you are all so powerful, then why didn't you…?

Does God sometimes shorten his arms to give us free will?

Some of us can relate to Mary.

We're just sad. We're just hurting. We love you, but we're just hurting. And we don't even know. It's not like verses are what we need.

We just need you to be there for us.

We need a ministry of tears, not truth.

Do you relate to Lazarus, where there are things in our life that are dead, that can't live on their own?

Lazarus can't come out, no matter how he tries.

You can't wake up from deadness.

You can't stir yourself up from deadness.

You can't pick yourself up from deadness.

Going to church doesn't help deadness.

Reading the Bible doesn't help deadness.

Only the voice of Jesus can raise deadness to life.

Jesus said some pretty outlandish stuff like I am the resurrection and the life. He who believes in me, though he dies, he shall live.

Who is Jesus?

He is the resurrection and the life.

But first, death.

You might have had a busy day, and someone comes and you're not working and you're thinking, *Don't you have a busy day?* You're like, yes, but first, coffee.

First, coffee.

That's serious business. I am writing this chapter about Easter. I want to close this chapter by pointing your attention to how powerful the resurrection is. But I wouldn't be doing a good job if I didn't say, *but first, death.*

But first, death, because the resurrection doesn't mean anything apart from death.

The resurrection means something to Carol because Jesus had to face death.

It's only necessary and only possible because of death. It's necessary because of your death and my death, spiritually and physically. You can die physically and you will, but you can also die before you die and spend a lifetime in the grave before your body spends a lifetime in the grave. Unfortunately, I have had some encounters with Mr. Death, and I know without a doubt that Mr. Death is at least three things.

Mr. Death is vicious.

Aren't you glad you are reading this?

Vicious.

Death is vicious.

It's a heartbreaker, not a hassle.

It's unfixable, at least this side of heaven.

What does that mean? Mister Death is cruel. It is capricious. It is unkind. Death is not like, oh, if I kill you, you don't have life insurance so your kids won't have a way to go to college or have rent paid next month? Ok, I'll let you live. We've all seen so many examples of how screwed up that is. Death is vicious. My first encounter with death was with 12-year-old Rich Aminsono. I was twelve years old. We (a group of neighborhood kids) had all just finished playing a game of pickup football and his mom called him home for dinner. He lived so close that we heard her call him. He got on his bike and pedaled home, ran through a stop sign, and was hit by a car. He flew over the car, hitting his head, and proceeded to get airlifted by helicopter in our street. When a helicopter lands in your street at 12, it's real. And then I remember the next time we gathered for backyard football and were picking teams and Rich was gone. Then his parents got a divorce, and they sold the house, and it was just vicious.

Isn't Mr. Death vicious? Yes. I didn't need to remind Carol in the AT&T store of the viciousness and cruelty as no parent should ever have to bury their child. That's not the way it is supposed to work. Then I remember my dad going to another AFB in fifth grade, and Adam, one of my fifth-grade classmates, got sick and had brain cancer and died. And just the hard reconciling of that little kid with his whole life in front of him having to go through brain cancer and unsuccessfully face the rigors and pain of chemo, and then eventually succumb to death. Mr. Death is vicious, isn't it? That's not cool. It's nothing if it's not cruel.

Mr. Death is also violent.

Death is violent in that many people die violent deaths. It's car accidents, it's machinery mishaps, it's something that goes wrong and it's a violent set of circumstances that leads to death.

It is not just violent in that many people die horrible deaths, but also violent in the way it feels to be left behind when someone you love dies.

That's violent too. That's what Carol was feeling. Grief is not linear. You get to the letter *H* in the alphabet and then, all of a sudden, you are back at *A*. When you lose someone that you love, you violently career through the different stages of grief, at times in no apparent order. You hear, oh, there's seven stages of grief, so you just assume it's going to be one, two, three. Goodness, I'm on four. Five has got to be better. It's not like that at all, at least in my experience. You can be in one season, and then all of a sudden, with almost a whiplash-causing snap of the neck, no airbags, no seatbelt, now you're in this stage, then you're back in this one. Grief is not linear, that's what you discover. *The intensity of sadness may wane, but you never get "over it"!*

Oh, you're feeling good for a while, and you think you're through it. Then all of a sudden, something sucker punches you and takes the wind out of you like an uppercut to the solar plexus. You hear that song or see a face that reminds you of his face, or smell that cologne, and you're left gasping for air, thinking you were already through that. Christmas triggers something, Easter hymns trigger something, something someone says, and someone you see. Every time Renee plays Easter songs on the piano, I think of growing up in church listening to my mom play these notes and how she gave me her faith. And it's violent to face death, no matter which side of it you're on. But it's not just vicious and violent:

Mr. Death is also vile. It's vile.

Why? To put it rather bluntly, after someone dies and is no longer living in their body, their soul leaves it and steps off into eternity and the body instantly begins to return to the state in which it was formed. The Bible says God formed us from dust, and we begin to decompose, whether it's through cremation and return to ash and dust very quickly, or it's through the decomposition of being buried. And that's vile. There's a smell to death. When my mom died, her wig was off and she was completely bald. It was a surreal experience to look at my mom sans her hair and see her lifeless body and to know I would never hear the words "I love you" this side of heaven.

When you're around really sick people, when you're around death, there's something unmistakable about it, and something wrong about it. And it's in the text we just read. I'm trying to be as delicate and as sensitive as I can, but in John 11, if we were to keep reading when Jesus finally got to the grave and said take away the stone, Martha objected and said to Jesus, no, *because it's been four days and there's going to be a smell.*

That's just heartbreaking and vile.

People tell you, oh, death is peaceful and it's beautiful and it's lovely. Let me tell you something, don't believe it for a second.

Death is your enemy, not your friend.

It's an atrocity. It's terrible.

It should sicken us to think of someone made in God's image being sown in dishonor.

That's how the New Testament describes it. It's a dishonorable thing to happen to a body that God lovingly, fearfully, and wonderfully made. It was never meant to happen. You were never meant to experience death. And don't you feel that when you're at a funeral and you sit there and you look in that casket? Doesn't everything inside you say, this is wrong, this is perverse, this is not how it should be? I get tired of people at funerals saying: "They look so peaceful. They look so good." Really? They look dead to me. They have got a bunch of makeup on, and the lighting is just right, but they are very dead. There's something very wrong here. And deep down inside, we sense the signature of God's hand on our soul telling us this was not what he intended to happen. He never wanted us to face death. It's a terrible thing. And eventually, we will not have to face it any longer.

So here's my outline. Death is vicious, death is violent, death is vile. And at this point, you should have seen Carol's face because she was like whoa! It got heavy quickly!

This is a lot to process.

She said, "Pastor John, I think you've given me a lot to think about."

I said to Carol, "Hold on a second, I'm not done. I realize you are looking at me like, geez, Pastor John has gone Donnie Darko pretty good here, but what I want you to understand is that good news isn't good if you don't get bad news first. And we can't just come and talk about resurrections without being honest about death! We can't be like, yay Easter, and isn't that great, if we don't understand our feet are standing in a cemetery, because that's what Christ rose out of. That was the circumstances under which the resurrection took place; people grieving, tears streaming down faces, people careening in and out of the stages of grief."

The resurrection is only possible and necessary because of death.

It's necessary because of your death, but the resurrection is possible because of Jesus's death.

Here's my whole chapter in a sentence: **He went into the grave to get you out.**

Jesus went in his grave to get you out of your grave.

That was the only way you were coming out. The only way I'm coming out is that he went in.

When you were left for dead, and some of you are there right now, he can go in and pull you out!

Some graves get dug for us.

Carol was in the grave of grief, drowning in sorrow and pain. We lose someone we love and we can get stuck in grief. Some graves we stumble into, such as depression. It feels so dark down in the hole we find ourselves in. We can't see the sun. There's a cloud following us. Some graves we dig for ourselves, right? Some of you have dug so many that your part-time job is a grave digger with the drinking, the drugging, the trying to fill that grave-like hole in your heart with sex or with distracting yourself with scrolling through your phone, or the grave of fear keeping you so trapped from living the life you were made to live.

You want to get out.

Radical prayer dares to believe that things can be different.

Radical prayer dares to say, "It doesn't have to be this way."

On Saturday, everyone said, "Jesus is dead; it is what it is."

On Sunday, God said, "It is what I say it is, because I am the Great I Am!"

There is a difference between knowing Christ and the power of his resurrection!

It's like the difference between knowing a person and resembling a person! Do you resemble Jesus in your life? Have you experienced some resurrections?

Shouldn't we see resurrections from a resurrection God?

You should see one in the mirror every day!

I once was lost, but now am found. Was blind but now I see.

I once was selfish, but now I am generous.

I once was a real piece of &$$#@, but now people like being around me; I am full of God's love.

I have seen some resurrections in marriages and prayed over them in my office.

The problem is that maybe you need to *practice the resurrection a bit.*

Resurrections of Christ should happen with our character, our values, how we spend our time, our money, and our demeanor. Are we rude and selfish, or are we loving and caring?

Resurrections should happen with and IN our relationships.

It's the story of Scrooge's friend, Charles Dickens. What did the old miser experience? A resurrection of his heart and soul!

I have experienced a resurrection.

Ask my wife: I once was a gorilla, but now I am a loving husband.

Look at the deadness in your life.

Look at the anger.

How is that going to be turned into forgiveness?

Look at the insecurity.

How is that going to be turned into confidence?

Look at the self-centeredness.

How is that going to be turned into compassion and generosity?

Look at the deadness in your friendships, your marriage, your family. How is that going to be transformed?

How?

The answer is that the dead stuff gets taken over by the Spirit of God. The minute you decide to receive Jesus as Savior and Lord, the power of the Holy Spirit comes into your life. It's the power of the resurrection, the same thing that raised Jesus from the dead!

But resurrections take time.

Even Jesus took three days. There's no hot water you can pour over your life for a quick fix, no pill for loneliness and deadness of the heart. There's no microwaving to weight loss, real love, or anything really good. Everything, even resurrections, takes time.

It's a process of taking your dead stuff to God's altar and seeking to be altered. It's why David prayed, "Search me, God, and know my heart; test me and know my anxious thoughts. See if there is any offensive way in me and lead me in the way everlasting" (Psalm 139:23–24, NIV).

This is a radical resurrection prayer! "Remove the offensive ways in me, O, God," David prays, "and replace them with your ways."

When the resurrection happens in our lives, His Ways become our ways; His thoughts become our thoughts; his love becomes our love.

That power, not just knowledge, is what changes you.

This belief is what allows me to stand at the casket of my mother and know I will see her again.

Power: We live and die; Christ died and lived!

Some of your marriages are in the grave. Some of your relationships with your family are in the grave. Some of your hearts and dreams are in the grave. So much so, have you ever been so lost, felt so lost, that you thought, I am dead?

Or maybe your friends and family have left you for dead. That's what the fear in your mind tells you "Give up. It's easy."

But you have got to fight.

I know, I know…Pastor, there are so many mistakes on top of my grave, you can never dig your way out.

The debt is too outstanding.

The pile of dirt called resentment has buried you.

The pile of regrets has buried you.

The lack of understanding from your partner has killed you and your heart.

Sometimes people get in so much legal trouble that they get left for dead in prison. One guy I know, Casey Diaz, was left for dead. We will come back to Casey!

Some people dig their grave with a bottle, and with every drink, you sink further into that grave. You can't relate to anyone because you're so deep in that hole of drinking they have given up on you and left you for dead.

You take another pill to ease the pain of all this suffocating dirt. You are buried in shame and guilt. You created this situation. You deserve to be in the miserable "Shih Tzu" you're in to atone for your sins.

You say I would be better off dead because I am already dead. You were left for dead.

Here's the Easter message, friends: Jesus was left for dead. But God didn't leave Jesus for dead. He brought him back to life and if God can raise Jesus from the dead, he can get anything in your life back to life!

Through God's power, I've gotten out of some of my graves. I've seen others get out of their graves. No, not on my own, but only after we invite Jesus to go into our graves do we go out because the deep truth about you is you need help!

Because when Jesus climbs into your grave, he always brings a ladder! He doesn't come with judgment. He comes with a ladder. He comes with some water. He comes with some food.

He doesn't bring a shovel. He brings a ladder, and he says, "I'll hold, you climb!"

Sometimes dreams can die in your graves.

Has anyone here ever thought I am too old? Too much time has passed for that dream to come true.

Sarah and Abraham thought they were too old for the dream to have a child. But they did and the first time God called them out of that grave they laughed, which is why they named their child Isaac, which means laughter.

On October 13, 2007, on a sunny Saturday afternoon, fifty-nine-year-old Mike Flynt, not as a coach or trainer, but as a player took the field for the Sul Ross State Lobos as a linebacker. Flynt had played for this Division III team back in 1970 but was forced to quit before his senior year. He never quite got over the regret of not getting to play. So thirty-seven years later, when he discovered he still had one more semester of eligibility, he sold his house, moved back to Texas, enrolled in school, and tried out for the team. Sports Illustrated called him *"the ultimate college senior." I guess so!* A grandfather, an AARP member, and eight years older than his head coach, he was capable of playing against guys one-third his age. He earned his spot on the roster like all the other players. He said, *"This opportunity is just a testament to what God can do at any stage of your life!"*[59]

We need to remember that many of our limitations in life are self-imposed. God never says you're too young, too old, too weak, too limited, or too anything to be used by him. He had a dream to play college football, it was as good as dead at 59 years old, but he did! He played! He was willing to jump in and try. But dead men don't jump. Are you dead?

Are you in a grave? If God is big enough to raise Jesus out of his grave, He's big enough to raise you out of your grave as well. God has a resurrection for you!

He wants to bring you out into the light again. He wants to bring you out of that tomb of oppression and give you a new start.

And listen—He has the power to do it. He can bring you back to life.

God has a resurrection for you!

---

59 Flynt, M. (n.d.). *Mike Flynt*. mikeflynt.com. https://www.mikeflynt.com/

Now that I've told you three things about your death, let me tell you three things about Jesus's death. Jesus's death, number one, was voluntary.

Voluntary.

I love that Jesus didn't have to die; he chose to die. Friends, it wasn't nails that held Jesus to that cross, it was love. It was love for you; it was love for me. "For God so loved the world, that he gave his only begotten Son, that whosoever believeth in him should not perish, but have everlasting life" (John 3:16, KJV).

You see this in that Jesus provoked the circumstances under which his death would occur.

What do you mean?

I mean raising Lazarus from the dead. It's not disconnected from Easter that we would talk to Carol about Jesus and Lazarus. This has everything to do with Jesus's death. What do you mean? I mean him calling Lazarus out, as great as it is, wasn't the big deal that day. I could prove it to you.

Lazarus had to die again.

I guarantee you, of all the happy people there at the tomb that day, Lazarus was the least pleased about this whole thing. He gets to heaven and thinks this is pretty good. He's just kind of settling into his new room. And all of a sudden, he's getting sucked out. He's like, I've only been here four days. What's going on? And then he's like, oh, I'm back in my arthritic body? This is the worst. Right? He's bummed. I mean, I'm sure he's happy. And then he had to die again. He's like, oh, this again?

This was the most public instance of Jesus doing a resurrection like this in his entire ministry. And the text specifically tells us in John 11:53 (NLT): "So from that time on, the Jewish leaders began to plot Jesus' death." Because now people aren't saying: Oh, he's a good guy. They're saying: He calls the dead out. We have to stop him. You know it's hard to keep people coming to your church when the pastor down the street is raising the dead! Jesus intentionally stood in front of that grave and said, Lazarus, come forth. Jesus raised dead people to life, and he still does. Can you see him standing in front of your tomb, where everyone left you for dead, and saying, "It doesn't have to be this way?"

You don't have to surrender your dreams, your life to a bottle, your marriage, your heart. There is life.

Jesus raised Lazarus, and he will raise you as well.

Jesus told Lazarus, come forth, come on out and live. Jesus knew that raising Lazarus would lead him to the cross! Yet he still chose to raise Lazarus from the dead! Jesus chose to do it. It was voluntary for you and me.

Secondly, it was also vicarious. It was vicarious. Jesus's death was vicarious.

Now, vicarious means *done for someone else or done through someone else*. A lot of parents live vicariously through their kids. And that can be sweet, but it can also be unhealthy. A father might say, "You have to go to Yale, Billy." "Why, Dad?" "Because I went to Yale. Every man in this family goes to Yale." He might be like, "Okay." A father might say, "You have to do gymnastics, Sally." "I want to play basketball." "Shut up and vault, Sally. Your mom was a great gymnast, and you'll be a great gymnast, so help me." It's like, ah. The job of a good parent is like the job of an archaeologist. We're to unearth what God put in, not to change what's coming out. We're just trying to sense and see what God put in our kids and coax that out. We're not trying to change the T-rex into a stegosaurus, right? We want our kids to walk in God's footsteps, not ours. We want our kids' mistakes to be their own, not ours. *It is the height of selfishness to try and live vicariously in a way that would distort our kids' calling as opposed to them just hearing God's voice and us being their biggest fan!* We would do well to have our kids know that we are pleased with them so long as they're doing what God put them on this earth to do and that we're going to cheer them on regardless of whether it's our career path or the sport we played or this or that or the other.

But when I say Jesus died vicariously on the cross, like I said, it's doing something for someone or doing something through someone. And both are kind of involved here because, listen to me, he didn't just die on the cross for you. *He died on the cross as though he were you.* That's what the Bible says in 2 Corinthians 5:21 (NIV): "God made him who had no sin to be sin for us, so that in him we might become the righteousness of God." As he hung there on the cross, he was vicariously dying for you, as God put all the sins that we've committed on him. *God treated Jesus like we deserved to be treated so he could treat us like Jesus deserved to be treated.*

It's a great exchange.

If you put your faith in Jesus Christ, God looks at you and sees the righteousness of God. And some days, you feel bad. Oh, I haven't been to church in a while. I haven't read my Bible in a while. And God's like, I don't know. You look like Jesus to me. And when you fall and feel lousy and like you haven't been praying, God says, I only see Jesus. I always see Jesus. Because as Christ hung there, he paid for your sins. He vicariously died for you that day, died as though he were you that day. His death was vicarious. And that's not all, because for the vicious and vile and violent death that we experience here on this earth, we have Jesus's voluntary, vicarious, and, praise God, his victorious death because he didn't stay dead. After he was taken off the cross, he was put into a grave, and on Easter Sunday, he rose out of that grave, and he lives today. He was dead, but he is alive. He lives forever. And he can offer the resurrection life to you so that, when you die, you'll know that your soul is in heaven! That's the totality of the

Christian faith, meaning we're not just following Jesus because he said nice things and did some miracles.

I think there's this kind of movement afoot to reshape Jesus into this just vegan-eating guy who said nice things, and man, that guy Jesus, he's the best, you know? It's almost like he's just Mr. Rogers with a beard. And to you kids, ask your parents or Google it to figure out what I'm talking about. But just a man with a cardigan who mainly just wants us to share more, you know? But that's not Jesus. Jesus was radical and wild and said ridiculous things like, I'm God. And if you believe in me, after you're dead, you can have life again. Now, if he's unable to deliver on that, he's not—oh, he's so lovely. No, he's a whack job if he didn't rise from the dead. But because he did rise from the dead and was seen by as many as 500 eyewitnesses who had no incentive or reason to follow him, John is a perfect example of this! John was Zebedee's kid and part of a prosperous fishing family. He had nothing to gain by following Jesus, but Jesus calls him, so he follows him. And it's pretty wild. He's seeing some things. He's like, man, this is great. Jesus is the guy. And so he thinks it's all going to go one way, but then Jesus gets killed. His disciples were horrified. He thought Jesus was going to be this epic Jewish messiah turned king and not get slaughtered. When he got slaughtered, they thought the party was over. They were all going back to their old life, back to fishing, and they're like that was a fun run, but it's done. And so they were mostly scared that they were going to get arrested too, and get killed, guilt by association. But then Jesus shows up and is like, "Wazzup." And they're like, "Ah!" And then he's like, "Touch me, feel me. Like, ahhh." And then they're like, "What can we do?" This guy's got the goods. He rose from the dead."

So what are the sermons in the early church? Read the Book of Acts. The first two sermons, they're just like "Jesus is alive. You killed him." That was not a good move, by the way. But he's alive anyway. He'll forgive you if you come. Five thousand people were saved in the first two sermons preached. Why? Because they were saying Jesus is alive, Jesus is alive. The resurrection of Jesus Christ is the very heart of the Christian faith. We cannot make too much of the death of Christ, but we can make too little of the resurrection of Christ. The resurrection is the power of our faith. He went into the grave to get us out of it. But don't miss this. The resurrection is meant to affect your eternity and your journey. Jot that down. The resurrection, what we're talking about, is not just meant to be something for—okay, I'll file that away for when I die one day. Because if you're honest, some of you are reasonably certain there is no God, but the only reason you're here is just to make sure in case you're wrong, and you're hedging your bets a little bit. You know what I mean? But to only think of our relationship with God in terms of life after death is to miss out on some of the best parts of what Jesus died for you to experience. And that's life during life. This very thing, pushing off of eternal things until just some distant thing, caused Jesus to give us the "I am" statement. When Jesus said, your brother's going to rise again, Martha said, I know, I know, he'll rise again one day.

Translation: I know heaven is a better place. I know that heaven stuff, yeah, that's great for then. And Jesus said no, you don't get it. I am the resurrection and the life. Present tense. The resurrection isn't some event for one day; it's a reality that changes your life today.

Resurrection: listen to me; it is not what he does; it is who he is. It's not some event he's going to get to someday, so when you die, that's great to know that heaven's there, like fire insurance. It's not what he does, it's who he is. And so if you're in a relationship with Jesus, resurrection is what he's constantly doing. He doesn't just want to resurrect your eternity but your journey. He wants to resurrect relationships. He wants dead things that have died because of shame and condemnation to live again. He wants the potential to blossom again. As you walk with Jesus, you can find anything in your life coming to life. You would think, I thought I would never get to see that. I've walked under this for so long. He says I am the resurrection. He wants you every day of your life to walk in this beautiful journey of experiencing bursts of resurrection as everything he touches springs to life. It's not a once-a-year holiday. It's a whole new, energizing dynamic reality that, every time you need a new resurrection, it's only a prayer away. **JESUS RAISED PEOPLE, AND HE STILL DOES.** Some of you don't believe this stuff happens today, but I am telling you Carol experienced the power of the resurrection and God's love in the AT&T store. **Resurrection means that the worst thing is never the last thing.** I mentioned Casey Diaz earlier. He was left for dead, rotting in jail. Casey Diaz was just a teenager when he became the leader of the Rockwood Street Locos, a street gang in Los Angeles. After years of vandalism, robbery, and violence, Casey was arrested and sentenced to thirteen years in prison for second-degree murder and fifty-two counts of armed robbery. In prison, he became a shot-caller. Do you know about a shot-caller? The shot-caller marks people for life or death behind the prison walls. Casey could randomly pick any other inmate in the prison and mark him for death, and someone in Casey's crew would kill them. When the warden discovered that Casey was a shot-caller, he sent him to solitary confinement. Inmates in solitary had almost no contact with other human beings. But one day, Casey heard a woman's voice outside his cell. She asked if she could speak to the young man in solitary confinement. The guard told the woman not to waste her time with him. He's been left for dead. She answered, "Jesus died for him too." Then she spoke to Casey from the other side of the steel door, "I'm going to pray for you. But there's something else I want to tell you: Jesus is going to use you. Every time I'm here, I will remind you that Jesus will use you." A year later, Casey was lying in his cot when he had a vision of Jesus carrying his cross up the hill to Golgotha, and just before he was crucified on it, he looked at Casey and said, "I'm doing this for you." Casey fell to his knees on the floor of his cell and began praying, confessing his sins. He began weeping. He called for a prison chaplain. The chaplain explained that Casey had just experienced salvation through Jesus, and he gave him a Bible. He began reading his Bible for hours each day. When he was finally released into the general prison population, Casey started telling other inmates about his new life as a follower of Jesus Christ. After completing his prison term, Casey opened a small business, and to the amazement of everyone who knew him in his prior life, he became a pastor. Casey says these words: "I marked people for death; Jesus Marked Me for life." Now, he spreads the message of marking others for a new life in Jesus Christ. Come on, that's resurrection. You can read about it in this amazing book called *The Shot Caller*.[60]

Jesus said I am the resurrection. Present tense. I will call you out of the graves where others left you for dead. The resurrection is not a sunset; it is a sunrise. God will not leave you for dead!

60 Diaz, C. (2019, April 22). *I Marked People for Death. Jesus Marked Me for Life*. ChristianityToday.com. https://www.christianitytoday.com/ct/2019/may/casey-diaz-shot-caller-marked-people-death-gang-leader.html

CHAPTER FOURTEEN

IF YOU ARE GOING TO MOVE A MOUNTAIN, START WITH SMALL STONES

Faith moves mountains, intelligence goes over them, wisdom goes around them, but love levels them.

—Matshona Dhliwayo

TRUE STORY: IN 1960, DASHRATH Manjhi was a common laborer from Gelhour Hills in Bihar, India. His community was somewhat remote, with limited access to vital services, because traveling involved going around a three-hundred-foot mountain between the towns. One day, his wife, Devi, was traversing the narrow path across the tall hills to bring her husband some water when she was seriously injured. The nearest medical facility was over forty miles away, and Devi perished shortly after her accident. *She died because he had to go around a mountain to get her to medical facilities. He loved his wife deeply, and his love did not die when she did.* People told him this would never change. You can't move a mountain.

It is what it is.

Right?

No, that's wrong.

You can't live right when you think wrong.

I know what you are saying: "Reality is what it is. You might as well accept it?"

No.

It's a *fatalistic expression* of "I am what I am!" "You knew who I was when you married me; you want me to change?"

"It is what it is…" So many times, people say it is what it is, but it's about a hassle, not a heartache. It's misreading and mislabeling a situation, including your ability to change yourself and your circumstances. Mountains can be climbed with our feet but moved with our souls! Mountains often appear like heartaches, but if you start with the small stones, they can become a hassle that is overcome.

It is what it is and what it will be. Wrong thinking leads to fatalistic living. Can you imagine Jesus looking at disease, death, or your brokenness and just saying: "Well, I was going to try and maybe do some healing, but it is what it is?" Often, *"It is what it should not be,"* and we are called to change it. God gave me the wisdom to know what is fixable and what is unfixable! God gave me the wisdom to know what I can and can't change!

It is what it is.

I mean, what does that saying even mean? People use it a lot in the workplace. I have heard it in the church office. I listened to it after the treasurer counted the offering. I have heard it about a kid's behavior. I have listened to it when a loved one dies. Ever since it came on the scene, it has irked me. I didn't quite know why. So recently, I started asking myself this question:

How can one phrase make me so annoyed and so very quickly?

When someone says this phrase, I hear a host of things behind it. Frustration, apathy, powerlessness, inability to make changes, fatigue. Some or all of these things often lead to the inevitable shrug, the heavy sigh, and the wistful "It is what it is" moment. But I also can't ever imagine Jesus looking at your life, your illness, your marriage, your weight, your problems, and saying, "Well, I know I am the Son of God. I know I cast the sun and the stars into space and know them by name, but when it comes to your life and your problems, sorry, it is what it is…"

You do realize on Saturday, when Jesus was in the tomb, everyone said, "It is what it is…" He's dead. The movement of God is gone. Peter even says, "I guess I will go back to fishing. Anyone want to go?" On Sunday morning, people began saying, "He is Risen," not, "It is what it is…"

If He has truly risen, anything, and I do mean anything is on the table for your life.

So, in the name of Jesus, let's unpack a few reasons why you should give up saying, "It is what it is," and instead say, "Well, if God raised Jesus from the dead, God can do anything in my life." If you believe this, it will change your life. Trust me, your life's quality will rise to your faith. It's why Jesus could not do miracles in his hometown; no one had quality faith in him, and their lives suffered accordingly. I live with the expectation that God is always working for the good, that God will show up, and that I will see evidence of His invisible hand. You know what happens? God always shows up.

How do you live?

So here we go, stop saying, "It is what it is," because:

It shuts down the conversation.

This phrase usually comes up when I have a concern or a complaint.

I have something I want to change, something that is causing me problems.

The person I am coming to has that "It is what it is" moment. I often hear it when the person is just done discussing things. So, where does that leave me in the conversation? If someone says, "It is what it is," what do I say? "No, it's not what it is?"

It conveys powerlessness. God is still on the throne. God is still alive. God is not powerless. **Every time God is portrayed in the Bible on the throne, He's sitting down. He's not on the edge of his seat, Nervous Nelly about what is happening.**

Sometimes, when people say this phrase, they express that there is little they can do. It's a "Sorry, kid. Greater things are happening, and I cannot do anything now." Maybe their hands are tied. I understand that happens sometimes in the workplace, especially in the corporate culture. But if you say, "It is what it is," you tell the listener they have zero chance to influence change. There is zero chance to do anything about it. There is zero chance to go to a higher level and make a difference. My view? That's not going to work for Christians. We worship a God who always has another move, another chance, another way to make a way when it seems there is no way.

It makes you seem tired.

Many people using this phrase have been at the job for a long time. They know the challenges. They know the impediments. This phrase nicely summarizes that they've been down this road; the dreaded "we've tried that before" sentiment. Churches say this a lot, right before they die!

It makes zero sense. I mean, really? Ever hear of circular logic? *It's a guy thing.*

Let's be honest. Close your eyes and think of those who always say this phrase. Do we have any estimates on the male/female ratio? I haven't conducted polling, but I think it is an 80 percent guy phrase. It is something guys say when they are just done. Whether it is because they are tired because they have tried before, because they are done with conversation, because this is a little uncomfortable…whatever the reason, they are done. It gives one person the right to pull the plug before the other is done talking! So, where do we go from here? Maybe next time you are conversing with someone, and they start to annoy you or tire you or present a fruitless idea, you can stop the tendency to shut down the conversation. Take that breath. Let it continue. Explore it a bit.

Maybe you can begin to say things like: "I think we should pray about this!"

I think God is the only way we can overcome this.

I think God will have to get involved if this is going to change.

If Jesus can be raised from the dead, anything is possible here.

As Christians, let's take every thought captive to Christ and see if it passes the smell test with Jesus.

I don't think this phrase does at all. I just can't see it, and then seeing Lazarus lying in the tomb, having been dead for four days, Jesus turned to Mary and Martha and didn't weep but said, "Sorry, ladies, it is what it is…" That's not what happened. Jesus wept. Jesus called Lazarus out of his grave. Jesus raised him to life. Jesus can do the same with your thinking. Who knows, you might just see God show up, when you retire this phrase.

What if we believed every mountain was climbable? Not all hills are heartaches. Dashrath Manjhi vowed that God is love, more potent than death, and *love never quits.* He would make sure that this accident would never happen again. Dashrath decided that his community needed *a road through the mountain.* Since no one else would do it, he decided he would. Climbing any mountain is going to cost you. He sold some goats to buy a hammer, chisel, and shovel and set out chipping at the hill daily after work. Sometimes it's not about the size of your shovel or the size of the mountain; it's about ongoing consistency. He started with the small stones first daily. He tapped into the power of a daily habit. Dashrath understood a fantastic principle that can change your life: *Ongoing consistency beats occasional intensity every time.* Have you ever tried to do one workout where you lose twenty pounds? We all have. But occasional intense dieting doesn't work long-term unless you like being a yo-yo. Ongoing, consistent life-style changes are what work long-term.

Consistency with the most miniature shovel can move the most prominent mountain. If you can find self-discipline and willpower in one area, it spreads to other places. So maybe this month, add one or two new habits that lead to health and life, and do that every month until you have 24-36 new habits at the end of the year. What have you become? Someone different!

Dashrath got home from his day job to do his God-given job. Can you relate? He and his little shovel went to work every day, rain or shine. He was ridiculed by his friends and family daily. So was Noah. So was Abraham. So were Mary and Joseph. So was Jesus. So was Martin Luther King Jr., and So was Nelson Mandela—his South-African apartheid-favoring captors would not allow him to wear pants for twenty-seven years because they didn't want him to feel like a man! The first day he wore pants, *he forgave them when he could have belittled them all.* Life-changers are constantly ridiculed. Do you think you can have a kid, Abraham? When did your last annual physical say your body is as good as dead at 100 years old? That's what the Bible tells us. Abraham's body was as good as dead, yet he faithfully (for the most part, minus Hagar) kept going toward God's plan for his life. Let's recall. This is pre-Viagra days, friends.

People will mock you when you begin to move your mountains. People will mock you when you don't accept your life the way it is, especially when it's the way their life is!

People will tell you it can't be done. They said Henry Ford what they needed was a faster horse. He built a car. People don't know what God called you to do!

Don't let your flames burn too low. Back in the 1950s, psychologist David Broadbent performed a relatively simple experiment. He set up several subjects with headphones that were putting out two messages simultaneously, one to each ear. Afterward, Dr. Broadbent tested the subjects' ability to retain the information. His conclusion? We can only listen to one voice at a time.[61] Have they ever tried to listen to two radio stations at once? It seems like this should be obvious, shouldn't it? Yet think of how much time we spend trying to listen to two (at least) contradictory voices simultaneously. I think more than two, like hundreds! Learn to recognize the voice of the one who made, sustains, redeems, and challenges you. Listen to the audience of the One! People called his plan foolish and said the project could never be completed, but he kept chipping away with his hammer and chisel and shoveling the mountain! He was so dedicated that they began to call him a *crazy mountain man.* He took the name as a badge of honor. Everyone is normal till you get to know them, right? Be weird. Being weird is a good thing. Ordinary people give up. Weird people don't quit. Be consistently weird.

Think about this—you are going to cut a tunnel through a mountain with a chisel, hammer, or shovel. 1960, chipping away. 1961, chipping away, shoveling away! Then people still ridicule you in 1962, 1963, 1964, 1965, 1966, and 1967. Let's fast forward to 1975, 1976, 1977, 1978, 1979, and 1980; it is still chipping away. 1981, chipping away. 1982—The project is finished. Ongoing consistency. He spent 8,030 days moving a mountain out of love for his wife. *Some of you still have 8,030 days left on this side of heaven. What mountains do you need to move?*

Noah built the ark for 120 years or 43,800 days without a drop of rain falling. Can you hear the taunts of the many voices? *Where are the clouds, Noah? That's a mighty big boat for zero rain in the last one hundred years!* The story of Dashrath Manjhi is of a man who single-handedly carved a road through an entire mountain that had been isolating his village from essential services. The road is thirty feet wide and cuts twenty-five feet deep into the rock. Now, instead of having to travel 55 kilometers for access to services, the people of his village need to travel only fifteen kilometers. *And it was accomplished by one man with a couple of hand tools.*[62]

One person with passion and commitment can change the world. Look at Jesus. Look at Mother Teresa. Look at Nelson Mandela. Look at yourself. What can you do with the next 8,030 days?

61 May, S. (2022, January 24). *The Power of Words Archives.* Steve May. https://stevemay.com/category/words/

62 Margaritoff, M. (2023, June 29). *The Inspiring True Story of Dashrath Manjhi: The "Mountain Man" Who Spent Decades Carving A Lifesaving Road Through a Treacherous Mountain.* All That's Interesting. https://allthatsinteresting.com/dashrath-manjhi

The mountain was a hassle, not a heartache. It was fixable. How will you ever know what you can do if you never invite God into your life and never reach beyond you? **If you only do what you know you can do and never invite God into the mix, so what?** The truth about you is that you don't see what you and God can do until you try.

Don't ask God to move mountains if you are unwilling to pick up a shovel. You can do it in twenty-two years when you reach for it every day and keep chipping away. There is no such thing as an overnight success or a long twenty-two-year night to success and significance! They don't call him crazy mountain man anymore. They named the road after him. Dashrath Manjhi Road.

Can you imagine living in such a way that they name a road after you? Are you willing to pick up a shovel? If I am being honest about my mountains, I think I am guilty of praying a few times: "God, can you help me, but sort of make it look like I did it all myself?" Why? I want the credit and the glory. But mountains I don't know how to climb or cut through help me realize how short I am and how tall God is. So we pray for what only God can do, but we also do whatever we can do. It was Frederick Douglas, the freed abolitionist and enslaved person who wrote three bestselling books on the *evils of slavery* and helped turn the tide of American opinion which once said, "I prayed that God would emancipate me, but it was not till I prayed with my legs that I was emancipated!"[63]

He prayed for God to give him freedom, and God said, "Okay, start walking!"

"Oh God, help me with this mountain."

God says: "Okay, where's your shovel?"

Have you started moving the small stones? Have you listened to other voices or the voice of one? Pray yes, with a shovel. Pray yes, with your feet. Pray as if everything depends upon God, work as if everything depends upon you.

Moving mountains is always a joint effort. Faith honors God and God honors faith. It takes faith to make God smile and to please God. Hebrews 11:6 (NIV) says, "And without faith it is impossible to please God." It takes faith to pick up a shovel and move your mountains! It takes faith to work on a project for twenty-two years and not quit. It takes faith when it doesn't rain for 120 years to keep building an ark. It takes faith to believe you are going to have a baby at one hundred years old without a little blue pill, and your wife is post-menopause. God is love. God never quits. If you invite God to the tabernacle in your heart, you become a person who never quits. If you take after your "Father in heaven," you will resemble your Father in heaven, and your ways will become more like His ways! 1 Corinthians 13:7 (NLT) says, "Love never gives up, never loses faith, is always hopeful, and endures through every circumstance!"

---

63 Quoteresearch, (2021, November 23). *I prayed that god would emancipate me, but it was not till I prayed with my legs that I was emancipated.* Quote Investigator. https://quoteinvestigator.com/2021/11/23/pray-legs/

What does it come down to then? How bad do you want it? That's the thought when others say: "It is what it is." How bad do you and God want it? There's one line with a bunch of people in it, and the banner above that line reads: Hungry to Win. There's another line with hardly anyone in it, and the banner above that line reads: Hungry to Do What Winning Requires. Everyone wants to win, but not everyone wants to win with the same intensity and the same fire. Some fires are burning too low.

Ever wanted to lose weight but didn't want it bad enough to do the things required to lose weight? Most of us don't need more knowledge. We need more power. We need more desire. How bad do you want it? How bad do you like the dreams God has placed in your heart?

The promises God has spoken to you will not come to pass without opposition, delays, or people trying to talk you out of it. There will be plenty of opportunities to get discouraged, to let your fire burn too low, and to think that it's not meant to be. But if you reach your destiny, you have to think right. *If you give up after the first time, the fifth time, or the thirtieth time, what that means is you didn't want it bad enough. There should be something you believe in that you are relentless about. You are not moved by how impossible it looks. You're not discouraged by how long it's taking. You don't give up because people tell you no. Your attitude is, "If I have to believe my whole life, I am not going to stop believing. I am not going to take no for an answer. I'm not going to settle for mediocrity. I'm going to keep pursuing what God put in my heart."*

No one does anything of significance with half of their heart.

Do you believe that if God can raise Jesus from the dead, God can do anything in your life? That is faith! Grab your shovel if God laid it upon your heart to change it. When people say you can't do that, say, "You didn't give me my medal. You can't take my medal away. God gives it to me!" Oh, Pastor, they always get my goat. Well, tie up your goat elsewhere. Quit letting others pop your balloon. Protect your balloon. Guard your God-given dreams. A person cannot be truly happy if they make only a partial commitment. Have you ever asked someone for a Snickers bar, and they take three bites out of it and then hand it to you? It happened to me on my mission trip. No thanks. I don't want a half-eaten Snickers bar, nor does God want a third or half of your heart. You don't move a mountain with a third of your heart! Love the Lord your God with your *whole* heart.

God is either everything or God is nothing at all.

How often do we hand God half of our hearts, half of our Snickers bar, and half of our attitude? Here's part of my life, God, just a bite or two. I want about two dollars' worth of God. No, that never works. You can't let God be part of your life. God wants your whole life. Dashrath heard God say to him, this mountain, it does not have to be this way. You can build a road through it. People don't have to die anymore!

Can you say it?

It doesn't have to be this way!

When you look at the number on the scale.

When you look at your finances or debt.

When you look at your marriage.

When you look at your relationship with your family.

When you look at your relationship with God.

When you look at the worries you carry.

When you look at the guilt and shame that weighs you down.

When you look at your health struggles.

When you look at your struggles with alcohol or drugs.

When you look at some toxic behaviors.

When you look at how you have given up on your God-given dreams.

When you look at never being able to answer some of the whys in life.

Remember this. Whatever you are not changing, you are choosing.

If God can change Jesus from lying dead in a tomb to the tomb being empty, anything is possible in your life. Your current reality doesn't always equal your future reality. It is not what it is. Jesus changed all that. There is always another move with Jesus. There is no checkmate! Jesus said, "Look, I am making everything new…" (Rev 21:5, NLT). Did you notice the present tense… *I am making!* You have got to start looking and working. No matter where you're starting from, change is possible. No matter how tall the mountain is, you can climb it.

I know what you are saying. "Wait, wait, wait a minute, sometimes mountains in our life are taller than 300 feet!"

Okay, let's talk about the tallest! How about 29,032 feet above the sea, a 29,032-above-sea-level problem, like a Mount Everest-sized problem?

We all have had some challenging problems and felt a little short. We all have looked at that problem, and instead of praying with your feet, you pray with your fears! You don't buy the shovel. You don't get the hand tools. You keep procrastinating and running from it, and fear makes the problem look taller and taller. When God told the Israelites to go to the Promised Land, ten scouts returned and essentially said, in Numbers 13:33, "We can't do it. We are like grasshoppers compared to those already living there." I know sometimes, when I look in the mirror, I see a grasshopper! Faith looks with a telescope to see what you and God can do. Even if you feel like a grasshopper, God and a grasshopper can hop over any mountain.

Faith says: You are not a grasshopper. You are a child of the King. You are made in the image of the God who makes the impossible—possible.

Think about what you think about. How tall are you? No, not your height, but in your mind. I am 5'11". But in my mind, in the objective reality where life is won or lost, I am a solid six foot seven and growing. How tall is your mind? Is it growing? I like what Russ, the rap singer, says, "I know I'm fine, but the money makes me handsomer… I'm 5'6" but the money makes me 6'5" (Russ, "Handsomer"). It's not often I get to quote rappers! Russ may have this wrong. It's not money that helps you grow taller. It's your *thought* life, your *faith* life.

Twenty-nine thousand thirty-two feet above sea level—that's how tall the tallest "problem" in the world was to Sir Edmund Hilary. In 1924, George Herbert Mallory and his team set out to climb the highest mountain in the world—Mt. Everest. This was the third attempt after the initial failure. They were very excited to reach the pinnacle of victory. They trained, prepared, and even secured funding, the best gear, and all the resources needed, yet the team failed. The mountain proved too tall for the team, and the conditions too rough. Mallory and several of his teammates died in the challenge. Only two of his colleagues survived. It took 75 years for his body to be recovered from the mountain!

Mount Everest 1, George Mallory 0.

When the survivors returned to England, the Queen held a welcome party for the two men who lived to witness the tragic failures, and it was at this point Sir Edmund Hillary's mind shifted, and he began to grow taller. He said with tears in his eyes: "That mountain cannot grow any bigger, but we can. That mountain cannot get any stronger, but we can. We can only become the individuals that will beat that mountain because that mountain cannot change, but we can!"

Imagine thinking that and saying that to the mountains in your life! Guess who climbed Mount Everest first? *Sir Hillary Edmund 1, Mount Everest O.*

What Sir Hillary discovered was that:

If you change your thinking, you will change your life. You can change your life. If you don't like where you are planted, move—you are not a tree. Suppose no one has your back; it's time to move your back. But, and it's a big old thing, quit looking for a life free of difficult circumstances. This is not heaven; this is Earth. Quit Star Trek prayers where you get "beamed up to heaven" and removed from life's challenges. Is that what Jesus taught? "Beam me up, God. Get me out of here. These people are nuts and want to kill me!" Everyone's world has mountains in it. Everyone is given a fire to tend. It rains on everyone's fire. It's your responsibility to feed the fire! There is no mountain-free life out there that you can find! Besides, you can't grow without climbing the mountain. No one wakes up one day a millionaire. No one wakes up a professional bodybuilder. No one wakes up on top of Mount Everest by accident. You have to train; you have to climb. Life with God is no different. There is no red pill that you can swallow to avoid obstacles. As a kid, I would scream and complain, "Dad, Dad, my sister got a bigger piece of the pie. It's not fair!" He would say, "You are right, it's not fair. Life is never fair: learn to deal with it." I think God says life is not fair. Learn to deal with it. Learn to change it, work at it.

As long as you have breath, you will have mountains. What can be different about you and distinguish you from others is your thoughts and attitude about your problems and mountains.

Once you think right, then you can live right.

A disciplined mind leads to a disciplined life.

Most Christians pray the wrong prayers, thinking the wrong thoughts.

They view problems as things God needs to change, mountains that God needs to move!

What if you quit praying for God to remove your problems and instead give you the strength to deal with your problems? What if God wants to change you through the circumstances you ask God to remove?

What if God knows the only way your "prayer legs" get stronger is by hiking the mountain? You are only one attitude adjustment away from greatness—the right thought. Think about the biggest problem, the biggest mountain in your life right now! How tall is it? Who can grow more: You or your mountain? The biggest advantage you have over the "Everest" in your life is that it doesn't grow any bigger, but you can grow taller, stronger, and better in all possible ways. Faith is always about vision and seeing what other people cannot see, thinking thoughts others do not. Faith is a telescope, allowing us to see what the human eye cannot.

Faith is not: See it to believe it! Faith is: Believe it, then you will see it.

Once Sir Hillary knew he could get more robust, be better equipped, and overcome the mountain, once he believed it, then he did it. You must see yourself climbing 29,032 feet before you will do it. We cannot close our eyes and minds and wish the mountains would move, *but we can grab a shovel.* Tony Robbins once said, "Problems are the gifts that make us dig out and figure out who we are, what we're made for, and what we're responsible for giving back to life!"[64] What if you viewed your mountains as lessons in how to trust God? What if you viewed them as moments to grow in holy determination? What if you said life without problems is like school without lessons? So, what are you waiting for? Time is not waiting for you! Dig your teeth right now into that mountain-sized problem, get your shovel out, start digging, and watch how your problems will have problems. You can't be passive and indifferent. You have to have a *holy determination.* It's more than just your will; it's a fire on the inside, "a knowing" that it's supposed to be yours. And when everything says it's not going to happen, instead of

---

64 Robbins, T. (n.d.). *Get Inspired. Get Motivated.* Quotefancy. https://quotefancy.com/

getting discouraged, you kick into a new gear. Normal people would give up. Ordinary people would settle, but you're not normal.

You are weird.

God is weird.

Be God-like.

You want it on another level. This is the abundant life Jesus came to give us. Jesus said it this way: I came so they can have real and eternal life, more and better life than they ever dreamed of. When David was seventeen years old, the prophet Samuel anointed him as the next King of Israel, but David didn't go to the palace; he went back to the shepherds' fields, where it was lonely. He was overlooked and mistreated by his family. When he finally goes to the palace to serve King Saul, Saul becomes jealous of David and tries to kill him. David had done no wrong, yet he had to live on the run, hiding in caves and spending time in the desert alone. But David would not let his fires burn low. He could have been discouraged and thought, "God, this isn't fair. You anointed me to be king. Nothing is working out!" But David didn't have a give-up spirit. He didn't feel sorry for himself. He didn't say everyone is always out to get me; I will never be king. He didn't let circumstances talk him out of it. He had a warrior mentality. His attitude was, "I am not quitting. I am not settling for mediocrity. I know there is greatness in me. I'm going to become who God says I am!" Most of the Psalms David wrote were in the darkness of those caves, which proves that our greatest growth and faith in God often grows in the dark times of our lives. One reason David took the throne is he wanted it bad enough. He waited fifteen years after being anointed king before he took the throne.

How bad do you want what God has put in your heart?

Bad enough to outlast the opposition? Twenty-two years of shoveling? Fifteen years of growing through the season you are in? Bad enough to overlook some insults? Bad enough to overcome three failed attempts to climb Mt. Everest? Is it bad enough to do the right thing when the wrong thing is happening? Do you want it bad enough to keep pursuing it even when circumstances say it won't happen? Many of the difficulties we face, the delays, the times it's not fair, that's simply a test. God is seeing how bad you want it. This is what weeds people out. If problems overcome you, you let circumstances push you down; people talk you out of it, and you won't have the strength or the courage to sustain where God is taking you. You have to be like David. I don't have a weak mentality but a warrior mentality. When my boys were little, I remember they would make guns out of everything. They would eat part of their Eggo Waffles and, with the rest of it, make guns out of it and run around the house "shooting" the pretend bad guys. Those Eggo guns are scary, right? My wife Renee comes to me all concerned. "What's wrong with our boys? Why can't they eat a waffle like a normal person?"

I told her, "Relax, that's what some boys and girls do. They have the warrior spirit within them." God has a warrior spirit within Him. They are made in the image of God. Exodus 15:3 (NKJV) says, "The Lord is a man of war; the Lord is his name." That's just the leadership qualities coming out in them. They want to tackle danger and be intrepid and strong. Let's not destroy that spirit. Let them run around like Don Quixote, galloping toward the imaginary windmills with their swords made out of waffles! They are going to climb some mountains! I love that spirit in them. We didn't teach them that. You don't have to teach kids that spirit, nor to say the word mine or no! Let's get them some more syrup and more waffles! You must dig your heels in and say, "I am in this for the long haul. I know what God has spoken to me. I will get well. I will accomplish my dream. I will become the right person until I attract the right person!" I will do it if it takes twenty-two years to carve a mountain road! God rolls with a crock-pot, friends, not a microwave. That means you should roll with the slow cooker. Play the long game. Play chess, not checkers! You're not moved by what's not working out, how long it's taking, or who's not for you. You know who is for you, the Most High God.

Faith sees and believes one important eternal fact: God is always with me, even when I can't see or feel God! I become stronger and braver when I become aware and see God working as I grab my shovel. It's making my Eggo into a gun. It's reaching for the small stones. I know a pastor in Lake Charles, Louisiana, who called me up and asked my church for some help after they got hit by a major hurricane. But he also told me God is slowly building a masterpiece out of the mess. He told me this story about a young Black woman in his church whose home was hit pretty hard. The power was out, houses were flooded, and roads were closed. At the Red Cross center at the local middle school, a distraught Black woman asked tearfully for six flashlight batteries. "My kids are afraid of the dark," she explained. "Sorry," came the answer. "Only two batteries to a family. However. if you have relatives living with you, you can have two more for each one." The woman stood there paralyzed, helpless, when Ryan Abel, a White stranger, piped up. "I'm a relative," he said. "So am I," announced a young Chinese girl nearby. The Red Cross worker said, "Oh, I didn't recognize your family at first," smilingly handing the woman six batteries. Love never quits. It's been said that the definition of insanity is to keep doing the same thing repeatedly, hoping for a different result. Someone then asked, "What's the difference between that and persistence? Isn't it irrational to keep trying, failure after failure, expecting this time the outcome won't be the same?" Business leader Seth Godin had something to say about this. "Persistence isn't using the same tactics over and over. That's just annoying. Persistence is having the same goal over and over."[65] There's a story in the gospel of John, after the resurrection of Jesus when the apostles spent the entire night fishing but caught nothing. Jesus called from the shore: "Cast the net on the right side of the boat, and you will find some. So they cast it, and now they could not haul it in because of the quantity of fish. Essentially, in John

65 May, S. (2019, January 7). *The How of Persistence*. Steve May. https://stevemay.com/the-how-of-persistence/

21:6, Jesus says something like: "Keep trying; just do it a little differently this time." The goal didn't change. The strategy didn't change. But they modified their method a little bit, and it worked. If you've been pursuing an elusive goal you know is worthwhile, the solution is not to give up. Instead, consider what you might do differently. Consider how you might approach things from a new angle. Instead of giving up, ask yourself: What would it mean, in this case, to cast my net on the other side of the boat? The how of persistence is not that you keep doing the same thing repeatedly, trying and failing, trying and failing, hoping for a different outcome. The how of persistence is that you keep pressing on toward the same goal, adapting as you go, because love never quits! Let me paraphrase some of Mark Chapter 10, Jesus was leaving Jericho, and a great crowd followed him.

There was a blind beggar named Bartimaeus on the side of the road. When he heard all the commotion, he started shouting, "Jesus, son of David, have Mercy on me." The people around him told him to be quiet. "You're creating a scene; he will get upset." They saw Bartimaeus as insignificant. "You're just a beggar. This man, Jesus, will not be interested in you. He's the hottest celebrity around. He's on TMZ every night." The more they tried to quiet him, the scripture says, the louder he shouted. About that time, Jesus stopped, turned, and looked at him. I can imagine what they thought: "We told you. You should've been quiet. He's annoyed. He's going to let you have it." Jesus smiled and said, "Tell him to come to me." They were amazed. They said, "Bartimaeus, he's not upset. He's calling you." They brought him to Jesus, and Jesus said to him: "What is it that you want me to do for you?" Bartimaeus said, "I want to see." Jesus told him, "Go your way. Your faith has made you whole." Instantly, he could see. Here's my point: There were other blind men on the road that day. Other sick people were in the crowd, yet Bartimaeus was the only one healed. Why? He wanted it more than they did. He wanted it so badly that he didn't let people talk him out. He shouted even louder when they tried to push him down and discourage him. If he had listened to them, he would have missed his miracle.

Are you letting people talk you out of what God put in your heart?

"You can't get well. You saw the report. You'll never get out of debt. You've reached your limits. You can't start that business. You won't accomplish your dreams. You have too much opposition." Let that go in one ear and out the other. Ignore what they're saying.

They don't determine your destiny; God does.

They said you will never carve out a road in a mountain with some hand tools. Twenty-two years later, who was laughing? If Bartimaeus had been passive, indifferent, and thought, "Hey, I'm blind. It's just a bad break. It is what it is"- he wouldn't have received his sight. He had this passion, this fire on the inside that said, "This is your day. This is your time." He rose and took that step of faith. If you're going to see what you believe in, You have to be willing to do what other people won't do.

Other people may not believe it when it looks impossible. Other people may settle where they are. They may get discouraged and tell you not to bother praying or believing, that there is no use in getting your hopes up, and that you're wasting your time. You have to do like Bartimaeus and say, "God, this looks impossible, but I know you can do the impossible. The odds are against me, but God, I know you are for me."

When the odds are against you, you have to want it on a new level. How badly do you want to get out of debt? Bad enough to not buy things you can't afford? Bad enough to not try to keep up with your friends? Bad enough to honor God by tithing your income? How bad do you want that promotion? Bad enough to get to work early? Bad enough to do more than what's required? Bad enough to take that online course to sharpen your skills? "I don't want to take another course. I don't want more work. I just want the promotion." You don't want it bad enough. You have to stand out in the crowd. The Scripture says Daniel distinguished himself. He was so excellent in his work, so sharp, and had such a great attitude that he stood out among all the other young men. The king put him in a position of outstanding leadership. But it doesn't say God distinguished him. God made him excel. God made him stand out—it says he distinguished himself. He was willing to do what the other young men wouldn't do. It wasn't so much that he had more talent and more skill, *it was the fact that he wanted it more than they did.* How badly do you want your children to stay on the right course? Bad enough to bring them to church each week? Bad enough to get them up and dressed on your day off and have them in Sunday School Class? Bad enough to tell them to put down their phones and eat dinner with you? We don't think twice about having to get our children up for school and have them dressed, fed, and ready sometimes by seven in the morning. Their schooling is incredibly important, but I could argue that their spiritual life is even more important. When they grow up learning to honor God, as a person of excellence and integrity, knowing that they are fearfully and wonderfully made, knowing that they are surrounded by favor, those seeds planted in them will affect them for the rest of their life. Every time you bring them, you are showing them by example to put God first place in your life.

How badly do you want your marriage and your relationships to work out? Bad enough to bite your tongue when you feel like telling them off? Bad enough to clean up a mess that you didn't make? Bad enough to grow and become a soulmate for your partner? Soul mates are not found like it's a treasure hunt. Soulmates are made. The day you get married you are committing to become, day by day, the right person for the other person. Your focus is on their happiness and making them happy. When you care more about their happiness than your own, then you know it's real, it's love, it is something beyond your belly button!

There are new levels in front of us, but much of it depends on how badly we want it. God is not going to do everything for us, we have to do our part. When Lazarus died, Jesus told his family, "You all roll away the stone, and I will do the raising." Jesus could have moved the stone, he's God. He wanted to see how badly they wanted it. Then Jesus told the crowd, you unbind him, you unwrap him. But Jesus, he smells. Yes, most people do. We all have messy lives, but it's our job to unbind people and help them to live and grow. You can pray, "God, help me to feel better. I don't have any energy. God I'm always so tired." Are you eating right? Are you exercising? Are you getting enough sleep? Are you living stressed and worried? If you roll away the stone, then God will do what you're asking. But you can't override natural laws and expect to live a blessed healthy life.

I am at Whataburger, and I see this guy and his family, and he's got like three number ones: Whataburger's double meat, double fries, onion ring, fried apple pie, and one large Diet Coke, because that will help! There is nothing on that table that can bless his body. But then I see him pray and I lean in to listen: "Lord bless this food to the nourishment of my body." It will take a miracle of God to bless the level of fat and salt that is before him. There is no such thing as a Dorito Tree. But there we are asking God to bless our Frito Pie, to the nourishment of our bodies, please Lord! There were no Oreo bushes in the Garden of Eden.

Do you want to get well bad enough to not drink eight Cokes a day and sleep three hours a night? Do you want to break that addiction bad enough to not hang around those people who are pulling you down, causing you to compromise? "Well, John I know these friends aren't good for me, but I like being around them." You don't want it bad enough. God is not going to free you until you roll away the stone. *When he sees you doing all you can, then he'll make things happen that you can't. But if you're not willing to do the natural, he's not going to do the supernatural!* Your destiny is too important to spend it with people that are not making you better. Who are you allowing to influence you? Are they challenging you, inspiring you, pushing you forward? You don't have time to waste with people who bring out the worst in you. You are hurtling toward death at lightning speed. This is not a dress rehearsal so get busy living your life! Start carving out your roads in the mountains!

But it's hard to shovel a mountain.

It's hard to bite your tongue, and not say what you feel, but that pain is less than the pain of having someone you love walk away. It's hard to lay off junk food, and things that are not good for you, but that pain is less than the pain of not being healthy. It's hard to break away from a friend who's pulling you down, but that pain is less than not reaching your dreams. And one of the saddest things is to come to the end of life and wonder what I could have become. What if I had not let those people talk me out of my miracle? What could have been me and my life? What if I had broken away from those friends who were causing me to compromise? Where would I be? What if I had treated my spouse with respect? What if I had decided to become what s/he needed instead of choosing my way? What if I had taken that step of faith in my career and not played it safe all the time?

You don't have to wonder anymore; you can start right now. Hear God permitting you to change your life today! It is not too late to become who God created you to be. The question is: Do you want it bad enough?

Love never quits.

There was a young man who was raised in a small town in Pennsylvania. Nobody in his family had ever left that area. They all stayed and worked there locally, but this young man had a dream to go to college. He knew he had more in him, but he came from a limited income. He didn't have the funds or the connections, but instead of giving up and accepting that as his destiny, he went to the local phone company and got the phone directory for New York City. That's where he wanted to go to school, but he had to find a job. He found a company that had 393 locations in the New York area. He decided to write each one of them a letter asking for a job. He didn't have a computer or a typewriter, but for the next month, he wrote about fifteen letters a week, telling the company that he would do anything from sweep the floors to clean out the warehouses. A month went by, and he didn't hear anything. Three months nothing, six months still nothing. He became discouraged. When he turned 18, he convinced his parents to let him take the train to New York City to follow up with that company. He arrived in Manhattan and went to one of their most prominent locations in Times Square. He told the person in charge who he was and how he had applied for a job and was wondering if they were interested. The person informed him that all the hiring took place at the corporate headquarters a few blocks down the street and that's where all the applications went. He walked into this big, colossal skyscraper, told the receptionist his name, and asked if he could see the person in charge of hiring. She called upstairs, and much to her surprise they said, "Yes, send him up." He stepped off the elevator, and they brought him to this sizable executive office with big, beautiful windows looking out. He was so nervous, so out of his element. He told the executive, "My name is so-and-so, and I was wondering if you received the letter I wrote asking for a job." The executive turned to his side desk, put his hand on a big stack of papers, and said, "Yes, we received your letter, all 393 of them. We knew you would be coming. You can start tomorrow." This young man did not only work his way through college, but when he graduated, he became a manager for a whole region of their stores. How bad do you want it? "Well, I put in four applications. They all turned me down." You have 389 left to go. Michael J. Fox failed and flunked out of high school because he wanted to be an actor so bad, that he had his dad drop him off in Los Angeles with a few dollars. But he had something many don't have—belief in himself and passion in his God-given dream.

The difference between a dream and a wish: A wish is something you just hope happens. A dream is something you put actions behind it. Pray with your feet. The Scripture says faith without works is dead. He could've wished he could get a job, wished somebody would hire him, wished he could go to school. Wishing isn't going to get you anywhere. He was willing to do what others wouldn't do. The people who succeed don't always have the most talent, the most education, and the most opportunity. Many times they simply want it more than others. You have to pursue what God put in you. Being passive and indifferent will keep you from your destiny.

Jesus said in Matthew 5:6 (HCSB): "Those who hunger and thirst for righteousness are blessed, for they will be filled." Here's the principle: If you're not hungering after anything, you're not going to be filled. Are you hungry to get well? Hungry to accomplish the dream? Hungry to meet the right person? You can teach people to have faith. You can encourage them to believe, but you can't make people hungry. *If you want a bonfire, you have to throw more logs on the fire.*

"Well, my business didn't make it, that's why I'm down." How do you know your next business is not going to make it? "The medical report says I'm not going to get well." There's another report and it says God is restoring health unto you. Did you know that the third leading cause of death after heart disease and cancer in our country is medical error?[66] No offense to doctors, but they are practicing medicine, they are not God. They don't know how much time you have left or what you can do with the time you have left. That's a G-O-D question, not a doctor's question. If you have been diagnosed with something, don't put all your faith and energy in a doctor, but in God, the one who made you and can remake you! Are you hungry for it? You may have had some setbacks, but you have to be relentless when it comes to what God put in your heart.

When I met Renee, I was madly in love. I thought this girl was one of a kind. I am not going to let her get away. I would do anything she wanted. I would go to the mall with her, follow her around, and hold her purse while she tried things on. I don't even like to shop. I didn't mind it one bit. I was with her. One time when we were first dating, she asked if I wanted to go work out at 5:30 in the morning. I thought, "No, I don't want to go to work at 5:30, I want to sleep." Without missing a beat, I smiled big and said, "I'd love to go work out at 5:30. I'll be at your house at 5:15." I was lying, but I was in love. Here I was driving down the road, 4:45 in the morning, as happy as can be, never complaining one time. I was about to see the girl of my dreams. When you want something bad enough, you'll do things that you usually wouldn't do. *If you think I wanted her that bad, you should've seen how bad she wanted me! I can't think of any examples, but I know she did.*

---

66 Sipherd, R. (2018, February 28). *The Third-leading Cause of Death in US Most Doctors Don't Want You to Know About*. CNBC.
https://www.cnbc.com/2018/02/22/medical-errors-third-leading-cause-of-death-in-america.html

You know what I am saying? Quit telling yourself it's too hard, it's too early or I've had too many setbacks. You can do what you want to do. **Quit saying: the mountains are too vast, the mountains are too tall. Tell your mountain you and God are coming with shovels.** Don't miss your destiny because you didn't want it bad enough. What God put in you is worth fighting for. It's worth being uncomfortable for a season. It's worth having to stretch, get up early, try again, and do what others aren't willing to do.

Let me tell you about my friend Chris and his grandmother. I first met Chris's grandmother in New Braunfels, Texas. She had a little farm and was a very feisty woman. She was a real character. She grew up way out in the country, and her husband, Chris's grandfather was very poor. They didn't have much education, but they were great people. But later in life, Chris's grandmother took up chewing tobacco. She liked to dip snuff. People used to tease Chris about his snuff-dipping grandmother. One time someone asked Chris if you could chew tobacco and go to Heaven. He said, "Yes, but you'll have to go to hell to spit." Now the funny thing is Chris's grandfather couldn't stand it. He begged her and begged her to stop. She said, "Jack, I just can't do it. I've tried everything, I'm hooked." This went on year after year, and nothing seemed to help, and Chris's grandfather was desperate. He finally told her, "Ellie May, I will give you $10,000 if you will stop dipping snuff." She wanted the money so badly. She tried everything she could, but still couldn't stop. Well, eventually Chris's grandfather died. He went to be with the Lord, but Chris's grandmother didn't like being single. Ellie May wanted to find herself a man. She met this man who was twelve years younger than her. She was so excited. He was handsome and had a great personality, more than she could imagine, but she started thinking, "If he finds out I dip snuff, he will never even ask me out on a date, much less marry me."

Do you know how long it took Ellie May to quit dipping snuff? Snap your fingers. That's how long it took. She did it instantly. She didn't go to Snuff Dippers Anonymous. She didn't have any withdrawals. What she couldn't do in years, she did in a split second all because her "want to" got big enough. The question is: How big is your "want to"? You can break that addiction if you want to. You can forgive that person that hurt you. You can make your marriage work. You can write that book. You can accomplish your dream if you want to bad enough. You can carve a road through a mountain if you want to, for twenty-two years. It is not the way it is because love never quits!

CHAPTER FIFTEEN

QUIT LIVING IN THE SHADOWS OF OTHERS

A heart at peace gives life to the body, but envy rots the bones.

—Proverbs 14:30 (NIV)

To be honest, I blame the tooth fairy. Have you ever been mad at the tooth fairy, Santa Claus, or the Easter Bunny? Now, just to be fair, how many of you have had the tooth fairy show up at your house when your kids were growing up? So, I had two boys growing up, four years apart. Two boys mean a lot of teeth. Now, I don't know about your house, but when the tooth fairy comes to our house, yes, I have been known to be rather conservative financially. Yes, maybe even tight. When my kids were growing up, the going rate for the tooth fairy to retrieve a lost tooth at our house was one dollar. Little did I know, the economy was a little bit better at some of your houses. Maybe with inflation, the going rate has gone up because when Zach, was around seven, he came home one day and said, "Daddy, you're not going to believe this." The day before he was happy with his dollar. "We only get a dollar for our tooth fairy, and Hosea my friend at school, told me that the tooth fairy brings him five dollars for each tooth." Zach was just beside himself and couldn't figure this out. He said, "Daddy, why, oh why, do we only get a dollar, Hosea gets five dollars?" And I said, "Oh, uhh, times are tough for the tooth fairy." And Jacob, being older, came to my rescue. He said, "Daddy, maybe we can find out which tooth fairy they use, and we can use that one too." Envy is like yeast; it swells the fortune of others.

People caught up in the sin of envy are constantly comparing themselves to others. I get one dollar, he gets five. They exaggerate the blessings others have and minimize their own. In other words: Envious people keep score. It affects all of us. If you have ever envied someone, say: Envy. I first learned about envy from the Disney Classic *Snow White*. I know kids today grew up with *Frozen* and *Let it Go, Let it Go, Let it Go*, but we grew up with a hot young damsel and the seven dwarfs, right? And what did we learn about envy from Snow White?

We learned the question that envy always asks; it's the same question we ask ourselves when we look in the mirror: *"Magic mirror on the wall, who's the fairest one of all?"* Snow White is safe as long as the mirror says the old evil stepmother queen. You remember the old queen, right? She's the queen who lives in a large stone castle that sits high atop a mountain. Her magic mirror hangs in a dungeon-like room with large pillars and ornate carvings. As the queen approaches the mirror to get her daily dose of affirmation, she summons the specter that has constantly and faithfully identified her as "the fairest one of all." This inferno or fire billows within the mirror gave way to a ghostly face. The beautiful but wicked queen inquires, "Magic mirror on the wall, who's the fairest of all?" Then, one day, the mirror responds, "Vain is your beauty, majesty. But, oh, I see a lovely maid. Rags cannot hide her gentle grace. Alas, she is fairer than thee." The queen's face contorts, and her eyes burn with anger. How could a maid, dressed only in rags, compare to the regal beauty of the queen? "Reveal her name!" demands the queen. The mirror tells the queen the name of Snow White. "A lash for her!" hisses the queen.

Now, the queen had the good life. She was the second prettiest in the land, with all the money and material goods she needed, but envy blinded her. Envy is blind to one's gifts and good fortune. The envious person may have some wonderful assets and abilities, but all he or she can see are the gifts or blessings or fortunes they don't have, but that another does. What another person has always seems larger or better or more special. Though she is a beautiful queen surrounded by royalty, her envy of Snow White consumes her. From that moment forward the queen seeks to destroy Snow White. The queen commands a huntsman to take Snow White into the woods and kill her, returning only with her heart. When this doesn't work, the queen attempts to kill Snow White by giving her a poisoned apple. Instead of just being ok, being the queen, and doing what a queen does, she can't be happy unless her competition is eliminated. Ultimately, the queen perishes, she is destroyed by envy. Socrates once said: "Envy is the ulcer of the soul."[67] It makes us ask the question: Mirror mirror on the wall, who is the best of them all? It doesn't matter where you are looking: pride, lust, greed, sloth, or envy.

It's a funny thing, Jesus addressed all seven wicked sins with a couple of sentences. "Love the Lord your God with all your heart and with all your soul and with all your mind and with all your strength," And, "Love your neighbor as yourself" (Mark 12:30–31, NIV). Essentially Jesus is saying: "Whenever you love the least of these, you are loving me." He was so right. Because when it comes to loving the least of these, I have no problem with it. Do you know who the least of these are? The least of these are the people you're most likely not to notice or, if you notice them, most tempted

---

67 Goodreads. (n.d.-b). *A quote by Socrates*. Goodreads.
https://www.goodreads.com/quotes/76088-envy-is-the-ulcer-of-the-soul

to avoid. They smell. They look funny. Jesus described it this way: They're beggars. They're prisoners. They're naked, and their nakedness is not attractive to you. They're hungry. They're needy. Those are the least of these people. You want to rush by; you don't want to make eye contact with the least of these. They are the guy begging for help on the street corner. They are a person whose life is a train wreck without the train. Everybody's passing these people by. It's so easy to blow by the least of these. Let me be brutally honest and maybe it's just me. I don't have any problem loving the least of these, because I always consider them lesser than me. The mirror on the wall always tells me, I am fairer than all! But I will tell you where I struggle with loving like Jesus tells me to love—it's loving the most of these! The most of these is the person *you're most likely to notice and resent.* The most of these is a person who does what you do and just does it better. They eclipse you. They leave you in their long shadow. It's your prettier sister. It's your more athletic brother. It's the worship singer that everybody gushes over, and they do it right in front of you, and you're a worship singer too. Most of these are that person who excels in the area in which you want to excel (and probably do); but they seem to excel a little more. We are most threatened not by those who are different from us. We're threatened by those who are most like us, just a little better. *"I am to love God enough to be contented; I am to love men enough not to envy."*[68] The queen was most threatened by Snow White, because she was a queen dressed in rags, and even in rags she looked better.

Science Fairs and Envy

Does anyone here remember Science Fairs when you were a kid? Does anyone here remember who you competed with in school? Rick Buessing was my guy. I hated Rick. I wanted to be like Rick while hating how good he always did. He was the kid who got back his math test and then said, "Did anyone else get a 101? I got the bonus question right." There I am looking at my sixty-seven, thinking maybe I can mow the teacher's lawn. Oh, Rick, athletic, tan, toned, and perfect in school. I hated Rick. For the Science Fair, we had to do a project with a cardboard display and visual aids. I worked for weeks. I was going to beat Rick in the Science Fair. I was in sixth grade and wrote over twenty-five pages about thunderstorms. My parents had hired me a tutor for school as they hated Rick as well.

My tutor helped me make a real-life mini-tornado. We used a vacuum and made four walls with two glass sides, two sides black wood sides, and about a half-inch gap at the four corners. We had a hot plate at the bottom to boil water and the vapor rose. The vacuum at the top pulled air in through the corners. This made an incredible tornado. How many sixth graders can create a tornado? Many hours of work, hundreds of dollars with a tutor, and I got a lousy B+. Are you kidding me—a B+? The tutor and I made

---

68 Spirituality, F. (n.d.). *Chapter 19 - True Spirituality by Francis Schaeffer.* The Transformed Soul. http://www.thetransformedsoul.com/about-the-book/chapters/chapter-2a-summary-of-the-boo19

a tornado happen! My teacher said I wrote too much; twenty-five pages was too long! Can you imagine me being too verbose?

The night before, Rick worked a couple of hours without a tutor and wrote four brilliant paragraphs about molecules. He took a saucer, a little water dish detergent, and a straw. He blew in the straw, made a few bubbles, and talked about how many atoms it took to make a molecule. He blew bubbles through a straw like a three-year-old and received an A+. I hated Rick. I still hate Rick. I wanted to be Rick. He had the perfect hair, house, family, and grades. When I looked in the mirror, I wanted to see Rick, but all I got was me. Can you relate? **Have you ever woken up, looked in the mirror, and said I want to be someone else? Have you ever felt like you grew up in someone else's shadow?**

As I am writing this chapter, it took everything I could not to try and look Rick up on Facebook this week. He's probably a preacher in some mega-church. LOL I am okay. I just re-signed up for more therapy. Ha! Is anyone here with me? Ever heard this? Why can't you be more like your brother or your sister? If you comb your hair that way, people won't see how prominent your forehead is compared to others! What happened to you? (As they look at the success of your family.) You were trying to shine your light, make it bright, but man that older brother's shadow was long or that older sister was hard to follow in her footsteps. I had a friend who had an older brother. No one knew his name. He was just "Kevin Bishop's brother." One day he said, "I have a name and it's not Kevin Bishop's brother!" I didn't want to live in Rick's shadow or anyone's shadow. I've got a light to shine!

When we compare ourselves to others, we are denying the uniqueness that God made each of us, and we are also forgetting that everyone is made out of mud. It's true. From dust you came, to dust you shall return. Kurt Vonnegut Jr. says it best: "*God made mud. God got lonesome. So God said to some of the mud, "Sit up! See all I've made," said God, "the hills, the sea, the sky, the stars." And I was some of the mud that got to sit up and look around. Lucky me, lucky mud. I, mud, sat up and saw what a nice job God had done. Nice going, God. Nobody but you could have done it, God! I certainly couldn't have. I feel very unimportant compared to You. The only way I can feel the least bit important is to think of all the mud that didn't even get to sit up and look around. I got so much, and most mud got so little. Thank you for the honor! Now mud lies down again and goes to sleep. What memories for mud to have! What interesting other kinds of sitting-up mud I met! I loved everything I saw!*"[69]

We are mud but "Holy Mud" because God has placed eternity inside our souls. What a difference it would make if we could see ourselves and others as "Holy Mud." Instead of throwing mud, we would cherish and value the mud all around us. But we forget this because my mud doesn't look like your mud. My mud might be a different color than your mud, and I don't like the color of my mud. My mud might not have the same skills

---

69 Vonnegut, K. (2010). *Cat's Cradle*. Dial Press Trade Paperbacks.

that your mud has, or different skills and I want what you have. Every September the mud comparison contest begins in schools all around our country.

In September, school will be cranking up, and parent/teacher conferences will be going on. What are the odds that parents in any-town USA will meet with a teacher and ask, "How is my kid doing?" The teacher says, "I'd say about average. Your kid is right in the middle of the pack." Then they go to their kid's soccer coach and ask, "How's my kid doing?" The coach responds, "Your kid is average. I'd say half are better, half are worse." Then they go to their kid's tutor who specializes in preparing 7-year-olds for the SAT and ask, "How's my kid doing?" The tutor says, "I think you can expect right about the fiftieth percentile." What are the odds that a parent will respond to that by saying, "That's great. I have a normal kid. My kid is average, right in the sweet spot of God's bell curve?" Not likely. It turns out when we ask the question, "How's my kid doing?" there's always a little rider attached, always the phrase, "Compared to the other kids." We have a way of measuring our performance, our identity, and even our value and worth compared to the other kids. How's my mud compared to your mud?

In fifth grade, we were assigned to math groups based on how well we could add, subtract, and multiply compared to the other kids. Now they would never tell you this, but you could tell because the groups were named for birds—the Eagles, the Robins, and the Pigeons. If you were assigned to the Pigeon group, you knew you weren't tearing it up math-wise. I can still remember: In second grade we had taken this big, standardized test, and my teacher posted on the blackboard the score my sister got a year earlier and then my considerably lower score. She then asked me in front of the whole class, "How come your sister did so much better than you?" I got so mad, but what is interesting is I didn't get mad at the teacher. Do you know who I got mad at? My sister, like she had deliberately done well on that test to show me up. I called her not long ago to talk about that. It turns out she did do well on that test just to show me up, but that's a whole other conversation to have with my sister. There's this weird thing. We have a way of identifying our worth, performance, and value based on how we compare with other people. Not that comparing itself is not a bad thing. It's an inevitable part of learning. That's how kids figure out, "This box is bigger than that box," "A cheetah runs faster than a turtle" or "I can get a better deal on jewelry for my wife's birthday from Dollar General than I can from Tiffany's." We learn by comparing, but when I start to compare myself with another person, my ego gets involved, and my ego wants me to be exalted over another person. My ego feels like, "I'm going to be diminished if another person is enhanced. My mud needs to be prettier and skinnier and better looking than your mud!" My ego starts to whisper to me about envy and jealousy and gets me competitive. When I compare myself with others, if I do better than somebody, I feel superior and puffed up, which kills love in me. If I grade myself worse, I feel inferior and unworthy, which kills my love.

As you look at your mud, you will always be able to find someone's mud that seems to be doing a better job than your mud (creating envy), and yet you will always be able to find someone's mud who doesn't seem as effective as your mud, creating pride!

Either way, envy or pride, both attitudes will rob you of your joy.

This is why comparison is called the thief of joy; it steals it from you! We do this to ourselves. It's not even teachers or parents doing it to us anymore. We do it to ourselves. *We make ourselves miserable by comparing our mud with other mud! Instead of cheering on other mud, we throw mud, belittle it, and say, that mud is that way because they have things my mud does not.* I don't want any of this chapter to be just abstract or hypothetical, I want to invite you to reflect for a moment on yourself and whether you ever do this. We'll just do a *muddy reading confession*: I'll run through a few categories. If you have ever compared yourself, I'm going to ask you to say to yourself: Yep, I have been that kind of mud. Have you ever compared yourself to anybody else based on looks, like "She's cuter than me" or hair, teeth, physique, anything like that, or intelligence, grades, or GPA? Have you ever compared your career to somebody else's career, your house to somebody else's house, your car to somebody else's car, your girlfriend or boyfriend or spouse to somebody else's, your kids, how you're doing as a parent, even your spiritual life? If you have ever in any way compared yourself to anybody else, say "Yes I am that mud!" That's what I thought. It's a sickness amongst everyone made of mud! Some of you might be saying right now: "Yeah, I have done that, but my mud is way better at it than most other types of mud!" We all want to know, "Am I in the Eagles or the Robins or the Pigeons?" How is my mud compared to everyone else's mud? This muddiness goes way, way back, and runs through the Bible and especially in American culture.

Now, where will you find envy? All different sorts of places. For you, you might have a bit of physical envy. Ladies, you might see a girl who's got a cuter figure than yours and you are going around saying, "Well, I wish my butt was smaller, my chest was bigger, my legs were longer." Guys, you might see some other guy and think, "Man, I wish I had some hair like that dude. I mean, look at his hairline. It's like still up front." You know, "I wish I had less hair on my back and more on my head." It could be relational envy. You'll see two girls. They are not married. They are good friends. They are having a blast. One girl gets a boyfriend who turns into a fiancé. The other one goes, "Uh! It's not fair. She got a boyfriend. She got engaged. Flapping that ring around like she's all that." There's this envy. You see it in a marriage, as well. "You know, her husband, he helps around the house, and he has this good job, and my husband, well, he's just a bump on a log."

Envy is congratulating your coworker for the promotion and salary raise she received, but then hinting to others in the office that she got it by providing sexual favors to the boss. Envy is giving a high-five to a teammate for an outstanding play but complaining to friends that he's the coach's favorite. Envy is putting out a contract to have the mother of your daughter's rival for the cheerleading team killed so that your daughter's competition will drop out. Then, technology is funny, because with technology, size matters. Right? "Oh, if I just had a bigger TV and a smaller phone." Bigger TV, smaller phone, remember when everyone wanted a smaller iPhone? The funny thing is the only time you'll ever hear a guy going up to another guy and saying he wants something smaller is with a phone. "Dude, man, yours is so small." "Man, I'd give anything if mine was that small." A phone is the only time a guy wants something smaller. Right?

This sin, comparing myself to others, is right at the root of the second sin in the Bible. Many of you will know the first sin—Adam and Eve eating the forbidden fruit from the tree. The second sin involves a couple of brothers, Cain and Abel. This is what we're told in Genesis: "In the course of time Cain brought some of the fruits of the soil as an offering to the Lord. And Abel also brought an offering—fat portions from some of the firstborn of his flock. The Lord looked with favor on Abel and his offering, but on Cain and his offering he did not look with favor. So Cain was very angry, and his face was downcast" (Genesis 4:3–5, NIV).

The first thing we wonder when we read this story is why Abel's offering was looked upon with favor, and Cain's not. Most likely, it goes back to the word firstborn. Abel offered some of the firstborns. We don't provide tithes regarding giving, generosity, or even tithing. We bring our tithes to God because they belong to God. God loves it when we make giving and generosity a priority. So, he would teach his people to provide not just some but the harvest's first fruits or the flock's firstborn. Right off the top, I first say, "God, here's the tithe. It's yours. I want to make generosity a priority." Abel does that. Cain doesn't. He brings some. The implication is he's doing it out of obligation with a grudging heart or because he thinks he has to. *Giving should never be, I have to… it should always be—I get to!* What if your prayer was this: God, help me become so financially stable that you use my full pockets to fill up others' pockets? What if God has blessed your heart so that you can bless others? Abel experiences what generosity does in a heart. He trusts and loves God and lives in the reality of God's favor and dependence on God. God loves that. God loves generosity. God is a generous God. Cain shuts himself off from that. Cain sees this joy in Abel, and it grates on him. It's so interesting. Cain gets angry, but not at himself. He didn't say, "Come on, Cain! You could do better." He gets mad at his brother Abel. He thinks, "If Abel weren't around, I wouldn't feel this pain." There's a comparison at the very beginning of the Bible. It's so interesting. God speaks to Cain: "Then the Lord said to Cain, 'Why are you angry? Why is your face downcast? If you do what is right, will you not be accepted? But if you do not do what is right, sin is crouching at your door; it desires to have you, but you must rule over it'" (Genesis 4:6–7, NIV). It's a fascinating story. God plays therapist to Cain. There were no therapists back then, so God is his therapist. He asks him, "Why are you so angry? Why is your face so downcast? If you do what's right, won't you be accepted?" Sin is crouching at your door. Sin always crouches and looks small before it crushes our life.

Crouching is what a lion does as he hunts an impala. The impala thinks it's just a bit of grass, and as the lion crouches, it doesn't look too big or intimidating, right? But then, boom, in an instant, the sin bounces on us, consuming us and turning us into someone we are not made to be!

In Mark Chapter 5 Jesus meets a man who is called Legion or filled with "many evil spirits!" We don't talk like that today, but we do say things like your mean girl is showing, or he's got multiple sides, not all of them good. Sin crouches and sin's control in your life will always be incremental. That is to say, the devil plays chess, not checkers, and so where your first move in the game, your first temptation in the game is always going to be justifiable. You'll always be able to talk yourself into it. You'll always be able to sort of rationalize it. If someone says, should you be doing that, and even your conscience flares up and goes, you shouldn't be doing that, what do you do? You say: *But no, you don't understand.* The enemy never comes to you right away with what, long term, he envisions you doing. It's just one drink. It's not you being buried in the grave all jaundiced from liver failure. I just buried a fifty-six-year-old this week. It started with one drink. It's just one drink! You should have seen his bride of thirty years pounding on the casket and screaming: "Was it worth it? One more drink and now look at you, dead, and I am all alone…" It's scenes like that at the funeral home that stay with me a lot longer than the 200 dollars they paid me to do the service.

Sin: It's always just the foot in the door, just a little bit more, and then you kind of say, well, that wasn't good but I did this, but I'm in control here. And you go, well, I'm not going to do that. At the beginning of his journey, in Mark 5, Legion ends up living in a cemetery and cutting himself with no friends. Whatever he told himself at the beginning of his sin journey, he would say, I'm never going to be naked on the cliffs cutting myself with stones. Like, why would I do that, right? Who wants to be howling out in pain coming off heroin? But I have seen it. They have sat on my couch. "I would never do that, it's just this small compromise, I'm not going to become a meth addict." "I am not going to become verbally abusive. It was just a couple of words I said to my wife."

Nobody sees what the enemy sees, and that is the end in mind that he intends. James puts it this way: "But each person is tempted when he is drawn away and enticed by his own evil desire. Then after desire has conceived, it gives birth to sin, and when sin is fully grown, it gives birth to death" (James 1:14–15, CSB). So that's where he wants to take you, one small compromise after another. Like the proverbial snowball rolling down the hill, it gets out of control fast. I would never cheat on my wife, but that friend at work who's fun to talk to, is it flirting, is it not? We're together sometimes. There's no doubt a connection and chemistry. This is how you torpedo your life, slowly.

Sin is incremental. It also divides. This man was split into pieces. What was his name? Legion. That's a number in the Roman army that means 6,000. That's a lot of demons. I figure anything over 4,000 is a bunch of demons. Why does the Bible tell us his name and that there are 6,000 parts of him? Because sin always splits the self. Now, I'm not saying you as a Christian are going to have a bunch of demons, and more and more of you. But the enemy does want to split you into pieces. And how does it work? Here's how it works. You give in to sin, and you do it but now you have to hide it, and now you must keep straight what you did that you hid. As Mark Twain once quipped: "If you tell the truth, you don't have to remember anything."[70] But when you lie, you better take good notes. And so, you're always in the moment thinking—now, wait, what did I tell who, and where did I say I was going to be, and what is it that I told my boss about this purchase, that it was business or personal?

James said that a man who does not believe in God does not walk in faith and is unstable in all his ways. He's a double-minded man. If you "unpack" the Greek text here, it is saying he is split-souled or fracture-souled. Now what are you doing? You're walking around. You're not just you, you're Legion for we are many. This is who I am on Sunday. This is who I am on Friday. This is who I am on Tinder. This is who I am on Facebook. This is loving husband John, but then there is also Volleyball John or over-competitive acts like a jerk Pickleball John and he's no fun! This is Pastor John, and sometimes, on Monday, I tie Pastor John up and put him in the closet, and Jerk John is in complete control. I am Legion for we are many.

It isn't very easy.

It isn't very clear.

It's exhausting.

Sin splits you into many people.

So, it's fascinating that David prays to God in the Psalms, "Give me an *undivided* mind" (Psalm 86:11, NIV). David said, "God, I don't want to be Legion. I want to be David. I want to be David at church, David in my marriage. I want to be David with my friends. I don't want to have to sort and sift through my mask closet and pick out the appropriate one to wear for the moment. I want to be David, forgiven, healed, anointed, called, marred, chosen, loved, broken, David." When we have an undivided heart, we will get to be comfortable in our skin, grounded and present in the moment which is why Parker Palmer said, "The divided life is a wounded life, and the soul keeps calling us to heal the wound."[71] In a backslidden state, when you think about going to church, you'll play these kinds of mental gymnastics.

I can't go because I haven't gone in a while, and I did all this. I'm not worthy. So, you'll think to yourself, I need to straighten some things out, get better, work on this stuff, improve this, and then I'm ok to go to church, which is to buy into the lie that church is

---

70 Twain, M. (n.d.-a). *Mark Twain - If you tell the truth, you don't have to...* BrainyQuote. https://www.brainyquote.com/quotes/mark_twain_133066

71 Palmer, P. J. (2019, November 26). *A Life Lived Whole*. YES! Magazine. https://www.yesmagazine.org/issue/healing-resistance/2004/11/09/a-life-lived-whole

a museum for holy people and not a hospital for broken people! Church is the island of misfit toys; the church is for the broken people. Church is here to break the hard-hearted and to heal the broken-hearted! But we do the same thing with prayer. I can't pray because I haven't prayed. The evil one is keeping you back from the cure; look, you can't do this because look at what you've done. Therefore, you might as well do this; now he will help you move on to the next thing. He also wants to alienate you, which is why you will not pick up the phone when your Christian friend calls you to check in on you because you don't feel worthy of the friendship or worthy of the love. **He's trying to alienate you and keep you out in the tombs and not receive help from people positioned to bless you. Sin divides you; healing makes you whole!**

God begs Cain to talk, but Cain will not answer these questions. Cain dehumanizes his brother and doesn't see him as a brother; he sees him as a problem. The real question God poses, and a good one for you and me when we start comparing ourselves is: "What do I want?" See, what Cain wanted in his best self, in his most authentic self, was to be a generous person. He should want to trust God. He should want to love his brother and be a good brother himself, but Cain doesn't want to deal with those questions. We're that way. In our best selves, we'd want what's noble, but over time we quit looking at our best selves. We stopped asking that question. It is so fascinating. We surrender to our lesser selves, the divided self.

The text says God asked Cain these questions, but Cain did not respond to God. Here's the next verse. "Now Cain said to his brother Abel, 'Let's go out to the field'" (Genesis 4:8, NIV). There's a world of hurt and sin in this line. Now for the first time, Cain has to deceive his brother. He has to say this like this is what brothers do. He has to teach his face the tone of his voice and his body to deceive his brother. "While they were in the field, Cain attacked his brother Abel and killed him" (Genesis 4:8, NIV). This theme of deception, falsehood and comparison runs all through the human race.

Neal Plantinga wrote an excellent book called "A Breviary of Sin" several years ago. He tells the story of two lovely, young women in Iowa, Cindy, and Sonya. They would sometimes compete in beauty pageants. Cindy was Miss Harvest Queen and Sonya was Homecoming Queen. They both liked the same guy, a guy named Jim. Jim ultimately rejected Cindy and married Sonya, and it just festered. It killed Sonya. She couldn't stand to think of her rival getting what she wanted and being happy. She took a leather belt, and one night Miss Harvest Queen strangled the homecoming queen, and the whole town was left devastated. One piece of mud took the life of another piece of mud. Sin.

All through the human race and all through the Bible runs this toxicity of, "How come you have what I want?" Two brothers, Isaac and Ishmael, are estranged from each other. Then the next generation, two more brothers, Jacob and Esau, are estranged from each other. This is what the text says about them: "As the boys grew up, Esau became a skillful hunter. He was an outdoorsman, but Jacob had a quiet temperament, preferring to stay at home" (Genesis 25:27, NLT). "And Isaac loved Esau, because he did eat of his venison: but Rebekah loved Jacob" (Genesis 25:28, KJV). There's a world of hurt and a need for counseling in that last verse. Isaac, the father, loved Esau. He was a man's man. He was the guy who went to Academy. Jacob was favored and loved more by Mom, Rebekah. Jacob was staying home and trading recipes on the best chocolate chip cookies! I have a strange association with Esau and Jacob. A couple of comedians were brothers a long time ago, the Smothers Brothers. My Dad bought their albums and still has them. Anybody here ever heard of the Smothers Brothers? When they got into a fight, Tommy would always say to Dickie the classic line, "Mom always liked you best." Their big comedy album was titled *Mom Always Liked You Best!* That's Jacob and Esau. Parents will do this weird kind of thing. "He's the athletic one. He's the outdoors one. He's the indoor one." Why would I craft one of my kids' identities based on what their brother or sister happened to be like? Then there's Joseph and his brothers, and envy and rivalry there. This runs all through Scripture.

Another vignette involves Israel's first king, Saul. We're told (another comparative phrase), "Saul, as handsome a young man as could be found anywhere in Israel, and he was a head taller than anyone else" (1 Samuel 9:2, NIV). He was the king. He named David to be a warrior, a general for him. They went out to battle, and the battle went well. Here's what happened next. "The women came out from all the towns of Israel to meet King Saul with singing and dancing, with joyful songs and with timbrels and lyres. As they danced, they sang: 'Saul has slain his thousands, and David his tens of thousands.' Saul was very angry; this refrain displeased him greatly. 'They have credited David with tens of thousands,' he thought, 'but me with only thousands. What more can he get but the kingdom?'" (1 Samuel 18:6–8, NIV).

Why did it gall him? Well, for one thing, it's a lame song. The lyrics are bad, and they sang it to the tune of "It's a Small World (After All)." "Saul has slain his thousands, after all. David has slain his tens of thousands, after all. Saul has slain his thousands, after all. David has slain his tens of thousands, after all. Sing it again!" Then they'd keep going. That would drive anybody crazy. I think another verse from Texas goes like this: *Saul bought a Prius, but David drove a Truck!* (smile) But that's not the reason it galls Saul so much. This is why it galls Saul so much. "Saul was very angry; this refrain displeased him greatly. 'They have credited David with tens of thousands,' he thought, 'but me with only thousands. What more can he get but the kingdom?' And from that time on Saul kept a close eye on David" (1 Samuel 18:8–9, NIV). The way the Hebrew language expresses itself is often very concrete and physical. So, Saul isn't just jealous; he keeps an envious eye. Comparison is that way. When I start to get jealous, I look at you differently. I don't see my brother. I don't see somebody I love. I know the person who creates pain in me. "Why are you so angry, Saul?" "I'm afraid. What more could he have but my kingdom?" Something precious is at risk. Nothing precious is ever at risk in the Kingdom of God with Jesus, but you'll find fear where there's comparison and envy. "Why are you so angry, Saul?" "I'm offended. They have credited David with tens of thousands but me with only thousands." "Are you kidding me, Saul? Who's they?" "Well, everyone." "Saul, what do you care what everybody thinks? You're the king. You're the man. David works for you. If he wins, you win." Saul is so consumed with envy that he eventually tries to kill David. Of course, this is so often the way it works in life. What Saul fears most is the loss of his kingdom, which happens precisely because of the grasping, clutching, jealous, and comparative way in which Saul lives. It'll kill you. It does all the time.

Students at Harvard University were asked to make a seemingly straightforward choice: which would they prefer, a job where they made $50,000 a year (option A) or one where they made $100,000 a year (option B)? Seems like a no-brainer, right? Everyone should take option B. But there was one catch. In option A, the students would get paid twice as much as others, who only get $25,000. In option B, they would get paid half as much as others, who would get $200,000. So, option B would make the students more money overall, but they would be doing worse than others around them. What did the majority of people choose? Option A. They preferred to do better than others, even if it meant getting less for themselves. They chose the option worse in absolute terms but better in relative terms. People don't just care about how they are doing; they care about the performance of others.[72]

Getting to board a plane a few minutes early is a nice perk of achieving premier status. But part of what makes this a nice perk is that you get to board before everyone else. Comparison kills contentment. We see this illustrated in chapter four of the book of Philippians. The apostle Paul is writing from prison, and he says: "I am not saying this because I am in need, for I have learned to be content" (Philippians 4:11, NIV). I have learned to be content. It's not like you just wake up one day and you're like, I'm good, I don't need anything. It's a learned process. I love what the apostle Paul writes there. I've learned to be content, whatever the circumstances. I know what it is to be in need, and I know what it is to have plenty. I have learned, again, the secret of being content in any and every situation, whether well-fed or hungry, whether living in plenty or want. I can do all things through Him who gives me strength. I've learned how to be content because comparison kills contentment. And contentment in life is simply accepting who God wants you to be, and not who you wish you were. I will never be Rick!

When I submitted my first book to be written, the publishers wanted to change it so much. It was way better than what I wrote, but I prayed about it, and at the end of the day, God said to me, you have to write the book I put in your heart, not the book some professional writer has re-written. You can have AI write a book now, but it won't be you! Friends, you must write your own story; no one else can write it for you!

---

72 Berger, J. (2013, February 26). *Jonah Berger Explains How A $50k Salary Is More Desirable Than $100K*. fastcompany.com.
https://www.fastcompany.com/3006318/jonah-berger-explains-how-50k-salary-more-desirable-100k

People would be happy to see you do better, but not better than them.

The problem with comparison is that you always feel better or worthless compared to someone else!

Comparing, then, is the root of all envy and the root of all pride!

In Luke 18, Jesus tells a story about a Pharisee, a religious leader, much like if I were to pray something we see recorded in Luke 18:11–12 (NIV): "The Pharisee stood by himself and prayed: 'God, I thank you that I am not like other people— robbers, evildoers, adulterers—or even like this tax collector. I fast twice a week and give a tenth of all I get." This guy is an ideal church member. Now we look on and think, I would never pray like that; that's ridiculous. You realize you just did what he did. You're prideful that you would never be that prideful. What are we doing: Comparing? I remember thinking I was a great parent. I'd go to Walmart and see all these people who didn't know how to parent their kids in Walmart as I saw kids having temper tantrums. Until one day, I took my six- and three-year-old boys to Walmart with me.

Then I found out it isn't that easy, especially in Walmart. Walmart brings out the evil in your children. C. S. Lewis, I love this, says this: *"We say that people are proud of being rich, clever, or good-looking, but they're not. They're proud of being richer, cleverer, or better looking than others. If everyone else were to become equally rich, clever, or good-looking, there would be nothing to be proud of."*[73] So true, right? If everything else were on a playing field, there would be nothing to be prideful about. Finding contentment in life is simply about accepting who God wants you to be, not who you wish to be.

The second thing **comparison can do is it can leave us jealous.** Proverbs 14:30 (NIV) states: "A heart at peace gives life to the body, but envy rots the bones." So, a peaceful heart leads to a healthy body. Doesn't that sound good? But, oh man, jealousy is like cancer in the bones. Bones are like the very structure of our body. It's what gives us form and shape. Our bones are the foundation, you could say. And the Bible is saying when you become jealous, it's like getting at the foundation of who you are. It's like cancer at your foundation, and it can leave you envious. Don't compare the size of your roof with the size of the sky.

Here's my chapter in a sentence: Comparison resents God's goodness in other's lives and ignores God's blessing in our own lives.

Read that sentence again and consider the blessings in your life. Are you using them to their fullest? Or are you wishing away and wasting what God has given you because God didn't give you what someone else has?

Don't make someone else's mud your benchmark for what your mud should look like or be able to accomplish.

---

73 Gentry, A. (2016, June 9). *Pride: CS Lewis.* Austin Gentry. https://www.austingentry.com/on-pride-cs-lewis/

Everyone's mud is different, but it is still mud!

Have you ever been scrolling on Facebook or Instagram and thought: Look at their life? Oh, my goodness. That's not my life. You are making their life your benchmark! I don't know how they took that vacation; that's ridiculous. They probably went into crazy debt. It's absurd that they did that, and I have no idea. How big is their house? What kind of car did they buy? They don't need another dress or another pair of shoes. I can't believe that they did that. You become the person you don't want to be. You resent God's goodness in somebody's life. And then you ignore the blessings in your life and the things God has given you. You ignore the fact that you have a car and can drive to and from, but you get in, you look at your friend's car, and you're like, this car looks like it just got detailed. My car looks like somebody dumped a box of Cheerios in the back, and then it's trying to dehydrate fruit. There is another way. There is a better way.

Have you ever tried to be someone you're not?

Have you ever been running in your lane, and then you start looking at someone else's lane and you think, *They are running so much better. So much faster. Look at their shoes, look at their job, look at their money, look at their purse, look at their house, their car, their marriage, their kids, I want to run in their lane...* Have you ever tried to be someone you're not?

I am at the gym on the elliptical, and I think I am doing pretty good. Got the resistance setting on 6 and incline on 10…and this lady three ellipticals down, in front of the whole gym, looks at my running and shouts, "You've been going a long time, same speed. What's your settings on, zero?" Zero? What? Have you ever been elliptical shamed at the gym? I have. I wanted to yell back, "Why are you comparing our settings, ma'am? Everyone has to decide their own elliptical settings. Everyone has to run in their own lane. Geez."

What if God is giving you permission to do it differently, to live the life God called you to live?

The challenge for a lot of people is sometimes you have to become something you have never seen before! It was Oscar Wilde who said: "Be yourself. Everyone else is already taken"!

Remember when David put on the armor of Saul and walked around for a moment? He has to fight Goliath, and he's like, "Give me whatever the guy who fights wears." Saul is like, "Here you go. You can wear mine." David walks around in them a little bit, and he's like, "This is heavy, this is weird, and this is not me right now. I think I would be better off with my slingshot, with what God called me to do. I know this is how you would fight, but I have to do it differently." David had to be something he had never seen before—I am talking about imposter syndrome, and it's real. How many of you ever felt imposter syndrome? Like the persistent feeling of "I am not good enough to do this job" or "I am not sure what I am doing in this area of my life"? It's low self-esteem, anxiety, depression over your life. You feel like you are faking it on the job or in your marriage or while preaching a sermon. (smile) Anyone? I read a study that said: Experts estimate that at least 80 percent of the general population experience impostor syndrome at some point in their lives, and the more successful you become, the worse the imposter syndrome is. After all, there's more to be exposed now. The expectations have been raised even higher! The fear of not being good enough is real for most of us! It's feeling like a bit of a *fraud*. I had someone ask me on the beach the other day at a wedding: "Are you a real pastor?" Meaning, "Are you ordained, or did you go online and get a certificate for seventy-five bucks to do a wedding?" Some of you are like, "That's not a bad idea for a little side gig." *Are you a real pastor?* If they only knew how often I've asked myself that question. Am I a real pastor? What makes one a real pastor? Are you a real teacher? Are you a real doctor? Are you a real husband? A real mom? The experience of looking around and feeling as though you pale in comparison to the talents of others is not unfamiliar to me—imposter syndrome is something that I still struggle with. The Bible says the same thing: "Make a careful exploration of who you are and the work you have been given, and then sink yourself into that. Don't be impressed with yourself. Don't compare yourself with others. Each of you must take responsibility for doing the creative best you can with your own life" (Galatians 6:4–5, MSG). Keep your eye on your own elliptical settings. Everyone has their own race to run!

Jacob had become envious of Esau's gifts from God. Jacob was never going to be a hunter or get his father's love, so he pretended to be something he was not to get what he felt he needed.

Validation.

Jacob should have been looking at God and asking God, "Who did you make me to be?" **Ask your creator who you are called to be, not other creations.** As God's children, there's no space for a spirit of comparison, because the thing is, if you constantly have your eyes on the people around you, a day will come when you eventually stop looking at God altogether! **If we keep trying to be someone we're just not meant to be, we'll never become who God wants us to be.** Come on, who am I writing to today, besides myself? Anyone? Elliptical shaming, lane shaming, always comparing how far along you are in life compared to others, that's exactly what the Adversary wants: *for us to be derailed and distracted from walking into our God-given destiny.* See, because now you are Jacob trying to run in Esau's lane. Now you are checking your elliptical settings against someone else's! *If we keep trying to be someone we're just not meant to be, we'll never become who God wants us to be!* Your path doesn't look like anybody else's because it can't, it shouldn't, and it won't. So who are you really? And who will you choose to be?

We're told in the New Testament: "There was a man sent from God whose name was John" (John 1:6, NIV). This is of course, John the Baptist. John the Baptist had one central message, and that was, "Turn around, repent, for the Kingdom of God is on its way." Then, one day, John sees Jesus and says to people who see him, "Look, the Lamb of God, who takes away the sin of the world!" (John 1:29, NIV). Then, people begin going to Jesus. Then the strangest thing happens. "They came to John and said to him, 'Rabbi, that man who was with you on the other side of the Jordan—the one you testified about—look, he is baptizing, and everyone is going to him'" (John 3:26, NIV).

John has disciples just like Jesus has disciples.

John is called "Rabbi," just as Jesus is called "Rabbi." John baptized people just as Jesus's followers are now baptizing people. John's disciples say, "Hey, remember? We used to be number one. We were the most prominent. Everybody was coming to see us. Jesus, the guy you baptized, is becoming more popular than you are, and everybody will see him. The more people who go to see you, the more important you are. We're your disciples, so if you're becoming less important, we will be less important. We don't like this, so you'd better do something to recapture market share." That comparison deal goes on even in spiritual arenas, even in ministry. A long time ago, when I was first starting in church ministry, I was at a pastor's conference, and during one of the breaks, there was a little group of three of us talking to each other. We were all pastors, and one of them said to the other one, "How is your church going?" For those who don't know, that's pastor talk for, "How many people go to your church?" That's pastor talk for, "How important are you? Will I get status if I hang out with you?" The first guy says, "A thousand people, something like that. How's your church?" The second guy said, "Twelve hundred people." I knew what was coming next. I was at a church of about 250 people. I immediately thought, "I'm going to say we're like 300 people because that will sound much more impressive than 250 people." Do you know how your mind works in a moment like that? I thought to myself, "Really? Really? I don't know these guys. I'm never going to see them again. Do I want to give up my integrity (which is all you have; that's reality) for the sake of status gained by fifty lousy people?" I said, "We run about 2,000." I figured if I sacrificed my integrity, I might as well make it worthwhile. I remember a bunch of churches in a denomination, old churches but larger than other churches in their denomination. They sometimes gathered and called themselves the "tall steeple churches." Has anybody noticed there are not a lot of steeples being built in the US these days? Combining grandiosity and irrelevance more succinctly in a single phrase would be hard. John the Baptist's disciples say, "We used to be a tall-steeple ministry, and now everybody is going to him." Superhuman. I know that feeling. John's response is unbelievable. Look at what John says: "To this John replied, 'A person can receive only what is given them from heaven. You yourselves can testify that I said, 'I am not the Messiah but am sent ahead of him.' The bride belongs to the bridegroom. The friend who attends the bridegroom waits and listens for him, and is full of joy when he hears the bridegroom's voice. That joy is mine, and it is now complete. He must become greater; I must become less" (John 3:27–30, NIV). This has a kingdom all over it. Don't worry about who's in the Eagles, who's in the Robins, and who's in the Pigeons. John the Baptist essentially says, "I know who I am, and that begins with who I'm not. I'm not the Messiah. It's not me." That's a perfect place to start, to look in the mirror and say: "I am not the Messiah!" John talks about who he is. He uses this remarkable picture. He essentially says, "I told you, I'm not the bridegroom; I'm a friend of the groom." He's using an image here from Hebrew weddings. There would be a character with an official role, like a best man in our weddings. The Hebrew word for this was called the Shoshben, a friend of the groom. He would provide many ceremonial functions that a best man would do. The final task of the Shoshben would be to stand in front of the bridal tent, where the bride would be inside at the end of the day's festivities. He would stand guard there so nobody got to the bride until the bridegroom came. It would be dark so that he would hear the groom's voice. When he heard the sound of the groom's voice, his final task was to step aside so the groom could go into the bride. Then he would have the joy of knowing, "I did my job. I helped my friend, and now the groom and the bride are together." John essentially says, "That's me. I'm not the groom. The bride belongs to him. The church belongs to Jesus. She's not mine. The people aren't mine. If I try to grab for the joy that belongs to him, I will not get his joy, and I'll lose my joy. So, don't you think when other people are going to Jesus instead of me, it's causing me to lose my joy? My joy is fulfilled. I'm the groom's friend and am so glad the groom is here. By the way, as a church, we want to reach every single person for Jesus Christ that we can, but somebody was talking to me about other churches once and said something about the competition. Other churches are not our competition. Thank God for every church in America that preaches Jesus. The more God breathes life into his church, whatever church it is, wherever the church is, the better it is. Then John has this amazing statement: "He must become greater; I must become less" (John 3:30, NIV). In other words, "My life is not centered on me." This is an essential thing to understand about the way life works. The more my ego is at the center of my life purposes, the more miserable I will be. It's this strange paradox. When I die to my ego and put God in the center of my life, the greater my life, the bigger my world. I must grow lesser; he must grow greater. That's the kingdom. That's life.

By contrast, there was a movie a decade or two ago called *Amadeus*. It's this amazing story of a court musician named Salieri. He's gifted and competent but recognizes that Mozart is a genius. Mozart is this obnoxious character, and it grates at him that God made Mozart the genius and not him. He's convinced God has done him wrong because he cannot be happy while Mozart is in the world. One piece of mud doesn't like another because his mud is prettier or more talented in his eyes. He says to God: "From now on, we are enemies, you and I. Because you chose for your instrument a boastful, lustful, smutty, infantile boy and gave me for reward only the ability to recognize the incarnation; because you are unjust, unfair, unkind, I will block you, I swear it." Salieri had amazing gifts that put him in the top one-tenth of 1 percent, an amazing privilege. His mud was gifted, but he couldn't stand it; it was not Mozart's mud. He also could have been given the gift of recognizing the greatness in Mozart and said, "What a great thing it is to live in a world where there's a Mozart and have the whole world listen to and love that music." But all he could see was, "I'm not Mozart. God has done me wrong." The idea that he might find joy in humbling himself and being able to applaud the greatness of somebody else never occurred to him. The end of that movie is just chilling if you've ever seen it. Salieri is with a priest, and he's making this accusation against God. He's convinced in his mind that it is unanswerable, that he is right and God has done him wrong. He tells the priest, "You are a mediocrity, but don't worry; I am your champion. I am the patron saint of mediocrities." Then he's wheeled out in this asylum for the insane and the wretched and says, "I absolve you of your mediocrity." We live in this crazy world. I have to compare myself. I have to be in the Eagles group. I must have done better than Rick at the science fair, but I am dying to love it when I think that way. So how do I live in another way? Maybe you can focus on letting your mud become a flower. "A flower does not think of competing to the flower next to it. It just blooms" (Zen Shin).[74]

A flower doesn't care what is next to it or what, when, why, or how it will bloom. It only worries about blooming itself and fulfilling its purpose. What about you? Are you busy blooming or busy comparing because you can't do both? The Bible gives us similar advice in Galatians 6:4 (CSB): "Let each person examine his work, and then he can take pride in himself alone, and not compare himself with someone else." Notice the Bible says first, you should "examine [your] own work." You should look at your past and learn from it. Next, you should "not compare [yourself] with someone else." As you examine your life, don't let your eyes wander to how God works in the people around you. Concentrate on what he's done in and through you.

There are plenty of reasons not to compare yourself to others. One, it denies the unique part of you that God made, that makes you, you! No one else has mud as you do! God will not judge you based on what God gave to others, only on what God put in your heart and your pockets. Examine your life: What are you good at doing? What do you enjoy doing? What do you do naturally without any external encouragement? Where do you see God's presence the most? Now, go back and look for patterns. It's in the patterns where you will find your mud can start to shine. You probably still are if you were good at something when you were younger. Where did you see God blessing your life the most during that time? Was it when you were serving others, giving others hope, loving others?

74 Quotespedia.org. (2020, July 13). *A flower does not think of competing to the flower next to it. it...* https://www.quotespedia.org/authors/z/ zen-shin/a-flower-does-not-think-of-competing-to-the-flower-next-to-it-it-just-blooms-zen-shin/

Most likely! After identifying patterns in your life, ask God what he wants you to do with this information. Maybe, just maybe, God wants you to use what God has made you good at to make up there come down here, a little bit of Heaven on Earth! In high school, I used to counsel people on the porch. My mom called me the porch counselor or porch preacher. I had no idea what that would mean for my life, but I do now! What did you do back then that God wants you to do now? If it involves loving and serving, get busy!

I'll share with you a very revealing confession. Whenever I compare myself to other pastors, it's not pretty. I can't do that. I need to be faithful to just who God called me to be. For example, this is something that virtually all of you would not know about because we never promote this kind of stuff. This isn't our style. But, about a year ago, they came out with this deal where they ranked the fifty most influential pastors in the country. Now, I was not on the list of the top fifty! Shocker. But then I began looking at the list, going really? How can that guy with a toupee and pyrotechnics be ranked ahead of me? Then I started wondering: Where am I on the list of preachers? How do I move up in the rankings? Can you imagine this happening? Of course, you can. So, I started researching this, and here's what I found: our country has between 385,000 and 400,000 senior pastors. As I do this, I write in a prayer journal, confessing my sin of envy. God told me, "Stop hating people for what they have; start working for what you desire." I won't tell you where I was ranked because I couldn't find where I was ranked; they quit listing after the top 1,000. We don't view people in hierarchies. It's simply wrong. We love people. Galatians 6:4, "Each one should test his actions without comparing himself to somebody else." No comparisons. That's what we are not going to do. What are we going to do? Two Biblically positive things. Instead of resenting God's goodness in other's lives, we are going to celebrate it. We are going to celebrate God's goodness to others. Romans teaches us this principle. God's Word says, "Rejoice with those who rejoice; mourn with those who mourn" (Romans 12:15, NIV). Envy and greed starve on a steady diet of gratitude and thanksgiving.

My grandma taught me this principle. She'd send my younger brother and me a card with a check every Christmas. Both of us would always get a twenty-dollar check. We'd be so excited, but I'd always mess with him since my brother, Greg, was younger than me. It's part of a big brother's spiritual call and duty. So, when I would get my twenty-dollar check, I would open it up and say, "Wow! One hundred dollars!" And he would get his check, expect a hundred, and open it up and say, "Twenty dollars?" He'd say, "Did you really…" "Yeah," and I'd put it in my pocket and walk away. And he would cry and get all upset, and I felt so good. This is why I need therapy. He was younger, so I did this to him year after year: "One hundred dollars!" One year, Grandma found out about this. That year, I opened my twenty-dollar check and said, "One hundred dollars!" Greg opened his one hundred check and said, "One hundred dollars!" And Grandma taught me to rejoice with those who get a hundred gifts. Someone else gets something you were hoping for; rejoice with those who rejoice!

Here are a couple of questions to work on. "Who am I comparing myself to?" I invite you to think about this one. I probably won't compare myself financially to Bill Gates or somebody such as Mother Teresa or Joel Osteen. It'll be a person down the hall, down the street, down the road, somebody quite close by. Just be honest about that. Who am I comparing myself to when it comes to being a better husband? A better preacher? A better Christian? Probably not Billy Graham. But God didn't make you to be them, and God won't judge you for not being Billy Graham or Mother Teresa. Ask those questions God asked of Cain. "Why am I angry? What is it I want? Who would my best self be?" Then ask, "What's the joy God has for me? What are the gifts God has given to me? What's the task God has assigned me?" God hasn't asked me to be somebody else. I don't have to be Mozart or David or Saul. I have to be me. God is just calling you to be you. What gifts am I ignoring by focusing on the gifts and blessings in someone else's life? I promise you there's joy in loving the people around you, doing the things God has called you to do, giving the gifts God has called you to provide, and stretching the gifts God has given you to stretch. I promise you there's joy.

Then, if you want extra credit work, does anybody want extra credit work? I'll give you some. Take that person you're most prone to envy and compare yourself to and pray that God will cause them to succeed this week like never before. Just say, "God, would you let that person soar? Would you unleash their gifts in unprecedented ways?" Then, of course, don't do this on your power. We don't do this on our strength. We're leaning on the kingdom. I ask Jesus, "Would you help me with this?" all the time. Every time I'm tempted to compare myself to somebody else that becomes a little prompt for prayer. By the way, Jesus knows all about envy. You may have never noticed this tiny little phrase here. This is from the story of Jesus. Speaking of Pilate, the Bible says: "For he perceived that it was out of envy that the chief priests had delivered him up" (Mark 15:10, ESV).

Envy is what killed Jesus.

"Everybody is going to him. That means they're not going to us. They're not cheering us on. We have to kill that guy." "Want to go out in the field?" It's the story of the human race. It would be best not to compare yourself to others, for you never know the truth about anyone else.

Let me close with this story. As a preacher, one of my pettier, envious thoughts is that sometimes I envy people who get the whole weekend off. I don't have weekends off but let me tell you what I have. It's amazing. I get Fridays off—one day a week off, and honestly, most people get two weeks' vacation. The church gives my family pretty much whatever we need, as long as it is reasonable. I can take a month off during the year if I need to and four weeks if I need to. I am thankful that God provides that for my family, period.

I envy those whose jobs end at five o'clock. You know what? I am grateful that instead of my biggest goal being making money or making somebody else money, or making widgets or whatever, *I get to make an eternal difference.* I am thankful that God has called me to do this, period. When I first got into ministry, there was a six-year-old girl who was dying, and we were praying for her. She continued to get worse. I went to see her in the hospital, and I just looked at this precious little girl. I said, "Sweetheart, what do you want? Anything. You name it. You name it. What do you want? Anything and I'm going to get it for you," and I never will forget what this little girl did. She looked at me. Her head was bald. She lost her hair after two treatments, and instead of saying, "Oh, I just want to play like the other kids or whatever," this six-year-old girl looked at me and said, "Well, I've got my mommy and daddy here. I've got my two favorite sticker books. I've got my dolly, and I've got Jesus in my heart. What else could a little kid want?" I hugged her and would not let her go because her response made me cry. I put that little girl in the ground. I buried her just a few weeks later. That one little moment with her will stick with me forever. I don't know how your story goes, but here's mine.

I get to serve the greatest God, and I get to do it full-time. I get to love and share His truth with the greatest people, which is my calling. I've got my best friend, who is my wife, who has used her body and sacrificed to give me two kids. I have the greatest friends that I could ever have. I have the strongest staff and Jesus Christ, the Son of God, in my heart. What more could any guy ever want? I celebrate with all of you that you have the weekend off, and I embrace God's goodness in my life. I hope you can do the same and never envy again because, in the end, Jesus is enough.

EPILOGUE

IT'S LATER THAN YOU THINK

The bitterest tears shed over graves
are for words left unsaid and for deeds left undone!

—Harriet Beecher Stowe

HAVE YOU EVER KNOWN ONE?

Or were you one?

Or do you still think you are one?

You went to school with them.

You grew up with them.

Maybe you live with them. Perhaps you even think you are married to one. They are easily identified by the labels that we put on them, such as *losers, rejects, nerds, geeks, or failures.*

They get mocked, bullied, ridiculed, and made fun of. They are ostracized and isolated. They are on the outside looking in, and nobody ever offers to let them in. You might say they are "On the fringe."

One of the most amazing things about Jesus is that He gravitated toward the people we run away from.

The people that repel us, He was drawn to like a magnet.

The people we overlook are the people He looked over.

The people we wouldn't give the time of day to, He gave almost every minute of His time to.

"Two others, who were criminals, were led away to be put to death with him. And when they came to the place called The Skull, they crucified him and the criminals, one on his right and one on his left" (Luke 23:32–33, ESV).

Interestingly, Jesus is crucified between two criminals. Usually, the centurion in charge would have put the two criminals next to each other and Jesus off to one side. Still, the Roman soldier did not realize he was fulfilling an ancient prophecy. In Isaiah 53:12 (NIV), he says that he would be "numbered with the transgressors." This was the only crucifixion in history that was ever prophesized.

Jesus will take us under any condition. You would think that Jesus would at least be crucified with people who were guilty of what we might call today White-collar crime. Not so. Luke calls them criminals. The better word would be *evildoers*. Matthew and Mark use a different term that means "violent robbers." These men had a rap sheet a mile long. They were bad to the bone. They were only caught because someone saw them on Jerusalem's Most Wanted. From the time they came out of their mother's womb to the time they were nailed to a wooden plank, you could write one word over their lives—*failure*.

They were so inconsequential and so on the fringe we don't even know their names.

They had failed at doing anything right and succeeded at doing everything wrong.

It looks like they have lived a wasted life, and they are going to die a wasted death, but then something changes.

One criminal knew he was guilty and thought, *I deserve to die.*

He looked at Jesus and thought, *He deserves to live.*

I am a sinner. He is the Savior. Forgiveness is precisely what I need.

I wonder if what He offered them, He would offer me?

Interestingly, even though Matthew and Mark both record Jesus dying between these two criminals, Luke is the only one who records this conversation. I'm glad he did because it is scripture's only recorded deathbed conversion.

You won't find anybody in the Bible or even an experience in a more desperate situation.

Brutally crucified, dying in agony for crimes he committed, a guilty man justly punished, deserving to die and knowing that death is just a little while away with no stay of execution, no last-minute reprieve, the sand in his hourglass has only a few grains left, and soon he will be dead.

He is as close to death as you can be and still be living.

At the last moment, most probably with his last breath (because we are not told that he ever said another word), he makes one final appeal to the Chief Justice of the Supreme Court of the Universe!

He is one of the most extraordinary examples of faith in the entire Bible.

In an instant, just before this man slips off the clothes of Earth and puts on the clothes of Eternity, Jesus answers this man's request and makes a reservation for him in Heaven.

All the man said was, "Remember me," because all he had to offer was himself.

He couldn't say, "Remember my good works" because he had none.

He couldn't say, "Remember my church attendance" because he never went.

He couldn't say, "Remember my offerings" because he never gave.

All he could say was, "Remember me."

"Remember me when you come into your kingdom."

Probably with not a lot of confidence, probably not even being able to look Jesus in the eye, but with fear and trembling, he makes this simple request, "Jesus, *remember* me when you come into your kingdom" (Luke 23:42, ESV).

He didn't say, "Lord, I want to be honored when you come into your kingdom," or "I want to be blessed when you come into your kingdom," or "I want to be rewarded when you come into your kingdom."

He just said, "I want to be *remembered*."

He didn't want to die the second death, the death of being forgotten.

Lord, will you remember me when everyone else has forgotten me?

Look at me—the ultimate failure.

Here at my death with no friends and no family.

My enemies didn't even bother to show up.

I have failed at life, and now I am even failing in death.

Jesus, will you remember me?

Will you give me what I need the most and what I deserve the least?

Would you give me forgiveness and a place in your kingdom?

If you know the story, you already know the answer.

You can figure it out even if you know nothing about Jesus.

This man needed what Jesus had to offer, but he couldn't provide anything that Jesus required or wanted.

He had no leverage, no bargaining chips, and couldn't make a deal.

Sounds a lot like us.

What is he going to say? "Jesus, if you will remember me when you come into your kingdom, I promise you I'll go to church. I'll be a better husband and a better dad. I won't cheat on my income taxes anymore. I'll even start tithing."

He realized he needed what Jesus had to offer, but he had nothing to offer Jesus.

If you are reading this right now and you feel like a failure or much of your life has been a failure, if you are the one that has blown it and you feel like there is no way that God would ever accept you, this crucifixion scene reminds us of an important truth:

There is more grace in God's heart than sin in our past.

Jesus will take us under any condition.

Sometimes Jesus comes to us in disguise.

No man ever looked less like a king than Jesus did at that moment.

Beaten to a pulp so severely you couldn't recognize Him; his only throne was a cross.

His only crown was made of thorns.

He wasn't covered with the robes of royalty.

He was crucified stark naked.

He had not met Jesus until that day.

He had not heard Jesus teach by the sea.

He had not seen Jesus heal the sick or raise the dead.

He had not heard Jesus tell one parable.

He had not seen Jesus perform a single miracle, yet he knew that this suffering Savior was not just a king but the King of all Kings.

Don't miss this.

This man was never baptized, never took the Lord's Supper, never went to confession, never joined a church, never went to church, and never gave one penny to the Lord's work, but robbed a lot of money from the Lord's workers. There wasn't one thing this man had done for Jesus, and there wasn't one thing this man could do for Jesus.

The only thing he had left was to accept what Jesus was doing for him.

What does Jesus say to him, to you, to me, before you give up…? Know this…

"And he said to him, "Truly, I say to you, today you will be with me in Paradise" (Luke 23:43, ESV).

I did something that fascinated me. I timed how long it would take for those two men to make those two statements to each other. What the thief said takes less than four seconds. Jesus's reply takes less than six seconds.

In less than ten seconds, this man went from being a criminal to being a Christian.

This man went from being a failure to a success.

This man went from being on the outside looking into the inside looking out. You say, "That's impossible!" "With God, all things are possible." If God can say, "Let there be light," and turn on every sun, every moon, and every star in the universe, He can say today, "Turn life on" instantaneously.

If you had been there that day and somebody told you, "What chance do you think that criminal has of going to heaven?"

You would have said, "He doesn't have a prayer."

A prayer is all he had, and a prayer is all he needed.

There is one thing we grasp at this moment.

Anybody can call on Jesus anytime, and He will always answer.

You won't get a busy signal, and you won't get put on hold if you say, "Remember me," and He will say, "I will."

This man was out of options.

Jesus said, "Before you give up your last breath, your last hope, your last chance…"

It was too late to turn over a new leaf, too late to pay everyone back, too late for a new beginning. It was too late for this man to get married, raise a family, get a job, be responsible, and live a decent life, but it wasn't too late to be saved.

It is never too late to trust Jesus because we can trust Jesus at any moment.

Friends, it's later than you think.

Are you living in or heading for failure? Do you know you are in trouble?

Have you been left for dead?

Don't fake a resurrection; live into one!

Know this before you give up:

You are only one prayer away!

You are only one step away!

You are only thought away!

You are only one friend away!

You are only "A New Way" away!

You are only one way of "love" away!

You are only one shovel away!

You are only one splinter away!

You are only one restoration away!

You are only one seatbelt away!

You are only one belief away!

You are only four seconds away from changing your life.

Don't live your life robbing yourself of what could have been if you had risked what was and what is, for what could and will be!

Whatever you are facing right now…

Before you give up…

Life-giving change begins by knowing that it doesn't have to be this way.

REFERENCES

21st century king James Version (KJ21) - version information - biblegateway.com. (n.d.).
https://www.biblegateway.com/
versions/21st-Century-King-James-Version-KJ21-Bible/

Association of American Medical Colleges. (n.d.). *Carl Allamby*. Students & Residents.
https://students-residents.aamc.org/career-changers/carl-allamby

Aurelius, M. (n.d.). *A Quote from Meditations*. Goodreads.
https://www.goodreads.com/
quotes/293726-think-of-yourself-as-dead-you-have-lived-your-life

Berger, J. (2013, February 26). *Jonah Berger Explains How A $50k Salary Is More Desirable Than $100K*. fastcompany.com.
https://www.fastcompany.com/3006318/
jonah-berger-explains-how-50k-salary-more-desirable-100k

Bilefsky, D., & Severson, K. (2016, February 1). *Benoît Violier's death shines light on high-pressure restaurant world*. The New York Times.
https://www.nytimes.com/2016/02/02/world/europe/benoit-violier-chef-dies.html

Brooks, J. (2018, January 20). You Can't Go Wrong With Ben Franklin's Wisdom. *Dayton Daily News*. Retrieved from
https://www.daytondailynews.com/news/opinion/
commentary-you-can-wrong-with-ben-franklin-wisdom/
Pf3cJhk4iGSKBMJoaDcDMK/.

Buffett, J. (n.d.). *Jimmy Buffett - It Takes No More Time to See the Good Side...* BrainyQuote.
https://www.brainyquote.com/quotes/jimmy_buffett_425230

Burkey, R. (2005, May 19). *Sharing Jesus in Practical Ways*. Sermon Central. https://www.sermoncentral.com/sermons/sharing-jesus-in-practical-ways-richard-burkey-sermon-on-evangelism-how-to-79253?page=2&wc=800

byquoteresearch, P. (2021, November 23). *I prayed that god would emancipate me, but it was not till I prayed with my legs that I was emancipated*. Quote Investigator. https://quoteinvestigator.com/2021/11/23/pray-legs/

Christian Standard Bible. CSB. (2019, July 15). https://csbible.com/

Contemporary English Version. CEV.BIBLE. (n.d.). https://cev.bible/

Curtain, M. (2017, October 24). *Winston Churchill's 12-Word Definition of Success May Just Change Your Life*. Inc.com. https://www.inc.com/melanie-curtin/in-just-12-words-winston-churchill-gives-us-a-definition-of-success-that-could-outlast-them-all.html

de Rooy, L. (2020, September 20). *Chapter V: Advice from a Caterpillar*. Alice-in-wonderland.net. https://www.alice-in-wonderland.net/resources/chapters-script/ alices-adventures-in-wonderland/chapter-5/

Diaz, C. (2019, April 22). *I Marked People for Death. Jesus Marked Me for Life*. ChristianityToday.com. https://www.christianitytoday.com/ct/2019/may/casey-diaz-shot-caller-marked-people-death-gang-leader.html

Einstein, A. (1999). *Autobiographical Notes*. Open Court.

Ellams, I., & Saint-Exupéry, A. de. (2020). *The Little Prince*. Oberon Books.

Ferriss, T. (2015, December 14). Derek Sivers on Developing Confidence, Finding Happiness, and Saying No to Millions . *The Tim Ferriss Show*. other.

Flynt, M. (n.d.). *Mike Flynt*. mikeflynt.com. https://www.mikeflynt.com/

Gentry, A. (2016, June 9). *Pride: CS Lewis*. Austin Gentry. https://www.austingentry.com/on-pride-cs-lewis/

Gibran, K. (2019, January 1). *The prophet*. The Project Gutenberg eBook of The Prophet, by Kahlil Gibran. https://www.gutenberg.org/files/58585/58585-h/58585-h.htm#link15

Glass, A. (2018, February 9). *Congress eulogizes Theodore Roosevelt, Feb. 9, 1919 - Politico*. Politico.

https://www.politico.com/story/2018/02/09/
congress-eulogizes-theodore-roosevelt-feb-9-1919-391633

Good news translation. GNT.BIBLE. (n.d.).
https://gnt.bible/

Goodreads. (n.d.-a). *A quote by Pablo Casals*. Goodreads.
https://www.goodreads.com/
quotes/194563-each-second-we-live-is-a-new-and-unique-moment

Goodreads. (n.d.-b). *A quote by socrates*. Goodreads.
https://www.goodreads.com/quotes/76088-envy-is-the-ulcer-of-the-soul

Harrington, D. J. (2022, July 26). *D.J. Harrington*. Recyclers Powersource.
https://www.rpowersource.com/2022/07/is-your-telescope-set-right/

Harrison, L. (2024, February 2). *Black History Month Clean Water Champion: Mari
Copeny*. Clean Water Action.
https://cleanwater.org/2024/02/02/
black-history-month-clean-water-champion-mari-copeny

Helen Rowland - a bride at her second marriage does not... BraomyQuote. (n.d.).
https://www.brainyquote.com/quotes/helen_rowland_385987

Helen Rowland - there are only two kinds of men; the dead... Brainy Quote. (n.d.).
https://www.brainyquote.com/quotes/helen_rowland_147607

Housman, J., & Dorman, S. (2005, September). *The Alameda County Study: A
systematic, chronological ...* Education Resources Information Center.
https://files.eric.ed.gov/fulltext/EJ792845.pdf

Hymn #100: O God Our Help In Ages Past. Semicolon. (2011, September 13).
https://www.semicolonblog.com/?p=5299

International Children's Bible (ICB) - version information - biblegateway.com. (n.d.).
https://www.biblegateway.com/versions/International-Childrens-Bible-ICB/

Jubilee bible 2000 (JUB) - version information - biblegateway.com. (n.d.).
https://www.biblegateway.com/versions/Jubilee-Bible-2000-JUB/

King, M. L. (n.d.). *A Quote by Martin Luther King Jr.*. Goodreads.
https://www.goodreads.com/
quotes/147771-not-everybody-can-be-famous-but-everybody-can-be-great

Klein, C. (2012, October 12). *When Teddy Roosevelt Was Shot in 1912, a Speech
May Have Saved His Life*. History.com.
https://www.history.com/news/
shot-in-the-chest-100-years-ago-teddy-roosevelt-kept-on-talking

Leatherman. (2017, April 18). *Tool Tales: Ice Breaker*. YouTube. https://www.youtube.com/watch?v=U_1cLoBIMK4&t=60s

Leatherman. (2018, July 16). *Made of Mettle: The Leatherman Documentary*. YouTube. https://www.youtube.com/watch?v=rvCgGgokH_E

Lexham English Bible - LEB - verses, online study tools. Bible Study Tools. (n.d.-a). https://www.biblestudytools.com/leb/

Lisitsa, E. (2024, June 25). *The Four Horsemen: Contempt*. The Gottman Institute. https://www.gottman.com/blog/the-four-horsemen-contempt

Living bible (TLB) - version information - biblegateway.com. (n.d.). https://www.biblegateway.com/versions/The-Living-Bible-TLB/

Liz, M. (2017, April 11). *Over nearly 80 years, Harvard study has been showing how to live a healthy and happy life*. Harvard Gazette. https://news.harvard.edu/gazette/story/2017/04/over-nearly-80-years-harvard-study-has-been-showing-how-to-live-a-healthy-and-happy-life/

Margaritoff, M. (2023, June 29). *The Inspiring True Story of Dashrath Manjhi: The "Mountain Man" Who Spent Decades Carving A Lifesaving Road Through a Treacherous Mountain*. All That's Interesting. https://allthatsinteresting.com/dashrath-manjhi

Mark Twain quote. AZ Quotes. (n.d.). https://www.azquotes.com/quote/812796

May, S. (2019, January 7). *The How of Persistence*. Steve May. https://stevemay.com/the-how-of-persistence/

May, S. (2022, January 24). *The Power of Words Archives*. Steve May. https://stevemay.com/category/words/

The Message bible. (n.d.-b). https://messagebible.com/

Morris, E. (2001). *The Rise of Theodore Roosevelt: Revised edition*. Random House.

Murthy, V. H., Our epidemic of loneliness and isolation: The U.S. Surgeon General's advisory on the healing effects of Social Connection and Community (2023). Rockville, Md; U.S. Public Health Service.

New Catholic Bible (NCB) - version information - biblegateway.com. (n.d.). https://www.biblegateway.com/versions/New-Catholic-Bible-NCB-Bible/

New International Reader's Version (NIRV) - version information - biblegateway. com. (n.d.).

https://www.biblegateway.com/versions/
new-international-readers-version-nirv-bible/

New International Version (NIV) - version information - biblegateway.com. (n.d.). https://www.biblegateway.com/versions/new-international-version-niv-bible/

New king James Version (NKJV) bible - search and read online. Bible Study Tools. (n.d.-b). https://www.biblestudytools.com/nkjv/

Nilsson, J. (2018, August 24). *Albert Einstein: "imagination is More Important Than knowledge."* The Saturday Evening Post. https://www.saturdayeveningpost.com/2010/03/ imagination-important-knowledge/

NRT Media. (n.d.). *God's got a bigger thing going on song lyrics | greater vision lyrics | Christian music song lyrics, Christian music | newreleasetoday.* New Release Today. https://www.newreleasetoday.com/lyricsdetail.php?lyrics_id=52709

Official king James Bible online: Authorized king James Version (KJV). (n.d.-a). https://www.kingjamesbibleonline.org/

Ortlund, R. (2009, January 6). On Our Watch. *The Gospel Coalition.* https://www.thegospelcoalition.org/blogs/ray-ortlund/on-our-watch/

Palmer, P. J. (2019, November 26). *A Life Lived Whole.* YES! Magazine. https://www.yesmagazine.org/issue/ healing-resistance/2004/11/09/a-life-lived-whole

Putnam, R. D. (2020). *Bowling alone: The collapse and revival of American community.* Simon & Schuster Paperbacks.

Quotes from Raymond Chandler's Writing. Chandlerisms - Quotes. (n.d.). https://www.shamustown.com/quotes.html

Quotespedia.org. (2020, July 13). *A flower does not think of competing to the flower next to it. it...* https://www.quotespedia.org/authors/z/zen-shin/a-flower-does-not-think-of-competing-to-the-flower-next-to-it-it-just-blooms-zen-shin/

Ralph Waldo Emerson - it is one of the blessings of old... BrainyQuote. (n.d.-a). https://www.brainyquote.com/quotes/ralph_waldo_emerson_105261

Ralph Waldo Emerson - the only way to have a friend is to... BrainyQuote. (n.d.-b). https://www.brainyquote.com/quotes/ralph_waldo_emerson_100740

Read the bible online. ESV Bible. (n.d.). https://www.esv.org/

Read the holman christian standard bible free online. Bible Study Tools. (n.d.-c).
  https://www.biblestudytools.com/csb/

Read the New Living Translation (NLT) Bible version online. Bible Study Tools.
  (n.d.-d).
  https://www.biblestudytools.com/nlt/

Read the New Living Translation (NLT) Bible version online. Bible Study Tools.
  (n.d.-e).
  https://www.biblestudytools.com/nlt/

Read the New Revised Standard Free Online. Bible Study Tools. (n.d.-f).
  https://www.biblestudytools.com/nrs/

Read The revised standard version free online. Bible Study Tools. (n.d.-g).
  https://www.biblestudytools.com/rsv/

Riis, D. (2019, March 18). *What Hitler got wrong about D-day*. History.com.
  https://www.history.com/news/d-day-hitler-germany-defenses-miscalculations

Ritter, W. (2020, April 20). The Race That Is Set Before Us. *RitterWrites*.
  https://www.ritterwrites.com/writings/2020/4/22/the-race-that-is-set-before-us

Robbins, T. (n.d.). *Get Inspired. Get Motivated*. Quotefancy.
  https://quotefancy.com/

Rubin, G. (2015, July 29). *Butter Scraped Over Too Much Bread*. Psychology Today.
  https://www.psychologytoday.com/us/blog/the-happiness-project/201507/
  butter-scraped-over-too-much-bread

Saint-Exupéry, A. de, Galantière, L., & Cosgrave, J. O. (1939). *Wind, sand and stars*.
  Reynal & Hitchcock.

Schweitzer, A. (2005). *The Quest of the Historical Jesus*. Dover Publications.

Shakespeare, W. (n.d.). *Speech: "Tomorrow, and Tomorrow, and Tomorrow" by...*
  Poetry Foundation.
  https://www.poetryfoundation.org/poems/56964/
  speech-tomorrow-and-tomorrow-and-tomorrow

Sherman, S. (2020, November 25). *How Much Is Enough?*. Mindful.
  https://www.mindful.org/how-much-is-enough/#:~:text=John%20D.,want%20
  things%20to%20be%20better.

Sipherd, R. (2018, February 28). *The Third-leading Cause of Death in US Most
  Doctors Don't Want You to Know About*. CNBC.
  https://www.cnbc.com/2018/02/22/medical-errors-third-leading-cause-of-death-
  in-america.html

Spirituality, F. (n.d.). *Chapter 19 - True Spirituality by Francis Schaeffer*. The Transformed Soul. http://www.thetransformedsoul.com/about-the-book/chapters/chapter-2a-summary-of-the-boo19

Sudhakar, S. (2022, September 19). *Cleveland Auto Mechanic becomes doctor at age 51, inspires others to pursue their dreams*. Fox News. https://www.foxnews.com/lifestyle/cleveland-auto-mechanic-becomes-doctor-inspires-others-pursue-dreams

Sunscreens, E. G. to. (2023, May 23). *Skin cancer: EWG's guide to sunscreens*. Skin cancer | EWG's Guide to Sunscreens. https://www.ewg.org/sunscreen/skin-cancer-on-the-rise/

Toler, S. (2009). *God has never failed me, but he's sure scared me to death a few times*. David C. Cook.

Top 500 abraham lincoln quotes (2024 update). Quotefancy. (n.d.-a). https://quotefancy.com/abraham-lincoln-quotes

Tsioulcas, A. (2016, September 14). *From trash to triumph: The recycled orchestra*. NPR. https://www.npr.org/sections/deceptivecadence/2016/09/14/493794763/from-trash-to-triumph-the-recycled-orchestra

Twain, M. (n.d.-a). *Mark Twain - Ff you tell the truth, you don't have to...* BrainyQuote. https://www.brainyquote.com/quotes/mark_twain_133066

Twain, M. (n.d.-b). *Mark Twain - if it's your job to eat a frog, it's best...* BrainyQuote. https://www.brainyquote.com/quotes/mark_twain_414009

The twelve steps. Alcoholics Anonymous. (n.d.). https://www.aa.org/the-twelve-steps

Victor Hugo quote: "man lives more by affirmation than by Bread." Quotefancy. (n.d.-b). https://quotefancy.com/quote/926480/Victor-Hugo-Man-lives-more-by-affirmation-than-by-bread

View all posts by Captain Quote ? (2017, January 17). *Girl gets answer to her prayer with Baby Cow (true story-report)*. Ofthestory. https://ofthestory.wordpress.com/2017/01/17/girl-gets-answer-to-her-prayer-with-baby-cow-true-story-report/

von Goethe, J. W. (n.d.). *A quote by Johann Wolfgang von Goethe*. Goodreads. https://www.goodreads.com/quotes/424596-if-i-accept-you-as-you-are-i-will-make

Vonnegut, K. (2010). *Cat's Cradle*. Dial Press Trade Paperbacks.

Watts, I. (n.d.). *Poets' Corner*. Poets' Corner - Isaac watts - Selected Works. https://www.theotherpages.org/poems/watts01.html

William Shakespeare - we know what we are, but know not... BrainyQuote. (n.d.-c). https://www.brainyquote.com/quotes/william_shakespeare_164317

Woodward, T. (2011, March 16). The Man Who Robbed Himself. *Albert's Sermon Illustrations*. http://aksermonillustrations.blogspot.com/2011/03/man-who-robbed-himself.html

YouVersion. (n.d.-a). *Download amplified bible, Classic edition: Ampc bible: 100% free*. YouVersion | The Bible App | Bible.com. https://www.bible.com/versions/8-ampc-amplified-bible-classic-edition

YouVersion. (n.d.-b). *Download the passion translation: TPT Bible: 100% free*. YouVersion | The Bible App | Bible.com. https://www.bible.com/versions/1849-tpt-the-passion-translation

ABOUT THE AUTHOR

Reverend Roberts serves as the Senior Pastor at Grace Presbyterian Church in Corpus Christi, Texas. His extensive ministerial journey has led him across various regions of Texas, Missouri, and California. With a history of service at five distinct churches, Reverend Roberts has cultivated a distinctive teaching approach that is engaging and inclusive for all members of his congregation. Outside his pastoral duties, John spends his free time with his wife of thirty years, Renee, and their two sons, Jacob and Zachary. If you would like to learn more, please go to www.revjohnroberts.com

Made in the USA
Coppell, TX
08 March 2025

46836116R00196